Atlas of Keystone Reconstructive Technique in Melanoma Management

Springer Nature More Media App

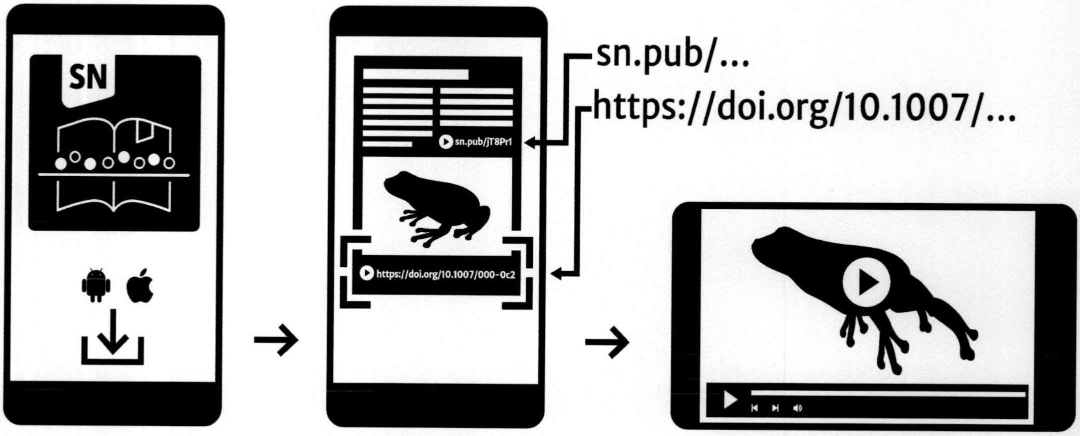

1. Download

2. Scan Link

3. Enjoy Video

Support: customerservice@springernature.com

Felix Behan

Atlas of Keystone Reconstructive Technique in Melanoma Management

Springer

Felix Behan
Department of Surgery, St. Vincent's Hospital
University of Melbourne
Melbourne, VIC, Australia

This work contains media enhancements, which are displayed with a "play" icon. Material in the print book can be viewed on a mobile device by downloading the Springer Nature "More Media" app available in the major app stores. The media enhancements in the online version of the work can be accessed directly by authorized users.

ISBN 978-3-031-39867-4 ISBN 978-3-031-39868-1 (eBook)
https://doi.org/10.1007/978-3-031-39868-1

This Springer imprint is published by the registered company Springer Nature Switzerland AG
The registered company address is: Gewerbestrasse 11, 6330 Cham, Switzerland

Paper in this product is recyclable.

Simplicity is the ultimate sophistication.

Leonardo da Vinci

Nature is pleased with simplicity.

Isaac Newton

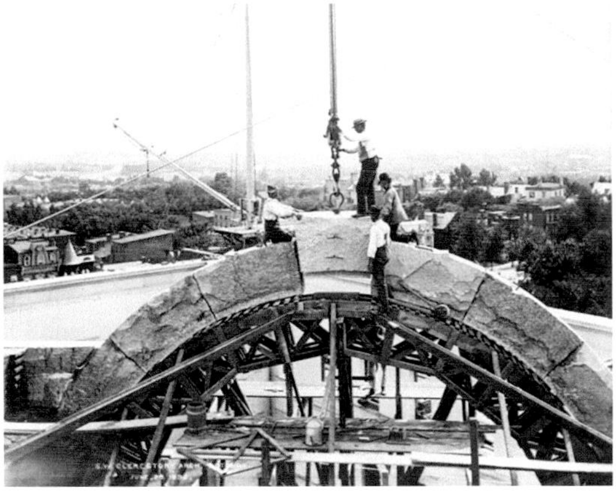

Men putting in place the keystone of the S.W. clerestory arch of the rotunda of the Library of Congress, 1892, Collection Building the Library, Library of Congress, www.loc.gov, Photograph under Public Domain

Foreword 1

As the unusual today seems to be the usual, so often by unintended means the pathways of a few are destined to crisscross. Such was the case with myself and the author, meeting for the first time a decade ago across the Pacific in Sydney where both of us had been invited faculty at the meeting there of the '17th International Perforator Flap Course' championed by Blondeel. To reinforce what I did not understand, Felix—as he always insists to be known—graciously took me aside and gave me a personal recapitulation of his lecture on the subject, what else but the 'keystone advancement island flap'. And ever since, near weekly emails and updates, no longer restricted throughout our world now blessed with technology.

I must disagree, and he would allow me to do so, that the circulation to these flaps is never 'random' at all; but arises from deep fascial perforators, whether via large calibre so-called 'true' perforators or more often diminutive 'capillary' or what we now both like to call 'nanoperforators'. Discrete, these never require specific identification, a major advantage over other forms of perforator flaps, which in general have now become the preferred soft tissue flap capturing the world's imagination. Indeed, the keystone island flap is a 'true' perforator flap, and more than deserved to be included at our initial retreat.

As I then found in my short time to know Felix, the past is always as important as the present which will soon be the future. After all, how did we learn to do what we do without having had our life experiences, so well related in the beginnings of this edifice by his personal historical precedence. This is followed by case reports encompassing all body regions, where variations in design or elevation are chosen to suit the circumstances, finished by absolute honesty in showing some adverse outcomes proving that complications, albeit rare, unfortunately occur with any surgical procedure.

May I end by how I, too, have adopted the acronym 'P.A.C.E.S'—*pain*less; *aesthetic* = plastic surgery; any *complications* are rare; *economic*, as time is more precious than money; and *sensate*—how we all communicate with our environment. Today, the next generation actively seeks any alternative to the complexity of microsurgical tissue transfers and the enigma of microvascular catastrophes. Therefore, it is imperative that all understand the role of the keystone advancement island flap as such a versatile local flap, an excellent choice no matter what the body region and so must never be overlooked.

Sacred Heart Division, St. Luke's Hospital
Allentown, PA, USA

Geoffrey G. Hallock

Foreword 2

I was fortunate to meet Dr. Felix Behan over 20 years ago in 2001 when I was in Australia as a travelling fellow of the Australia-New Zealand Chapter of the American College of Surgeons. Felix was a most gracious host and arranged for me to visit his clinic where he and I saw several of his post-operative patients who had undergone keystone flap reconstructions for a variety of defects in the head and neck, the trunk and the extremities. I will admit that I did not fully grasp the concept, or the power, of the keystone flap during that visit. When I returned home to the United States, I read Felix's articles, asked Felix for advice and eventually tried my first keystone flap. The patient had a distal-third foreleg defect from a sarcoma excision and dogma prescribed a free flap reconstruction, to which the patient was very opposed. Having presented a keystone flap to the patient as an option for which I had little enthusiasm and that I advised would likely fail, they were anxious to proceed. Short story, the keystone flap reconstructed the defect perfectly, the patient did extremely well, and I quickly became an early-adopter and advocate of the keystone concept, to the point that my American reconstructive surgeon colleagues would poke fun at me about it. Over the past 20 years, I have used the keystone concept in dozens and dozens, if not hundreds, of reconstructive surgery cases, I have presented the keystone concept and our outcomes at many national and international meetings, and we have published in the peer-reviewed literature as well. Most importantly, I've seen the keystone concept become adopted widely among American reconstructive surgeons. That's not surprising because the keystone flap concept is beautiful; it is based on sound anatomic principles allowing flaps to be supplied by multiple perforating vessels, it is robust with a wide margin of error, it does not require a separate, distant donor site, it employs the aesthetically favourable v-y concept, it is versatile, and it is straightforward and expeditious in execution. Put another way, the keystone flap can, with a low probability of failure, successfully reconstruct complex defects via straightforward and short operations, avoiding long, complex microsurgical or single-perforator flap operations that are technically more demanding and that risk complete flap loss.

Although it's often said that the essential core of Plastic Surgery is innovation, most of us can enact only small, incremental changes. With the introduction of the keystone flap concept, Dr. Felix Behan has enacted a major change to the reconstructive paradigm for patients with extirpative defects almost anywhere on the body. This enormous contribution that has benefited thousands of patients marks Dr. Behan as that rare colleague among us: a true innovator.

William M. Kuzon, Jr., MD, PhD, FRCSC, FACS
Reed O. Dingman Collegiate Professor of Surgery
Section of Plastic Surgery, University of Michigan
Ann Arbor, Michigan, USA

Foreword 3

Felix Behan's 'Keystone' technique of wound closure has now found an established place in the tool bag of modern reconstructive surgeons. This intuitively implausible flap which creates a secondary defect bigger than the primary, and which is itself closed by simply stitching it back from whence it came, defies logic and surgical convention. For some time and for good reason, sceptics were in the ascendency, for to commit meant a considerable leap of faith without a parachute. Safer to be a coward than have egg on your face. But the keystone is indeed a refreshingly original core concept, divined slowly during a period of baron creativity in plastic surgery when most were dreaming of more exotic breakthroughs such as benign immunosuppression for universal transplantation and tissue engineering as our next frontiers.

Keystone facilitates the closure of tight wounds and extends the limits of conventional flap reach so that grafts and free flaps can be avoided. In so doing it brings back the lost art of plastic surgery, the local flap, which respects like for like, cosmetic units and crease-line camouflage. It redistributes tension and contour. Melanoma and cutaneous malignancy defects are ideally suited to this repair as the depth of excision is to the level of deep fascia, and local flaps which are elevated in the same layer restore exact contour, colour and texture. Ugly branding with standout dinner-plate skin graft concavities and bulbous bullseye deformities from the regulation ALT free flap, an aesthetic foreigner but a universal fail-safe of the surgically stultified, should be a thing of the past for melanoma, especially for facial reconstruction.

The myriad clinical examples with superb photography and dermatome explanations highlight the versatility of the keystone for all reaches of the body. Such is the daring of this flap that in some cases the observer has cause to hold his breath in the expectation of certain failure only to see the post-op view bid fair to its success. Seeing is believing. The flap is variably tortured and twisted from basic keystone skin designs through Greek alphabet-shaped manoeuvres but all respecting Behan's principles of dermatome alignment, islanded with fascial release, one third attached, and closed with distributed tension. The writing is typically Behanesque, and the explanation for the flap's manoeuvrability and survival largely remains speculative but no doubt relates in some way to the complete skin islanding and fascial release, which result in a shift from supra-fascial horizontal perfusion, intolerant of tension, to the more robust vertical perforator one. There are some locations more favourable than others for its application because of tether and blood supply, and no doubt confidence and success in its execution increase with experience. There is a perennial delight in seeing something totally novel and unexpected, a magic trick, and wondering how was it done? This atlas is filled with delights as well as the magician's secrets. It should become the bible for the sorcerer's apprentice.

St Vincent's Hospital Melbourne
Fitzroy, VIC, Australia

Wayne Morrison

Department of Surgery
St Vincent's Hospital, University of Melbourne
Melbourne, VIC, Australia

Adjuncts

I had the great fortune to meet Assoc. Prof Felix Behan when as a newly minted young surgical oncologist I was appointed to the Peter MacCallum Cancer Centre which was just starting to undergo its transformation from a radiation institution to a fully-fledged comprehensive Cancer Centre. Felix had a special interest in melanoma and as the field began to develop our paths crossed. We found common interest in management of cutaneous malignancy, and he was always most helpful with assisting in reconstruction after major oncological extirpative procedures. Over a short period of time, we developed a symbiotic relationship or as Felix would say hand in glove. I was extraordinarily lucky to witness the development of the Keystone concept and even more lucky that Felix would share his vast experience with his colleagues regardless of their professional discipline. His enthusiasm and ability to teach meant that he rapidly became the go to for complex reconstruction and eventually shared this responsibility with several of his colleagues. The robustness of the keystone concept meant that well-trained surgical oncologists could perform the procedure safely and effectively. The procedure is now taught to all our surgical oncology trainees and the reasonable effectiveness of the procedure means it has been adopted by many of the major melanoma centres around the world.

Michael A. Henderson

Division of Cancer Surgery
Peter MacCallum Cancer Centre
Melbourne, VIC, Australia

Department of Surgery
St Vincent's Hospital, The University of Melbourne
Melbourne, VIC, Australia

Adjuncts

Excision of large head and neck cutaneous malignancy provides a significant reconstructive challenge. Often the defect would be repaired with tissue transfers which resulted in significant cosmetic and functional impairments. I was indeed fortunate to meet Felix over 25 years ago, when he was developing and refining his ground-breaking Keystone flap, a flap which achieved repairs which were perfectly contoured, colour matched and pain free. The repair was accomplished in a fraction of the time taken to perform reconstructions previously, the patients were far more comfortable, healed quickly, experienced minimal morbidity and were discharged far sooner than had been the case. The versatility of the flap was highlighted by its success in heavily irradiated tissue, where the flap even seemed to result in an improved blood flow to the surrounding tissues. Felix exemplifies a surgeon who 'thinks outside the box' and the Keystone flap exemplifies this thought process. Most importantly, it is the patient who has benefited most from this major advance in head and neck reconstruction, but the Keystone reconstruction has also resulted in significant reductions in theatre time, hospital stays and patient morbidity. In this Atlas, Felix has produced a clear demonstration of the technique and applications of the Keystone flap, a flap which he has shown is simple to learn, which has a myriad of applications and which should occupy an important place in any reconstructive surgeon's armamentarium.

Department of Otolaryngology
Royal Melbourne Hospital
Parkville, VIC, Australia

Andrew M. Sizeland

Acknowledgement

I have to acknowledge Professor Andrew Sizeland and Professor Michael Henderson who have been asked for their editorial assistance.

Contents

About the Author

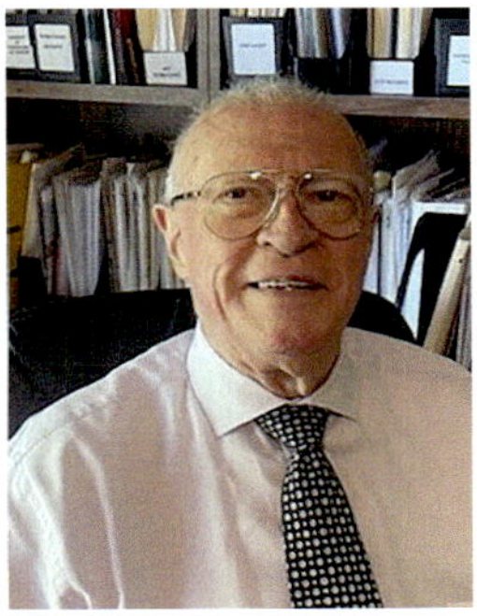

Felix C. Behan has a wide experience in Plastic and Reconstructive Surgery following his surgical training and clinical attachments in London at the St George's, Royal Marsden and Westminster Hospitals. He has continued in this facility in Head and Neck cancer surgery at the Peter MacCallum Cancer Institute where his appointment in the Head and Neck service extended from 1977 to 2014. He was instrumental in establishing the Melanoma Unit at the Peter MacCallum Cancer Institute, which is now part of the Department of Surgical Oncology. He was formerly Head of Unit in the Plastic and Reconstructive Hand Surgery at the Western Hospital from 1988 where 50% of the work relates to Hand Surgery with cases numbering in the thousands totally per year. He was instrumental in establishing the reconstructive loco-regional flap called the Keystone Perforator Island Flap—KPIF, which has been the main reconstructive tool as an alternative to microsurgical procedures. The first publication of this principle occurred in the ANZ Journal of Surgery in 2003 and its applications since it has resulted in over 35 further peer-reviewed publications applying the principles all over the body, even in irradiated tissue. He established in this clinical record of over 3500 flaps over 20 years. The characteristics which are so clinically relevant in Reconstructive Surgery synopsised by the acronym P.A.C.E.S.—almost Pain free, satisfactory Aesthetic match, Complications of a vascular nature are extremely rare and Economic in terms of theatre time in the 2-h timeframe compared with the microsurgical alternative and Sensory recovery in usually 3–6 months over the island flap with resolution of oedema, even after a chronic long-term injury. His full-time commitment in surgery was in the public service domain.

Principles of Keystone Reconstruction

1

Contents

Core Messages

- Clinical observation translates into good research.
- In the reconstruction of melanotic defects after resection, careful design of the Keystone perforator island loco-regional flaps will avoid the need for microsurgical free flap transfers and deliver a superior aesthetic outcome.

1.1 Keystone Technique and Characteristics

It is an established fact that the main management of melanoma, still 85% of cases are treated surgically quoting John Thompson in the Balch publication in the sixth edition of 'Cutaneous Melanoma'. The Keystone management in melanoma has made an important contribution in the surgical repair of major defects. Some have even asked 'is there such a thing as scarless surgery?' This case series below of a melanotic lesion in the calf in a 65 year old, treated with clearance and a Keystone island flap repair produced the following results (Figs. 1.1 and 1.2):

Another example of the Keystone principles delineated by the V2 area of the face as an island.

Supplementary Information The online version contains supplementary material available at https://doi.org/10.1007/978-3-031-39868-1_1. The videos can be accessed individually by clicking the DOI link in the accompanying figure caption or by scanning this link with the SN More Media App.

F. Behan, *Atlas of Keystone Reconstructive Technique in Melanoma Management*, https://doi.org/10.1007/978-3-031-39868-1_1

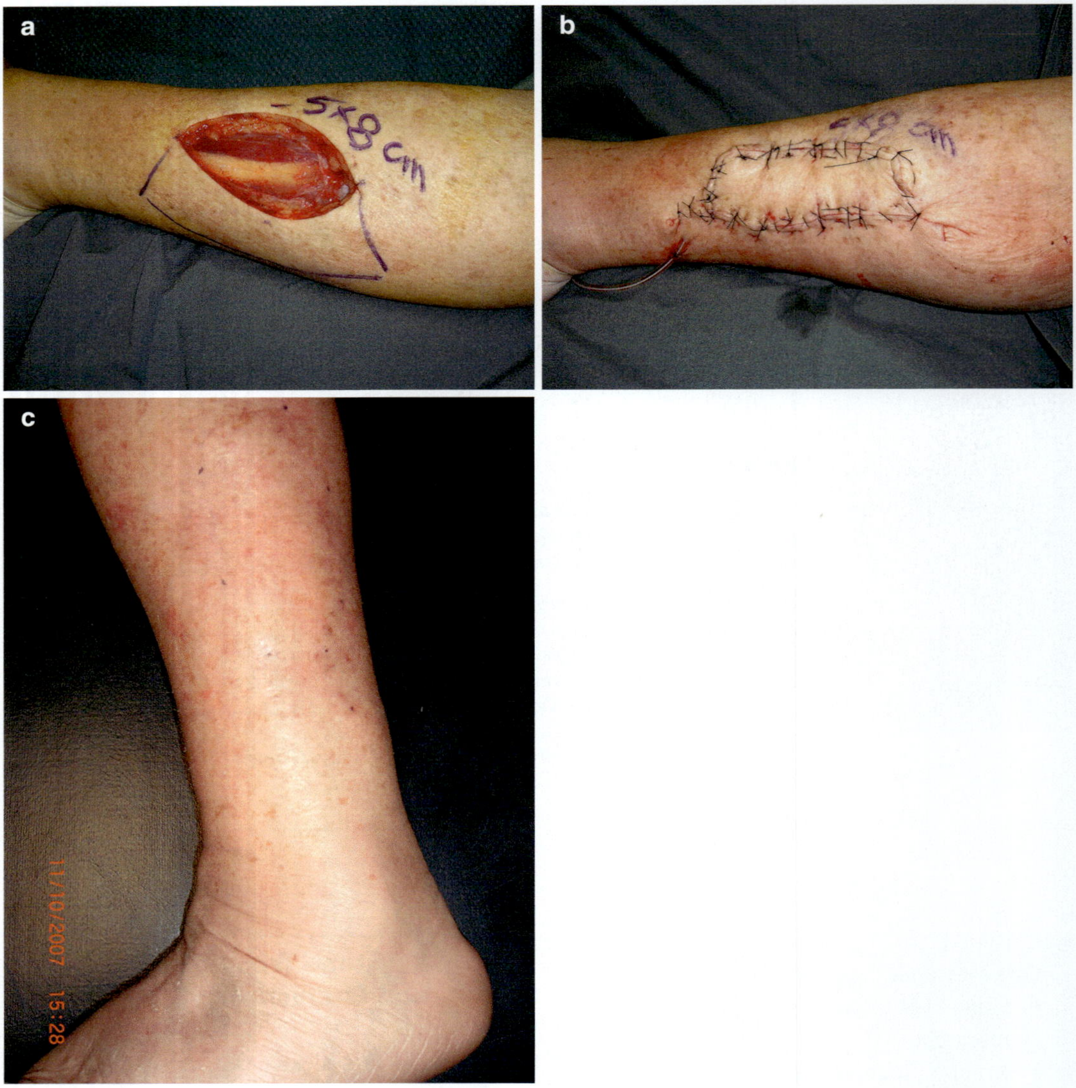

Fig. 1.1 (**a**) Clearance. (**b**) Closure. (**c**) Conclusion

The margins of clearance, according to guidelines, become forever complex because of statistical and research investigations.

My clinical practice following the teaching in the 1970s in Brisbane by Professor Hughes had a rule of thumb in which Level I melanoma received a 1 cm clearance, Level II a 2 cm clearance and Level III a 3 cm clearance, as tumour thickness has a direct correlation with local recurrence and therefore survival [1–3]. Current treatment regimes suggest a 1 cm clearance for a 1 mm Breslow and a 2 cm margin for a 2 mm Breslow [4–6]. Other experts like Gupta suggest a 1 cm margin for in situ melanoma and a 2 cm margin for less than 1 mm and a 5 cm margin for larger than 1 mm. In the latest Balch text on melanoma, multiple series are referenced but a minimal 1 cm clearance either side creates a defect which is easily mastered by the Keystone Flap and it can be almost universally applied as the text will reveal.

Formerly, the standard surgical clearance and the size of the defect ushered in a realm of split

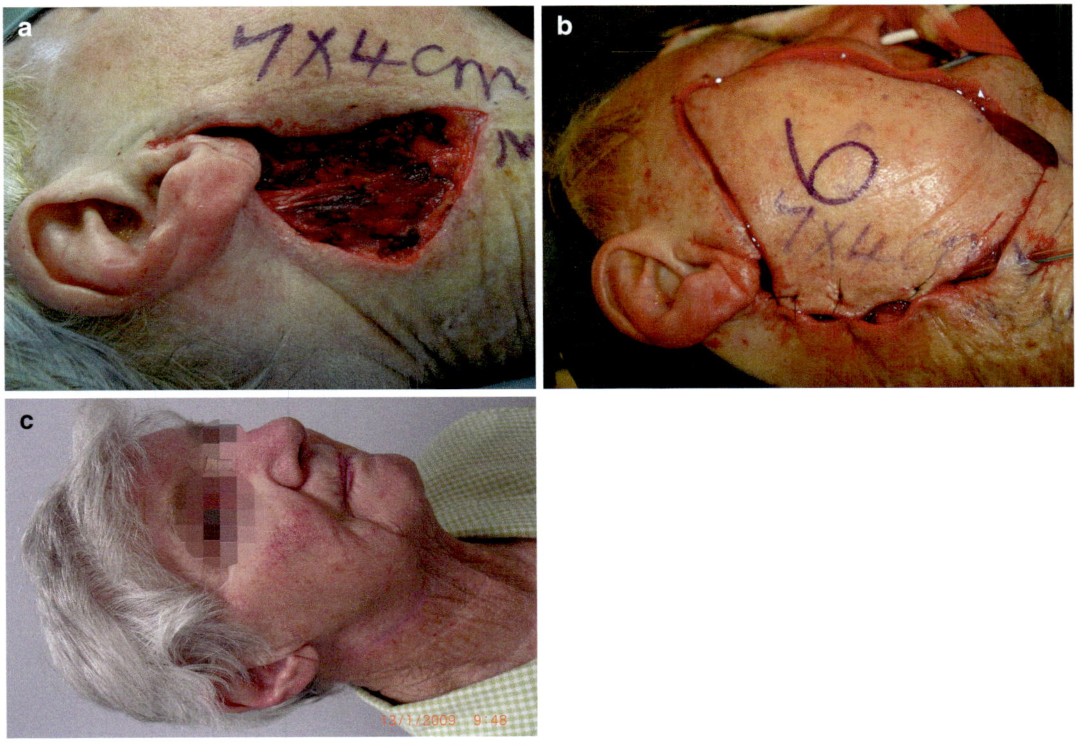

Fig. 1.2 (**a**) Clearance. (**b**) Closure in 6 min. (**c**) Conclusion

skin grafting for large excisional defects. As neurovascular island flaps came into prominence in the 1990s and with the introduction of the Keystone concept, first published in the ANZ Journal of Surgery in 2003, this island design of reconstruction entered a new phase.

My experience since 1995 over 20 years of over 3000 Keystone flaps universally applied all over the body, with a strong focus on melanoma, is the basis of this publication. Additionally, non-melanotic cases are included to show wider applications of the Keystone where their underlying pathology was not melanotic – they are included on the basis of completeness to show the almost universal application of the Keystone flap, which is really a conjoined V-Y flap of Dieffenbach fame [7] of the 1850s. This surgical experience, documented photographically, is the basis of the surgical applications of the Keystone island perforator loco-regional flap for patients with advanced melanoma from head to toe.

As long as these reconstructive principles apply in raising the Keystone, there should be universal success.

1.1.1 Keystone Flap Technique

1. **Fascial lining**: This is an absolute pre-requisite to line the deep surface of the Keystone, the source of the perforator supply, including neurovascular support and the accompanying autonomic, somatic and lymphatic supply. The division of the deep fascia allows the unit to swing in a collateral method and this single Keystone flap closes this double defect (the lesion and the flap) under tension.
2. **The dermatome roadmap – a random source of perforators**: The Keystone is designated within the dermatomal mark out and an axiomatic rule applies as random perfora-

tors embryologically follow the neural patterns of the dermatome, thus ensuring viability. Embryologically if there is a nerve supply there must be an accompanying blood supply and lymphatic support.

3. **Undermining is contraindicated beneath the Keystone**: Undermining the Keystone arc is totally contraindicated as this is the source of the random perforators. Even when undermining is necessary for a loco-regional repair, one third of deep attachment must be maintained to achieve a viable outcome. However, a drain tube in a U-shaped formation can lie within both defects, while discretely placed beneath the island.
4. **Like-for-like**: This reconstructive principle of using like-for-like, acknowledging Gillies contribution, is thus continued to optimise the aesthetic outcome.
5. **Three-phase suturing technique**: The single layer closure using a locking mattress nylon suture at the points of tension stay in situ for 3 weeks. The ordinary mattress sutures to complete the wound closure stay in situ for 2 weeks, and the epidermal closure with seal is done with a continuous nylon to provide perfect wound seal and these can be even cut from the seven day period. Absorbable sutures are avoided because of their unreliability in closing under tension and wound breakdown is a more common occurrence when they are used. Additionally, the absorbable sutures often leave a subcutaneous line of wound healing reactions which tend to be permanent.

The emergence of microvascular surgical repair concepts has played an important part since Ian Taylor's [7] publication in 1973. However, when the Keystone island flap concept is used, cognisant of its listed characteristics, compares favorably when tissue match, low complication rate, a shorter operative timeframe, with recovery of sensory somatic supply in an aesthetic outcome; thus, its value is continuing to be reassessed as an alternative.

The clinical characteristics of the Keystone are summarised by the acronym P.A.C.E.S. as an aide memoir:

Pain	The pain-free characteristic is a remarkable finding in the Keystone application in its postoperative phase. In simplistic terms, this may be explained that the cutaneous somatic supply divided around the arc of the Keystone creates an anaesthetic unit which recovers in some weeks as has been experienced in the past with any longitudinal incisional wound when operating. The only symptom the patient notices is a feeling of tightness which is one of the keynote features when wounds are closed under tension.
Aesthetics	The Gillies principle of using like-for-like is standard reconstructive idea entrenched in history and producing outcomes which are most satisfying to the patient, particularly on exposed sites. The normal attractive appearance of the integument is lost when large defects are grafted or microvascular free flaps, without tissue match, fill the oncological deformities.
Complications	Complications and adverse outcomes are rare. Wound breakdown when tension sutures are removed prematurely by an outside clinic may occur. Vascular complications are rare because the perforators are not individually skeletonised. Such technique may strip away the filamentous autonomic, somatic and lymphatic supports along the axial channels. Irradiated tissue is not a contraindication in the Keystone applications. In the diabetic lower limb where the microcirculation is the centre of pathology, the elements of partial necrosis have occurred in type II diabetics and as a consequence closure must be done without tension and a generous use of skin grafting.

Expeditious in execution	Time is money is a Benjamin Franklin quote from Fisher's book of 1748. If one can operate in a reduced timeframe, this has benefits for all modalities in the treatment and care of patients, particularly the elderly. It has also an economic factor and theatre throughput, whereas long reconstructive sagas may produce an adverse alternative. The implications for staff numbers need no elaboration in microsurgical procedures. We need not repeat that the longer the operative procedure, particularly with microsurgical techniques, then pressure areas amplify the co-morbidities.
Somatic recovery and swelling with the resolution of oedema	These final characteristics of the Keystone go hand in hand. As in any surgical wound, the division of the filamentous cutaneous branches creates a temporary anaesthetic field around the operative site. This may recover in the weeks that follow when the integument has healed and the scar is maturing. A final characteristic in observation is the resolution of swelling and oedema which goes hand in hand over this recovery period of up to 8 weeks.

Thus, clinically in any applied reconstructive situation, anything that offers advantages listed above is worthy of consideration.

Acquiring the technique, as in the author's experience, takes time hence the video supplement of cases explains the background to the thinking behind this technique.

Start small and then metamorphose into larger cases. The one area of limitation is major defects of the skull because the underlying bony substrate is best handled by microvascular procedures and other areas in the body where size becomes an important determinant. However, in the main, the Keystone can cover the majority of defects in the head and neck, trunk and limbs.

In the various sections, 80 cases from the preoperative to the postoperative phase will illustrate the applications and unifying principles of reconstructive surgery using the Keystone – simplicity in surgery is always welcome – the Keystone is simple to apply once mastered. Satisfaction becomes evident at the patient level, including that for the operator. This benefit of looking almost normal has a psychological benefit as well in cancer management.

My experience in melanoma surgery as a plastic and reconstructive surgeon goes back to my mentor Sir Benjamin Rank in the 1970s and my colleagues in London, Ian Wilson and Charlie Westbury at the Westminster, Marsden and St George's Hospitals, London.

The standard skin grafting technique for large excisions led me to develop island flap reconstructions and based on my research, the Bezier island flap was published in 1995 as a curvilinear ellipsoidal V-Y flap in the Dieffenbach manner. For larger defects in the lower back, one day, I doubled the size of the V-Y flap and ended up with a curvilinear arc flap, all based on random perforators. This arc flap came under the terminology of a Keystone (thanks to Alan Briedel). Geometrically, when one joins the opposite points of the curvilinear flap, it represents conjoined double VY flap and with excellent vascular reliability based on non-specific fascial perforators, suprafascial and infrafascial perforators [8].

1.1.2 The Melanoma Clinic at Peter MacCallum Cancer Institute

I commenced this clinic in association with Jill Ainsley and Michael Millwood and a combined consultation factor was the means of optimum treatment with a combined opinion of these specialist groups. The melanoma clinic was subsequently taken over by the Department of Surgery under Professor Richard Bennett. The clinic has mushroomed in size and now with dermatological input as well this combined force was the instigation for my development of the Keystone flap.

Without the combined input of Professor Michael Henderson and Professor David Speakman in the general management of difficult melanoma cases and my colleague Professor Andrew Sizeland in the field of head and neck, this ended up as a DUET performance in surgery. The case series illustrated in this Atlas reflect the value of this DUET surgery. Without the input of their combined referrals of complex cases needing complex reconstructions, the range of case in the melanoma atlas would be insignificant. The majority of the 80 cases are all melanoma but where other malignancies show additional advantages of the Keystone management technique, these have been included with editorial permission.

All photographic illustrations are my own preoperative, intraoperative and postoperative phases and the advantage of the simple photographic digital camera allowed me to discuss cases during the intraoperative phase. My London experience with Ralph Hutchens, the Chief Photographer at the Royal College of Surgeons in the early 1970s, was the basis of this photographic record which continued subsequently in Melbourne with the photographic department at Peter MacCallum under Charlie Frewin and Arthur Wills.

Thus, in conclusion, the melanoma cases from the Peter MacCallum Cancer Institute and the contributions from my surgical colleagues and the photographic departments, local and internationally, have been the basis for the text.

With the increasing range of melanoma cases with an increased difficulty in various anatomical sites, there has been evolution in the Keystone concept to its multiple oncological variations. This evolution of the technique has had two basic advantages, initially the oncological management and the subsequent aesthetic outcome which is always pleasing to the patient. The necessities of the skin graft technique have been mainly replaced by the Keystone design and the loco-regional Keystone flaps provide an attractive aesthetic alternative with its diverse architectural variations but still an island flap and perforator based, aligned within the dermatomes.

1.2 How the Keystone Island Flap Evolved

The basis of the Keystone originally began with the Angiotome concept [9] of flap vascularity based on neuro-dermatomal alignments. This is defined as a system of linked axial pattern flaps using the dermatomes as an aide-memoir. This developed from research into flap vascularity at the Royal College of Surgeons in London in 1971 when the importance of the fascial layer in locoregional flaps became evident. The study of the blood supply of the integument led to certain anatomical conclusions of the importance of this fascial layer concept in loco-regional reconstruction. This was presented to the 6th International Congress of Plastic and Reconstructive Surgery in Paris, 1975, having the support of the international surgical community including Professor William Manchester.

The pioneering German surgeon Dieffenbach (1792–1847) in 1845 [7] established the principle of the V-Y flap and this became the hallmark of a lot of the reconstructive flaps used in clinical practice in the 1970s. The V-Y advancement loco-regional flap concept has been refined and I developed the Ellipsoidal V-Y variant which I call the Bézier Flap [4] to facilitate tight closures, particularly in the Management of Melanoma. Bézier [4] curves – this is an ellipsoidal V-Y flap. The Keystone is a conjoined architectural shape of two V-Y flaps with V-Y points at either extreme (joining the diagonals produces the shape). I had my arc flap, fascially based, totally islanded and leaving any communicating venous links where possible all based on supra and infra fascial random perforators. My original terminology of the curvilinear arc design was superseded by the word Keystone thanks to my colleague Alan Briedal FRACS of Melbourne. This name with its architectural connotations has led to the development of observational findings from the point of view of clinical applications, even closing under tension because of its reliability. Even design variations, as illustrated in Fig. 1.3, from squares to rectangles have been used but always governed by the oncological defect. But, the principles of varying the design are still based on the dermatomal precincts as the neurovascular supply is based on embryological findings and deep attachment of at least one third of the flap size. Specific vascular investigations of perforators with angiotomes have not been found necessary if the above rules are followed in carrying out the

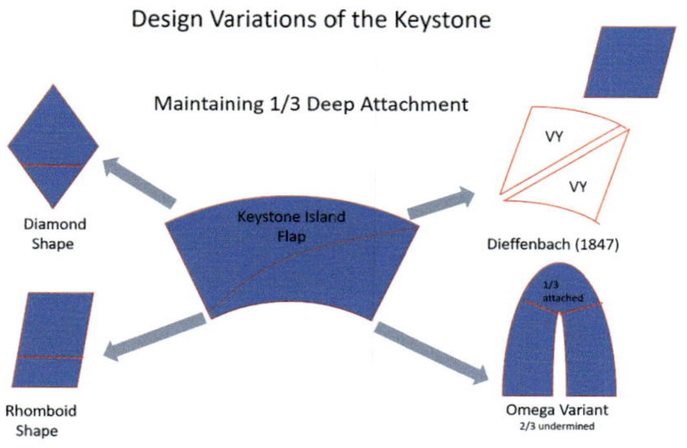

Fig. 1.3 Design variations of the Keystone Flap governed by the oncological defect

Keystone reconstruction. Such is the reliability of the vascularity, closure under tension is an accepted norm and even undermining, retaining the fascial base ensures its viability as long as there is one third of deep attachment retained throughout and as long as there is an intact nerve supply aligned within the dermatomes, there must be a vascular support system accompanying the nerves. In the Omega variant, the middle third deep attachment follows the same rule and allows the arm of the Keystone to close variations in anatomical sites. Another clinical observation as summarised below is the hyperaemic phase if these design precepts are followed where the Red Dot Sign is a characteristic finding of all Keystone closures in spite of wound apposition under lines of tension. The cases below, which illustrate these points, will be noted. As the perforators are not skeletonised and therefore not stripped of fine elements of autonomic and somatic nerve supply and lymphatic drainage support one can only assume hypothetically these factors support the clinical findings as evidenced in the postoperative results.

Some of these design variations originated from a wide experience in reconstructive surgery with use of the V-Y island flap (of which the Keystone represents a duplicated version) and earlier work on the Limberg Flap [10] and its designs on the flap integumentary surface.

The reliability of the Keystone is its main characteristic and the main limitation of the technique is closure under tension but the use of supplementary grafting on appropriate bed overcomes this problem. Lack of adherence to such principles, as enunciated here, has led to necrosis, as I have observed with other operators. Presumably undermining and disturbing support from the supra fascial and infra fascial perforators. In all reconstructive techniques, venous drainage must be maintained and in particular in the head and neck region, damage to the jugular veins is repaired rather than ligated. The hairline vascular perforator supports are thus embedded in the fascia and the depths of the Keystone (Fig. 1.4).

In the original dermatome mark out published in 1900 [11] using the virus infiltration by Herpes Zoster to establish the dermatomal mark outs and as viruses follow the nerve patterns Extrapolating from this on an embryological basis, if there is a nerve supply, there must be a blood supply and arterial flows create their own venous exit as they expand into the final developmental design. The vessels that grow with the nerves must have autonomic supply to control their dilation as well and likewise a somatic input allows their tactile sensation (e.g. an L1 spinal cord dysfunction creates an anaesthetic patch below the inguinal ligament on the anterior thigh) (Fig. 1.5).

A demarcation of perforators with their angiographic definition has not been a pattern in this reconstructive compilation of over 3000 Keystone flaps. However, the aide memoir in raising the flap within the dermatomes has been the basis of this clinical success because if there is a dermatomal blood supply embryologically, there must be an accompanying blood supply with these neural mark outs. The Keystone is really an umbrella of tissue expanded to cover various surgical defects with V-Y points at their apices. The random pattern of the perforators is the source of vascular supply to ensure Advancement, Rotation and Transposition (ART) of Keystone island flaps is possible as long as one third of deep attachment of the cutaneous island flap is maintained. I repeat, the gamut of vascular changes in the Keystone Island Flap come from observational findings not experimental investigations and the usual restrictions one observes in closing large defects enables wound apposition. However, the Keystone principle, as these are fascial based,

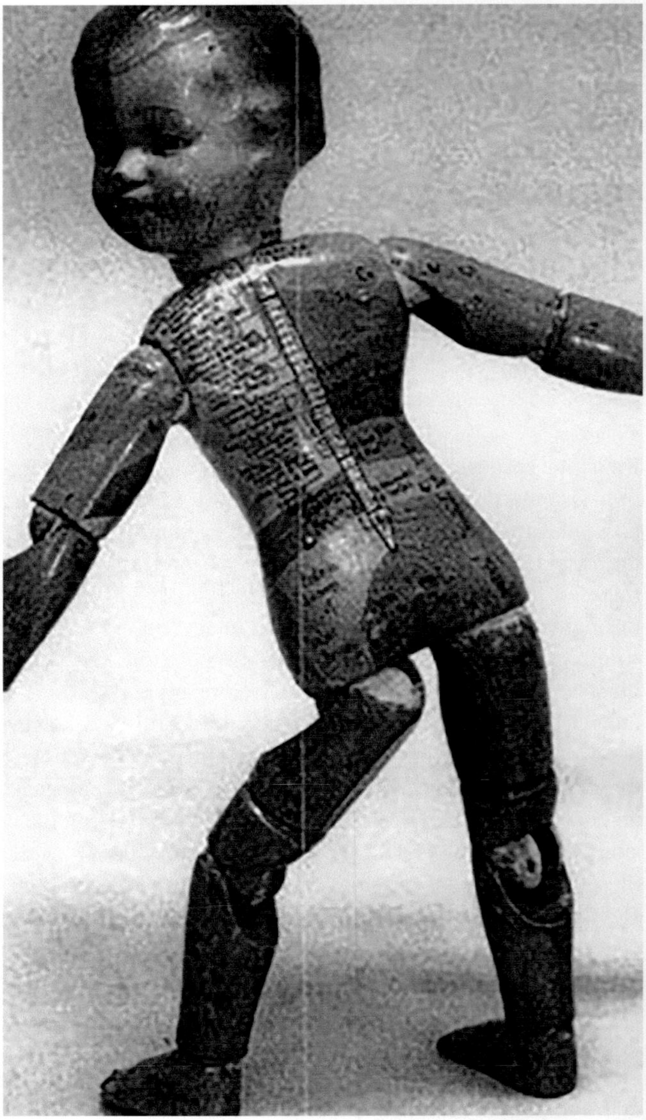

Fig. 1.4 The baby doll of the 1930's shows the dermatomes which were taken from Sir Henry Head's publication in 1900, '*Brain. The Pathology of Herpes Zoster and its Bearing on Sensory Localisation*'. (Reproduced with permission from the 2016 autumn catalogue by antique book library Alain Brieux, Paris, and from Henry Head, A. W. Campbell, 1900, Macmillan and Company)

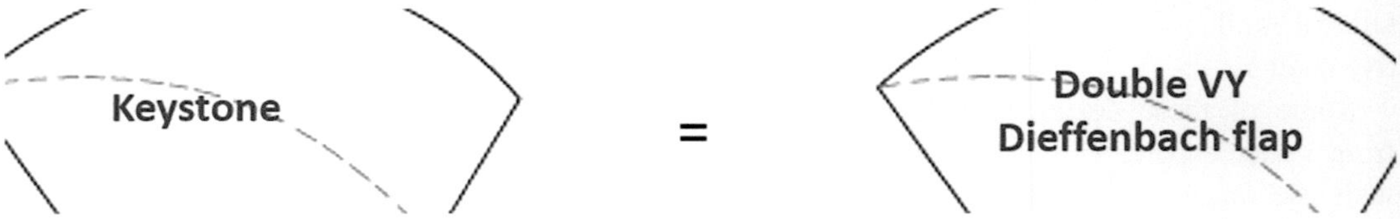

Fig. 1.5 The Keystone flap is a conjoined Double V-Y Dieffenbach flap [7] joining diagonally opposite points which may help to explain its success

allows one to close under tension – breaking one of the mandated rules of plastic surgery. Why is this possible or to quote the late Sumner Millar 'Why is it so?' Again, observationally there are two aspects to this vascular perfusional increase we call reactive hyperaemia [12], it is the same as a lumbar sympathectomy effect, creating a pink foot in due course to assist healing in the elderly diabetic with distal perfusional restraints. This reactive hyperaemia takes 10–15 min to reveal

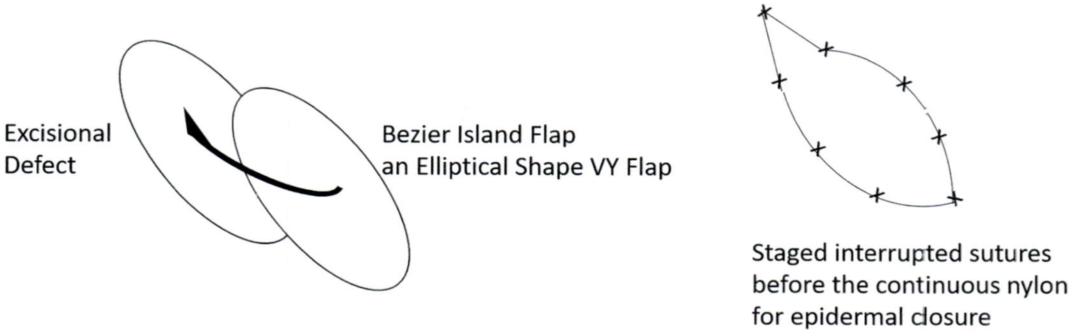

Fig. 1.6 Illustration of the Bezier curvilinear V-Y island flap

itself when using the Keystone island flap repair. However, others have observed that the island principle creates a hydrostatic barrier to perfusion forcing the venous exit to the line of least resistance down the perforator stalks. These findings are somewhat cyanotic from an observational point of view thus, if we have a combination of two hypotheses working out a combined outcome the hyperaemia causes the Red Dot Sign – the suture point site of exit through the Keystone is arterial red not cyanotic bluish which seems to convey there is an arterial factor in preference to a hydrostatic factor.

The Keystone experiences began in 1995.

The origin of the Keystone, being a double V-Y island, comes from my experience in using V-Y island flaps in many reconstructive options. As a preamble to the Bezier design, an ellipsoidal V-Y island flap – as illustrated in the diagrams, variations in the triangular design arise by joining the opposite extremes of the rhomboidal shape. The next stage in island flap design – the Keystone – is when this arc flap is a combination of two V-Y island flaps conjoined. In other words, this elliptical shape allows an easy apposition without tension in the closure of a surgical defect, one of the limitations of the straight V-Y flap (Figs. 1.6 and 1.7).

Any reconstruction based on a defined perforator may experience interference with their somatic, autonomic, lymphatic or humeral supply. The Keystone concept retains these neurovascular supports at the arterial, venous, somatic, autonomic and lymphatic support which has clinical applications in reviewing the postoperative effect of the Keystone.

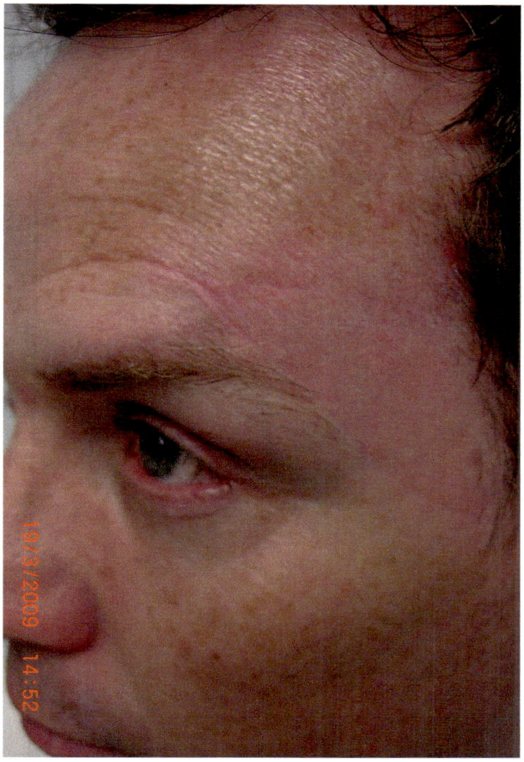

Fig. 1.7 A clinical example of the Bezier curvilinear VY island flap – appearance at 6 months

The Science Behind the Keystone Flap: All Observational Findings

William Osler (1849–1919) the influential Canadian physician said that *'observation is the basis of scientific advancement in medicine'*. My observations of the behavior of various islanded local flaps led me on to search for the physiological basis for these findings. This was inspired by other research published in the surgical literature on angiogenesis, the increased blood supply in tissue-expanded flaps, concepts in endothelial stress and facial nerve repair. These observations have not been the subject of pathology investigations to date but to quote Carl Sagan the Physicist who said 'The absence of evidence is not the evidence of absence' [13]. We have repetitive observational findings with the Keystone.

The challenge was how to come up with good research projects confirming the clinical findings which have been observational. The Cheng paper [12] on vascularity of Keystones is the only one referenced about these tissue findings confirming the increased vascularity in island flaps - a sympathectomy effect.

The Clinical Characteristics of the Keystone: All Observational Findings

The acronym P.A.C.E.S. becomes a natural application:

Pain	The pain-free characteristic is a remarkable finding in the Keystone application in its postoperative phase. In simplistic terms, this may be explained that the cutaneous somatic supply divided around the arc of the Keystone creates an anaesthetic surface which recovers in some weeks as has been experienced in the past with any longitudinal incisional wound when operating. The only symptom the patient notices is a feeling of tightness which is one of the keynote features when wounds are closed under tension.
Aesthetics	The Gillies principle of using like-for-like is standard reconstructive idea entrenched in history and producing outcomes which are most satisfying to the patient, particularly on exposed sites. The normal attractive appearance of the integument is lost when large defects are grafted or microvascular free flaps, without tissue match, fill the oncological deformities.
Complications	Complications and adverse outcomes are rare. Wound breakdown when tension sutures are removed prematurely by an outside clinic may occur. Vascular complications are rare because the perforators are not individually skeletonised. Such technique may strip away the filamentous autonomic, somatic and lymphatic supports along the axial channels. Irradiated tissue is not a contraindication in the Keystone applications.
	In the diabetic lower limb where the microcirculation is the centre of pathology, the elements of partial necrosis have occurred in type II diabetics and as a consequence closure must be done without tension and a generous use of skin grafting.
Expeditious in **e**xecution	Time is money is a Benjamin Franklin quote from Fisher's book of 1748. If one can operate in a reduced timeframe, this has benefits for all modalities in the treatment and care of patients, particularly the elderly. It has also an economic factor and theatre throughput, whereas long reconstructive sagas may become an adverse alternative. The implications for staff numbers need no elaboration in microsurgical procedures. We need not repeat that the longer the operative procedure, particularly with microsurgical techniques, then pressure areas amplify the co-morbidities.
Somatic recovery and **s**welling with the resolution of oedema	These final characteristics of the Keystone go hand in hand. As in any surgical wound, the division of the filamentous cutaneous branches creates a temporary anaesthetic field around the operative site. This may recover in the weeks that follow when the integument has healed and the scar is maturing. A final characteristic in observation is the resolution of swelling and oedema which goes hand in hand over this recovery period of up to 8 weeks.

Dermatomal Precincts

The dermatomes are the aide memoire to define random perforators. This avoids the costly investigation of angiography, which has not been

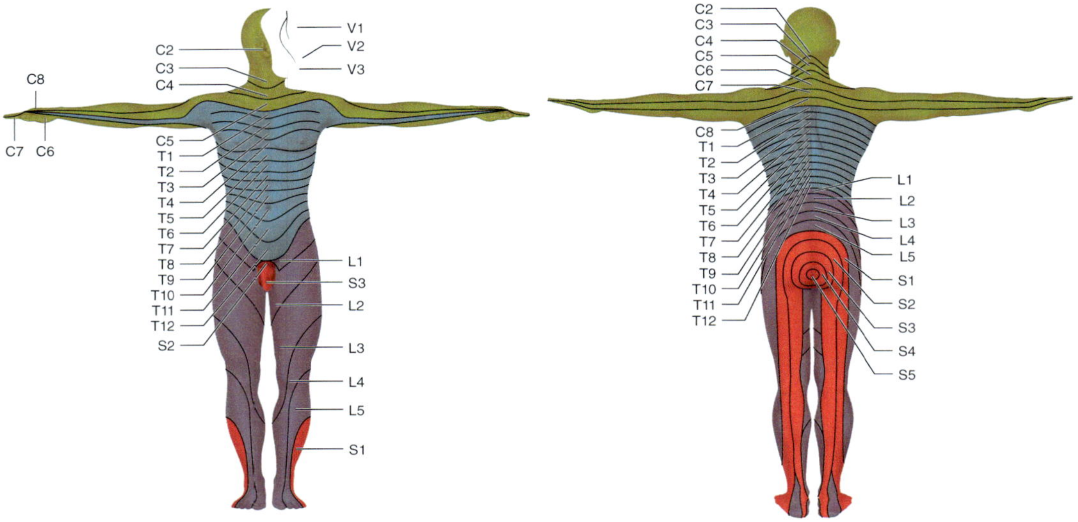

Fig. 1.8 The dermatome precincts

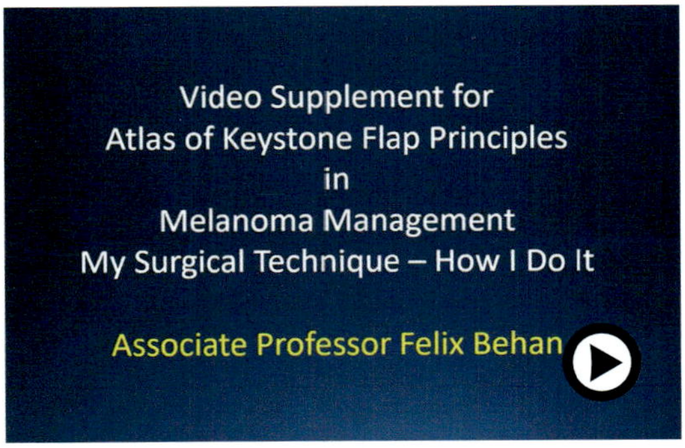

Fig. 1.9 Principles of the keystone (▶ https://doi.org/10.1007/000-b4j)

applied to any of these Keystone cases. Intact nerve supply indicated intact blood supply. The universal dermatome designs are the basis for Keystone orientation and then elevated with a fascial substrate. It is essential for undermined flaps when Advancement, Rotation and Transposition are necessary to leave one third attached near the main perforator axis. These dermatome precincts are illustrated in Figs. 1.8 and 1.9.

Synopsis of Surgical Principles for Raising a Keystone Island Flap

1. The dermatome alignment is an absolute prerequisite in the flap location.
2. The standard Keystone repair is a single unit straddling two surgical defects which are closed under tension.
3. With advancement, rotation and transposition of the fascial based Keystone, it is raised in a distal to proximal direction, clipping any fascial perforators but leaves one third of proximal attachment in any therapeutic repair.
4. The flap consists of skin/fat/fascia and longitudinal anatomical structures in the vicinity, e.g. any venous line as well as neural are all retained.
5. Two thirds undermining is a valid technical modification to facilitate rotation, with the remaining proximal one third attached for random perforator perfusion allows closure under tension.
6. The case images used with times and dates allow us to be specific about documented data.

1.2.1 Traditional Teaching

Keystone management has broken certain management rules in the reconstructive field allowing us to continue the Gillies dictum of like-for-like in any reconstructive saga. Governed by the need for success, let alone aesthetic outcomes multiple descriptions of techniques plague the literature with various anatomical and architectural designs. The Keystone incorporates most designs from a reconstructive point of view. The value of pedicle flaps, a follow on from microsurgical repair, has been the vogue and the Blondeel book [14] is the latest update summarising such applications. Because in the Keystone principle, specific perforators are not defined and based on random perforators, this avoids the angiographic investigation and its cost saving implications. Most of us in the reconstructive domain have used these throughout our career and like melanoma the extent of wider excision is related to the Breslow thickness (REF treatment of primary melanoma). Generous margins in the initial treatment of melanoma are a natural consequence when there is almost no concern about closing of the surgical defects, as reflected in the use of the Keystone and a skin graft can always supplement the closure.

1.2.2 How the Keystone Universalises the Clinical Outcome at Most Sites

As the possibility of long-term outcome and the patient's wish for an aesthetic outcome, this is where the Keystone seems to unify all the variables and as described above, the P.A.C.E.S. acronym is synoptic. Another advantage of this expeditious means of reconstruction is governed by the patient's co-morbidity status and the concerns with complications from mismanagement aggravate the morbidity factor in the elderly. Thus, if radical removal of groin mass can be done by a simplified technique, this is where the Keystone application becomes pre-eminently successful.

1.2.3 Arteriovenous and Lymphatic Communications in the Perforator Support Passing Through the Deep Fascia

The advantages of a non-complicated surgical repair need no elaboration and the Keystone has one preeminent characteristic, that is neurodermatomally based within embryological mark outs. This has the accompanying arteriovenous, autonomic and somatic supply. All Keystones must be fascial lined for advancement, rotation and transposition and for more awkward locoregional repairs they can be safely undermined two thirds while preserving deep attachment to the remaining third over the neurovascular perforator supports including lymphatic drainage. This embryological background has been the basis for the clinical characteristics synopsised by the acronym P.A.C.E.S. covering Pain, Aesthetics, vascular Complications, Expeditious in execution and the subsequent recovery of Sensation with the resolution of oedema, presumably dilating lymphatic channels. Again, these are all observational phenomena gleaned over the 3000 cases done to date in oncological management. The DRAPE [15] procedure (Delayed Reconstruction After Pathology Evaluation) while awaiting pathology clearance is another important clinical additive in the management of melanoma, particularly Hutchinson's melanotic freckle.

1.2.4 Microvascular

We have all been victims of metamorphosis through the reconstructive perspective from Ian Jackson's work with Gwynn Morgan and the groin flap leading to Taylor and Palmer of 1987 had a microsurgical perspective and the quote for success ranged from 95% but there can be adverse findings, particularly aesthetically and I refer you to the Figs. 2.266–2.268 in the head and neck section. Here aesthetics and function have been found wanting as that applies to many microsurgical applications. None of the cases in this series needed microsurgical reconstructive input as a backup. Another plastic surgical edict that has been questioned is the use of the Keystone in irradiated tissue which happens frequently in head and neck cases and is the domain for microsurgical repair in most units – as in Case 23. However, the Keystone is not contraindicated in irradiated tissue.

The Lamberty [16] classification of vascular perfusion may need to be revamped because of these ongoing clinical findings and not latex injection studies in cadavers. I repeat, the success of the reconstructions has a clinical viewpoint without experimental vascular speculation. Perforator flaps need reassessment as the Keystone has proved its clinical value by not skeletonising perforators presumably stripping them of somatic, autonomic, lymphatic support. The Keystone preserves the integrity of all random perforators suprafascial and infrafascial. As I stated above, its success is based on fascial lining with a deep third attachment always retained and the variations of the Keystone design, as discussed above, observes and respects the integrity of the random perforators.

1.2.5 Closing Under Tension—Another Edict of Plastic Surgery Called into Question

This basic dictum of general surgical principles applied universally is part of our surgical education because closure under tension produces epidermal necrosis. However, the Keystone has reorientated the thinking of this concept because of the redirection of vascular flow—the vertical infrafascial and suprafascial perforator support have hydrostatically superior to that of the horizontally orientated subdermal plexus. For example, comparing fire hydrants and garden hoses. All the cases illustrating the hyperaemic effect in the text have all been closed under tension. Absolute white lines of tension are a warning to realign and replace the sutures but in the main the vascular flow on the fascial base to the microperforators eventually creates the dynamic effect of hyperaemia and the Red Dot Sign of the blood at the suture site of the flap confirms this dynamic, bleeding more on the flap side than the receiving side – under tensional closure we have increased flow. Variations on the design like Hatchet flaps completely miss the point of this dynamic perfusion concept and all gleaned from over 3000 cases of experience. It is mentioned here merely to dispel the clinical applications of such variations and this reflects erroneous thinking – however based on tradition from the times of Baron and Emmett [17]. From experience, the Keystone on lax tissue for example the Keystone in the lateral peroneal compartment will cover defects close towards the anterior tibial line but do not base Keystones on the resistant tissue of the underlying bone of the shin – doomed to failure. Discretion must always operate and when an area like the anterior tibial wall is needed for repair site, it is wiser to use a loco-regional Keystone to cover any bony defect from the lateral L5 dermatome, with or without grafting over muscle.

References

1. Breslow A, Macht SD. Optimal size of resection margin for thin cutaneous melanoma. Surg Gynecol Obstet. 1977;145:691.
2. Balch CM, Murad TM, Soong SJ, et al. Tumor thickness as a guide to surgical management of clinical stage I melanoma patients. Cancer. 1979;43:883.
3. Zeitels J, LaRossa D, Hamilton R, Synnestvedt M, Schultz D. A comparison of local recurrence and resection margins for stage I primary cutaneous malignant melanomas. Plastic Reconstruct Surg. 1988;81(5):688–93.
4. Behan F, et al. Island flaps, including the Bezier type in the treatment of malignant melanoma. ANZ J Surg. 1995;65(12):870–80. https://doi.org/10.1111/j.1445-2197.1995.tb00579.x.
5. Vollmer RT, Seigler HF. Using a continuous transformation of the Breslow thickness for prognosis in cutaneous melanoma. Am J Clin Pathol. 2001;115(2):205–12.
6. Veronesi U, et al. Thin stage I primary cutaneous malignant melanoma. Comparison of excision with margins of 1 or 3 cm. N Engl J Med. 1988;318:1159.
7. Behrbohm H. History of facial plastic surgery in Europe. European Academy of Facial Plastic Surgery, 2017.
8. Rodriguez-Unda N, Abraham J, Saint-Cyr M. Keystone and perforator flaps in reconstruction. Clin Plast Surg. 2020;47(4):635–48. Elsevier
9. Behan FC, et al. Vascular basis of laterally based forehead island flaps and their clinical applications. In: Transactions of the 2nd Congress of the European Section of the International confederation of plastic and reconstructive surgery. Madrid, 1973. The Angiotome concept.
10. Limberg AA. The planning of local plastic operations on the body surface. The Collamore Press (Toronto) version. Originally published in 1963 in Leningrad, U.S.S.R.
11. Head H, Campbell AW. The pathology of herpes zoster and its bearing on sensory localisation. BRAIN Part III, 1900.
12. Lo CH, Nottle T, Mills J. Keystone Island flap: effects of islanding on vascularity. Plast Reconstr Surg Glob Open. 2016;4(2):e617.

13. Anon. (2019) Absence of evidence is not evidence of absence. Quote Investig 2019-09-17.
14. Blondeel P, et al. Perforator flaps: anatomy, technique and clinical applications. Missouri: Quality Medical Publishing.
15. Behan F, et al. Oncologic clearance with preservation of reconstructive options: literature review and the 'delayed reconstruction after pathology evaluation (DRAPE)' technique. ANZ J Surg. 2012;82(11):780–5.
16. Cormack GC, Lamberty BG. Cadaver studies of correlation between vessel size and anatomical territory of cutaneous supply. Br J Plast Surg. 1986;39(3):300–6.
17. Barron J, Emmett A. Subcutaneous pedicle flaps. Br J Plast Surg. 1965;18:51–78.

Major Head and Neck Regions Using the Keystone Technique

2

Contents

2.1 Case Presentations

Head and neck reconstruction is a formidable challenge [1].

The Keystone flap allows one to close large tissue defects under tension as they are all random perforator based and have no contribution from any input from the subdermal plexus where islanding creates an umbrella of tissue circumventing tension in the subdermal plexus which produces necrosis. The neurodermatomal pattern is the basis of its success in the design format.

Reconstruction utilising the principles of subunits does not apply because the Keystone allows one to reconstruct the surgical defect based on the oncological site and region. Hence, facial and grimace lines are all respected and that adds to the approximation to a normal appearance from the scalp, forehead, nose, cheeks, periorbital and perioral regions. Called sub-units by some specialists [2, 3], I call then anatomical units for the Keystone.

Supplementary Information The online version contains supplementary material available at https://doi.org/10.1007/978-3-031-39868-1_2. The videos can be accessed individually by clicking the DOI link in the accompanying figure caption or by scanning this link with the SN More Media App.

F. Behan, *Atlas of Keystone Reconstructive Technique in Melanoma Management*,
https://doi.org/10.1007/978-3-031-39868-1_2

Loco-regional flaps, part of the standard plastic surgical repertoire, are listed in every textbook embodying reconstructive techniques in an oncological setting.

2.1.1 Lip

Some of these go back to the time of Gillies [4] and the Karapandzic (REF) with its retained innervation, particularly in lip reconstruction. Our own Keystone variant of the lip in an oncological case shows the value of dermatomal alignments based on embryological principles. The value of such a system it embraces fully the Gillies concept of like-for-like.

The suturing technique employs the standard 3-phase single layer elements of:

- Locking mattress sutures with deep fascial involvement at the points of tension which stay in 3 weeks.
- Ordinary locking mattress sutures close the wound in a single layer to align the epidermis that stay in 1–2 weeks.
- The continuous surface nylon suture to achieve epidermal seal which are cut at 7 days creates a perfect line.
- Absorbable sutures are avoided because of their unreliability in closing under tension and wound breakdown is a more common occurrence when they are used. Additionally, the absorbable sutures often leave a subcutaneous line of wound healing reactions which tend to be permanent.

Every case illustrated is repaired by this 3-phase mechanism without the use or need of deep dermal sutures.

Skin grafts are rarely used except in sites of extreme tension like the case of the nasal reconstruction where a full thickness graft was used in Case 19.

Loco-regional flaps from Bi-lobed [5] to rhomboidal [6] to transpositional [7] to hatchet [8] have all been superseded by this Keystone reconstructive design – island flaps are safer when there is deep attachment of only one third of their dissected base following the undermining of up to two thirds. The design of the Keystone overcomes loco-regional reconstruction types and when a diagonal is drawn from the opposite corners, this really represents two V-Y flaps conjoined.

Free tissue transfer is not part of the design requirements with the Keystone except where large scalp defects preclude its effectiveness and the use of a Lat-Dorsi free flap becomes a necessity.

Jaw reconstruction cover: The Keystone flap may play a part in facial contour soft tissue reconstruction overlying any exposed mandible. There are no cases in this series relating to microsurgical jaw replacement.

Bony defects of the face, for example in the vicinity of the ethmoid complex, where standard teaching creates mucosal replacement by skin grafting the deep surface of any reconstruction flap. As we know mucosa 'grows like grass' and to have a mucosal replacement over an exposed sinus avoids the crusting problems of skin grafting the deep surface of the flap.

In the scalp melanoma case illustrated using the island flap, not quite Keystone in design but reflecting the Keystone characteristics without skeletonising the posterior occipital artery is advanced into the defect while retaining all the peri adventitial components of the neurovascular stalk. We see the resultant outcome of tightness in the postoperative phase without pain, aesthetic match, no complications, expeditious operating timeframe and the return of sensory function. All defects in the Melanoma series were repaired around those specific axes of named vessels but I repeat, skeletonising them for ease of mobilisation detracts from its overall usefulness.

Multiple other variations like Bi-lobe flaps, rotational flaps and pinwheel flaps are just name styles to incorporate design variations.

Forehead and temple reconstruction as in Case 5 shows the value of the island flap reconstruction based on the V2 area of the infraorbital neurovascular structure but created into an island to embrace the Keystone principles of hypervascularity in a tissue plane on a single neurovascular stalk – the infraorbital neurovascular complex. Advancement and rotation techniques are part of the island flap utilising established Keystone characteristics to optimise closure and repair.

The Keystone application in ear reconstruction relates to complex issues like reconstructing the conchal fossa. The case illustrated here shows the advantage of the C2, C3 cervico submental flap from the neck, undermined containing cervical fascia but leaving one third proximal area attached over sternomastoid to retain perforators. The island Keystone closes the conchal defect with a deepithelialised bridge allowing reconstruction of the conchal defect and the helix margin to be reattached.

The Keystone closure of parotid defects has been a valuable contribution and a quick solution, particularly in the elderly, in this area of reconstruction, normally the province of free flap repair. It needs no elaboration on the aesthetic outcome using loco-regional repair when compared with microvascular tissue borrowed from an external source. The aesthetic outcome reflects the patient's satisfaction because at clinics that have not used this Keystone reconstructive method, the constant story of the patient's dissatisfaction is not unique. They have become a social outcast, hiding from society, wearing a beanie as a disguise for any public appearance. The Keystone provides an alternative option and the technique is easily mastered when the technical refinements are followed – dermatomal alignment, fascial based, totally islanded leaving one third deep attachment at the point of rotation and retaining all venous links. The direct closure of the secondary defect of the neck under tension requires the stabilising buried mattress sutures to be left in situ for 3 weeks.

Nasal reconstruction: The aesthetic units of the nose are respected and the applications of the Keystone and its variants at three sites facilitate nasal repair. The side of the nose and a V-Y island flap (hemi-section of a Keystone) provides in a recurrent mitotic lesion, skin closure, pain-free, aesthetic appearance without complications, an expeditious timeframe with full sensory recovery. This V-Y principle based inferiorly adjacent to the lobule can be advanced, rotated and transposed to reconstruct nasal tips by advancing the tissue without skeletonising vascular axes to reach the nasal tip.

The nasal tip procedure by a collateral Keystone is advanced from the side of the nose, teased with blunt dissection with random branches from the facial artery and nerve supply from the infraorbital complex used to cover the defect.

The Keystone variant for the total nasal cover reconstruction employs a forehead flap principle Keystone variant design and placed along the bridge of the nose to meet the nasal tip. It is based on supraorbital and supratrochlear neurovascular structures which achieves soft tissue cover. The lateral side of the nose was covered with a full thickness graft to give an acceptable aesthetic outcome.

The Keystone application in the cheek reconstruction is a fairly simple procedure as detailed in the cases below. In the one of the Malar eminence down to the mid-section, over the angle of the mandible in a 97 year old, and a massive 6 × 5 cm in an Hutchinson's Melanotic Freckle in a 76 year old. However, the aesthetic balance in reconstruction of the cheek is evident but the Keystone characteristics evident in all flaps are illustrated again:

Pain-free postoperative outcome.
Aesthetically acceptable method of reconstruction.
Complications are rare in wound problems.
Expeditious in execution and compares favourably with microsurgical sagas.
Swelling is rapidly resolved, confirming lymphatic drainage and presumably dilation of the lymphatic trunks in a similar way to the vascular trunks and somatic recovery is achieved.

Irradiated fields which usually preclude standard forms of loco-regional reconstruction because of the subdermal vascular insufficiency created by radiation treatment, the Keystone reconstruction overcomes any restriction in irradiated fields. In this case the slightly variable appearance of the hyperaemic phase is noticeable with the predominant circulation in flare over the posterior margin adjacent to the auricular temporal perforators with facial artery branches involved in the anterior section of the Keystone. Again, healed without necrotic complications.

And finally, the Keystone has sound applications in the elderly when the expeditious nature of the repair is of paramount importance in this

97 year old, and the exposure time of 60 min is very relevant in this age group.

The lip reconstruction for an Hutchinson's Melanotic Freckle involving 2–3 cm of the vermilion margin is a simple surgical exercise when direct closure is standard practice. This has one drawback, when he shaves, he has to shave along the line of the lip and its new vermilion alignment with the hairs often a source of irritation along the oral margin. This simple technique of doing a mucosal island flap from the inner surface of the lower lip in a Keystone design and with blunt dissection this can refashion the lower lip and returns the lip to normal function and the mucosal defect in the buccal sulcus is allowed to mucosalise, healing by secondary intention without any surgical closure of the secondary defect. Otherwise, the vermilion inversion would occur with beard irritation along the margin.

The two thirds excision of the lower lip and its subsequent closure using the V3 dermatome for the external repair and a mucosal island at the region of the L modiolus creates normal lip apposition without any effect on masticular articulation, drinking or even mastication.

In the neck the applications of the Keystone along clavicular perforators and intercostal perforators are all random, leaving one third of the Keystone attached ensures viability, hyperaemia and an aesthetic match like-for-like closure, without complications, expeditiously sound in principle with full sensory recovery. I repeat, we achieve these outcomes all based on embryological mark outs.

Each of the cases below substantiates the findings, and accompanied by slides with a video PowerPoint supplement in the operative procedure and the outcome achieved.

In summary, the Keystone is a universal technique with applications in most sites of the body and in this head and neck section, it seems to supersede all the eponymous names of loco-regional designs over the years when this very simple idea in terminology – the Keystone – is based on embryological principles with dermatomal alignments and with wide applications.

2.1.2 Scalp

The applications of the Keystone on the scalp based on neurovascular supply at various sites, but closure under tension is almost the norm. The mismatch of free tissue transfer is an obvious aesthetic disadvantage but often a necessity because of the nature of the reconstructive challenge and the malignancy [9, 10]. Sometimes skin grafting is a necessary accompaniment to the Keystone because of tensional closure restrictions and restraints over the bony vault.

Advancement and rotational flap techniques all apply, often with delineation of various defined neurovascular structures (superficial temporal neurovascular structures, postauricular and occipital neurovascular structures). Microvascular variants from fascio-cutaneous latissimus dorsi flaps and rectus abdominus flaps have not been part of our reconstructive repertoire [11, 12].

2.1.2.1 Case 1: Scalp Melanoma Level II 1.5 cm

Melanoma of the vertex of the scalp (see Figs. 2.1, 2.2, 2.3, 2.4, 2.5, 2.6, 2.7, and 2.8).

In summary, the pain-free postoperative phase and the absence of necrosis, and that characteristic of increase in hair growth of the Keystone in the scalp was not compromised by complications. Expeditiously executed is the keynote here – the timestamp confirms the 1 h timeframe with sensory recovery in 3 weeks.

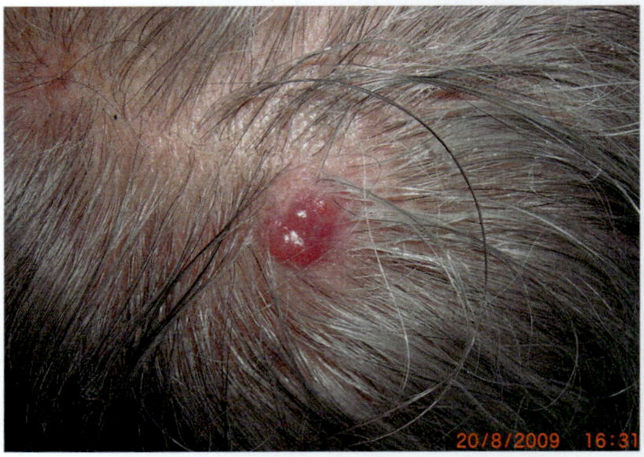

Fig. 2.1 The melanotic lesion

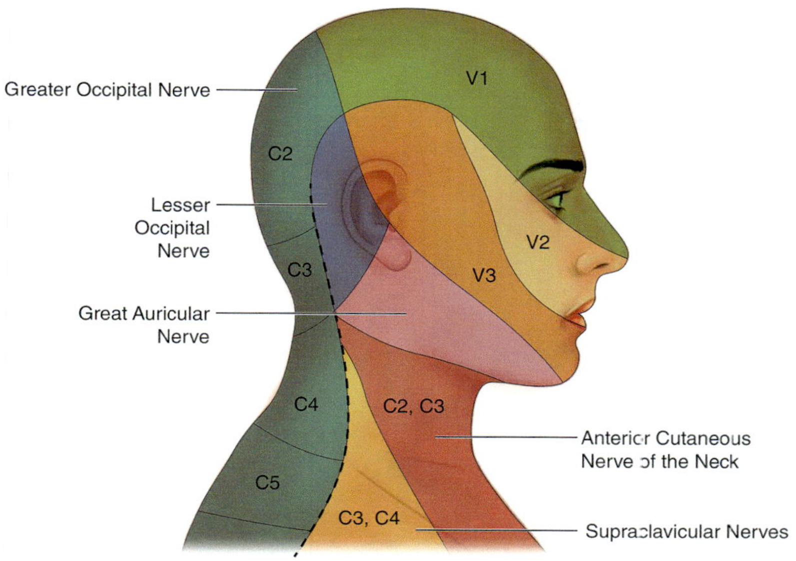

Fig. 2.2 The dermatomal mark out is the guide for the location of the random perforators accompanying the fascia

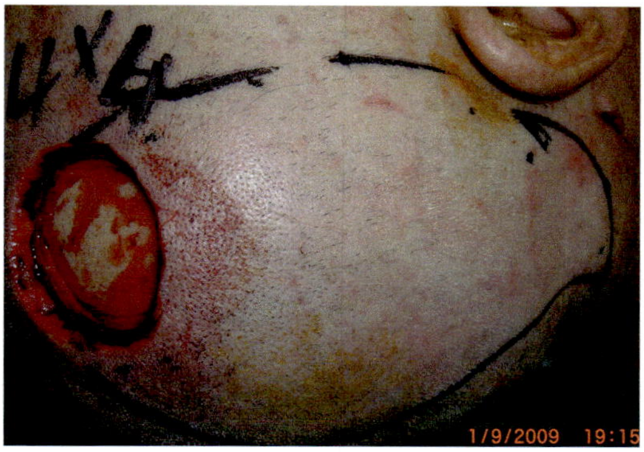

Fig. 2.3 4 × 4 cm clearance including pericranium. The mark out of the island flap design sits in the region of the occipital branch of the postauricular artery in the C2, C3 origin

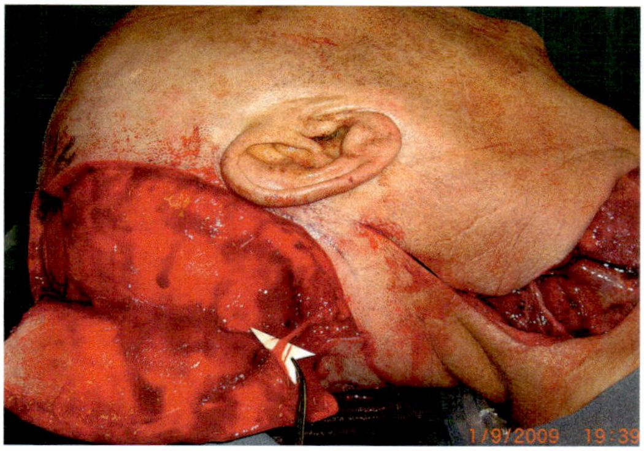

Fig. 2.4 The neurovascular axes supporting the flap are freed from the surrounding tissues but the structures are not skeletonised to maintain autonomic, somatic and venous support to the arterial stalk of the occipital branch of the posturicular artery (arrowed)

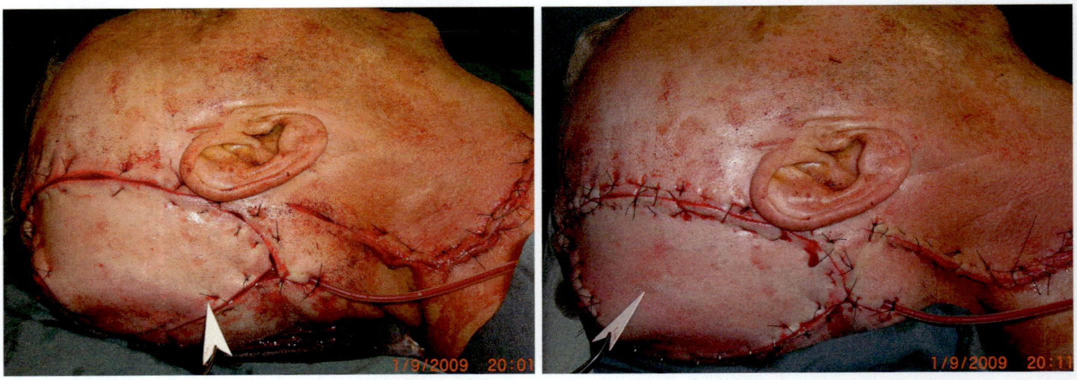

Fig. 2.5 The 3-phase suture closure technique with locking mattress at the points of maximum tension, mattress sutures to close the wound and a continuous nylon around the periphery for epidermal seal. The lines of tension at the key points are mattress locking sutures. The remaining loose neck in the skin is trimmed accordingly. The hyperaemia, a Keystone characteristic, is evident in the island flap

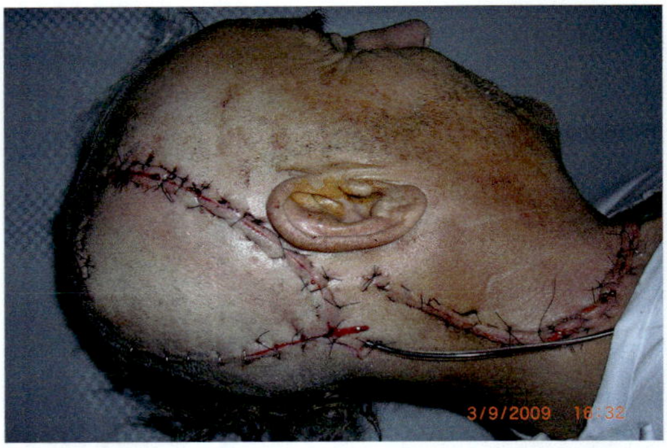

Fig. 2.6 Appearance at 2 days with drain tubes functioning

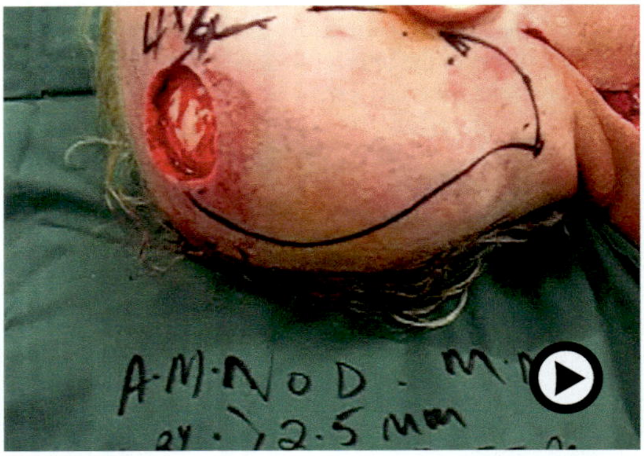

Fig. 2.7 Operative sequence (▶ https://doi.org/10.1007/000-b5g)

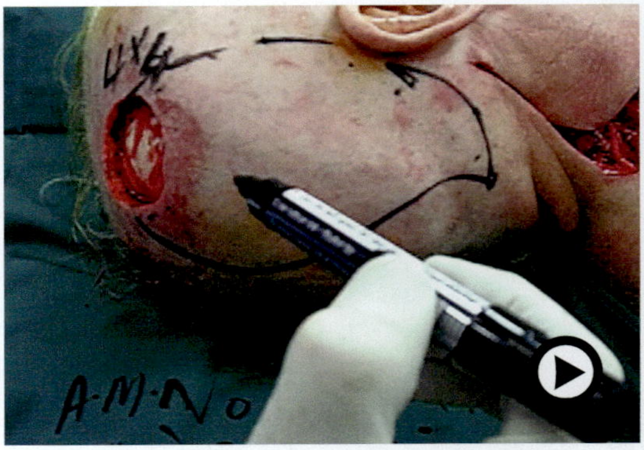

Fig. 2.8 Operative sequence (▶ https://doi.org/10.1007/000-b4m)

2.1.2.2 Case 2: Mitotic Lesion Recurrence Involving Outer Table of the Skull

The tumour defect on the vertex of the scalp produced an oncological clearance of a defect 8 × 8 cm (see Figs. 2.9, 2.10, 2.11, 2.12, 2.13, 2.14, 2.15, 2.16, 2.17 and 2.18).

In summary her aesthetic result without complications is an acceptable outcome. All the P.A.C.E.S. characteristics were evident throughout.

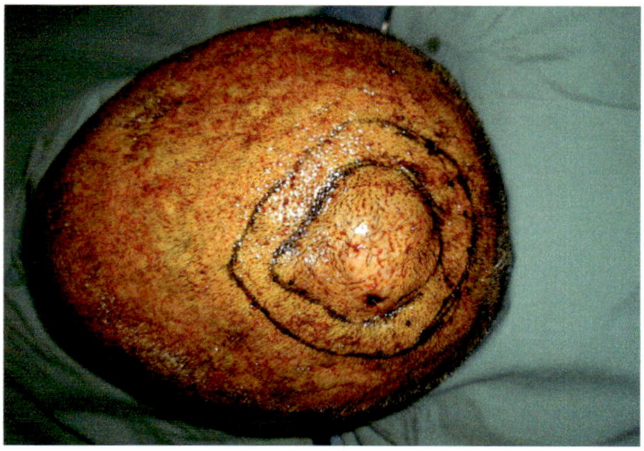

Fig. 2.9 The mark out of the tumour macroscopic and the 2 cm peripheral clearance of 1 cm into the outer table of the scalp

Fig. 2.10 The dermatomal mark out is the guide for the location of the random perforators coming through the fascia

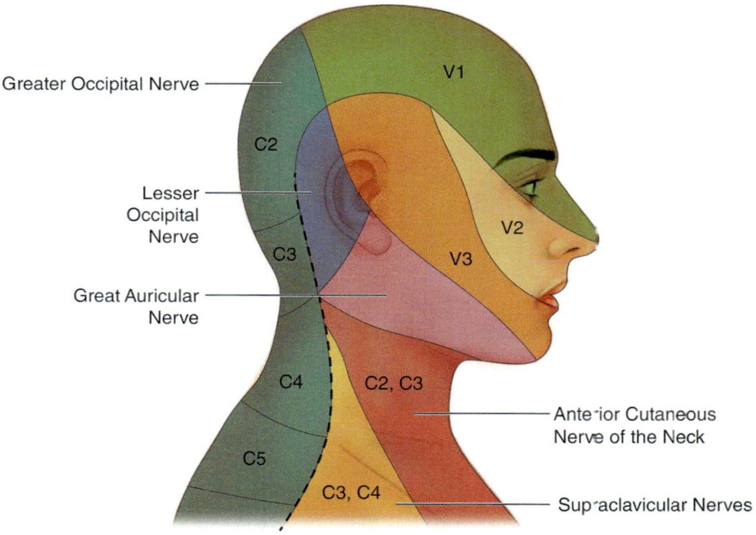

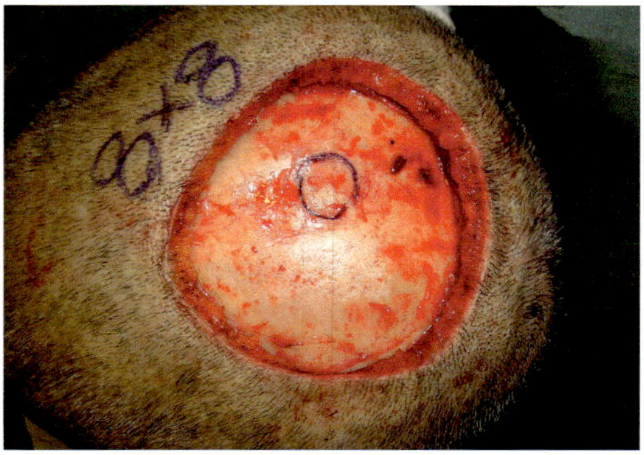

Fig. 2.11 The peripheral clearance before additional removal of the outer skull table producing a scalp defect 8 × 8 cm

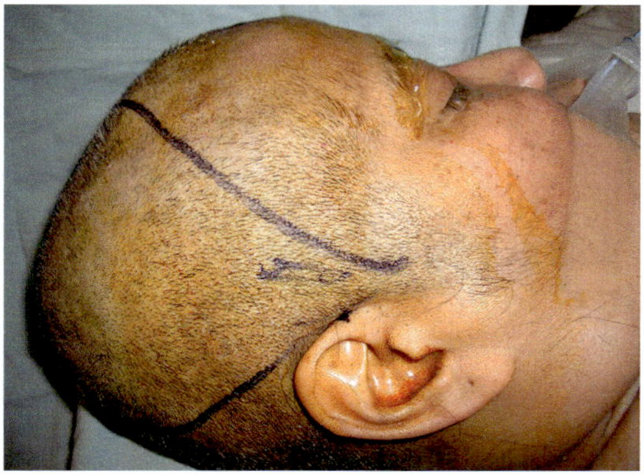

Fig. 2.12 Superficial temporal artery mark out. The flap is raised retaining and not skeletonising the axial neurovascular structures. This retains periadventitial tissue to ensure autonomic and somatic input

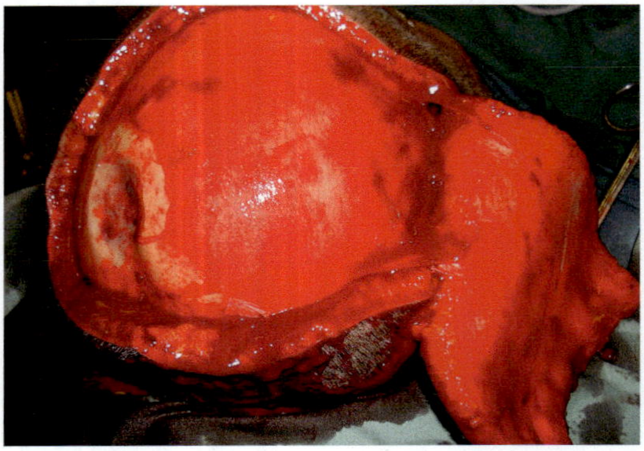

Fig. 2.13 Raising the flap using blunt dissection once the integument is divided around the periphery

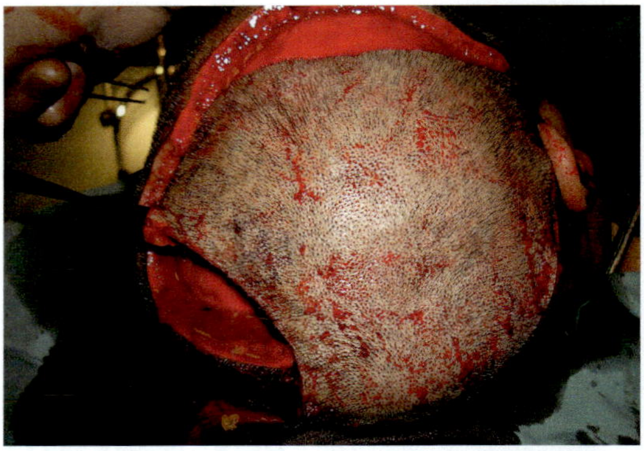

Fig. 2.14 Staged closure sequence

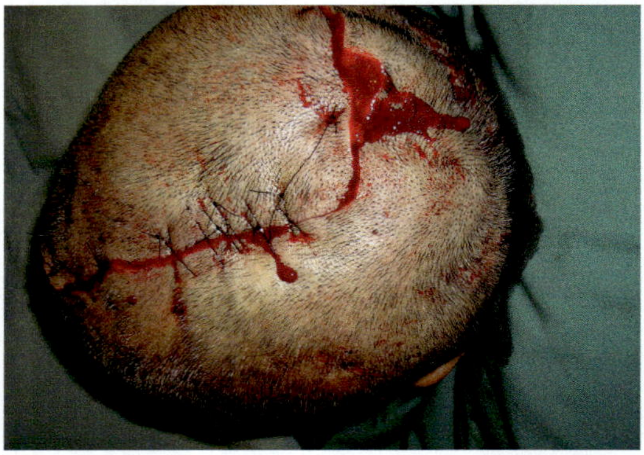

Fig. 2.15 The locking mattress sutures at the points of maximum tension to close the defect before ordinary mattress sutures produce wound closure

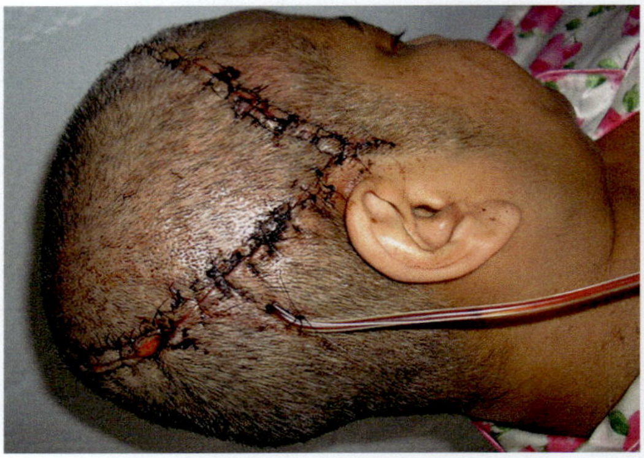

Fig. 2.16 On completion with Redi-vac drainage. Note the hyperaemic flare in this Keystone style island flap compared with the image of the surrounding scalp at the drain site

2.1.2.3 Case 3: Local Recurrence into the Occipital Glands

Level II melanoma of the scalp in a golfer. Secondary melanoma of the R neck – (T2N2) and occipital nodes in this 62-year-old male. Tumour-free interval 15 months (see Figs. 2.19, 2.20, 2.21, 2.22, 2.23, and 2.24).

In summary, islanding in the Keystone manner has hypervascularised the flap to close successfully a large oncological defect of secondary melanoma. All the P.A.C.E.S. characteristics were evident throughout the procedure indicating the Keystone principles apply in this reconstruction.

2.1.2.4 Case 4: R Occipital Mass Unknown Primary

Secondary melanoma dissemination into the posterior neck over the mastoid in a 77-year-old male following a scalp excision of the melanotic region 12 months earlier (see Figs. 2.25, 2.26, 2.27, 2.28, 2.29, and 2.30).

In summary, all the P.A.C.E.S. characteristics were evident throughout the procedure. Done as a DUET procedure with Professor Andrew Sizeland at the Peter McCallum Cancer Institute.

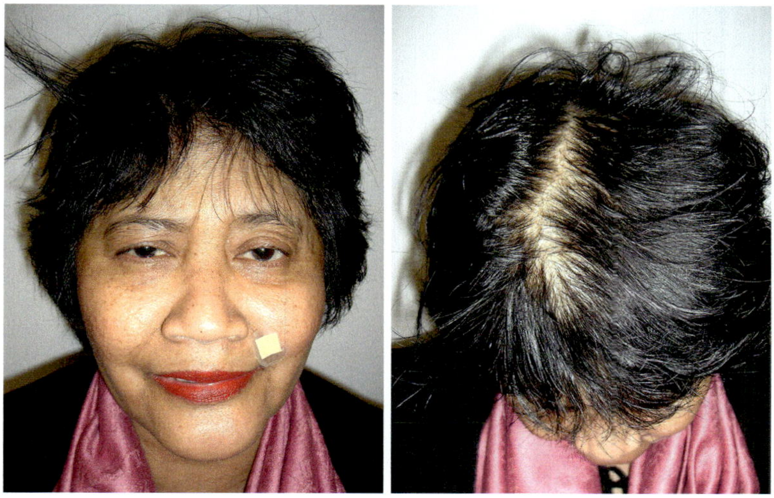

Fig. 2.17 The appearance 6 months later and I bring to your attention the patient's observation of the increased hair growth and thickness. Again, a clinical outcome of hypervascularity in the scalp

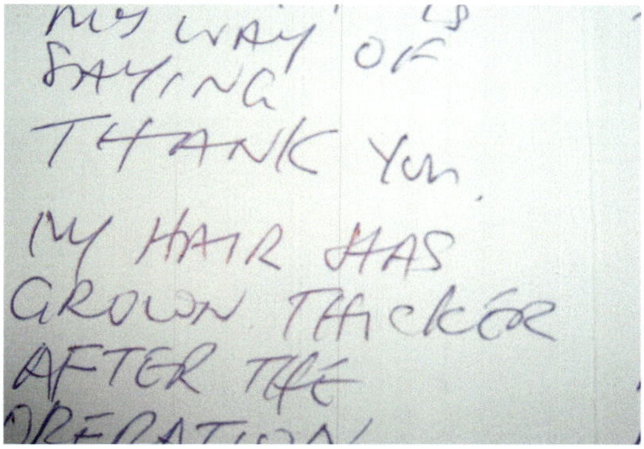

Fig. 2.18 Her Christmas card thanking me for the surgical procedure and stating that her hair is now growing thicker as a result of the Keystone reconstruction

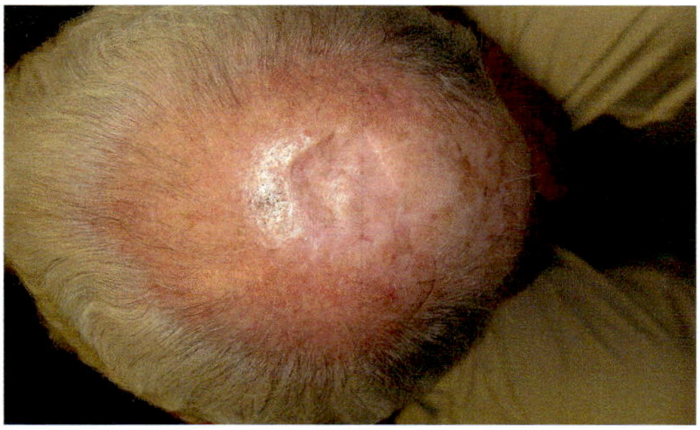

Fig. 2.19 The postoperative melanoma appearance of a graft on the scalp prior to regional dissemination into the R occipital glands

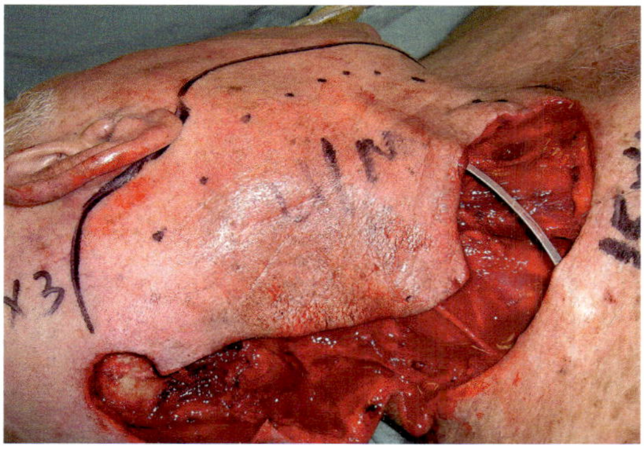

Fig. 2.20 The surgical clearance of the occipital glands and levels II, III and IV neck glands. The dissection created a defect 15 × 3 cm over the occiput and 15 × 4 cm in the neck performed by Professor Andrew Sizeland of the Peter MacCallum Cancer Institute
The flap undermining is defined by the Redi-vac tubing (arrowed) in situ and the distal incision leaving a third of deep attachment guarantees the flow at the fascial level and the hyperaemic vascular apperance.
This leaves 30% of deeper attachment along the chin and anterior neck, supplied by the facial artery and branches, but lying within the C3, C4 and C5 neuro-dermatomes. Without the skin incision to create the island of skin and subcuataneous tissue, the reflex hyperaemia would not occur and flap viability would be questionable. This simple idea of incising the skin then closing the wound surgically creates this biological phenomena of hypraemia to ensure the absence of necrosis in flap reconstruction.

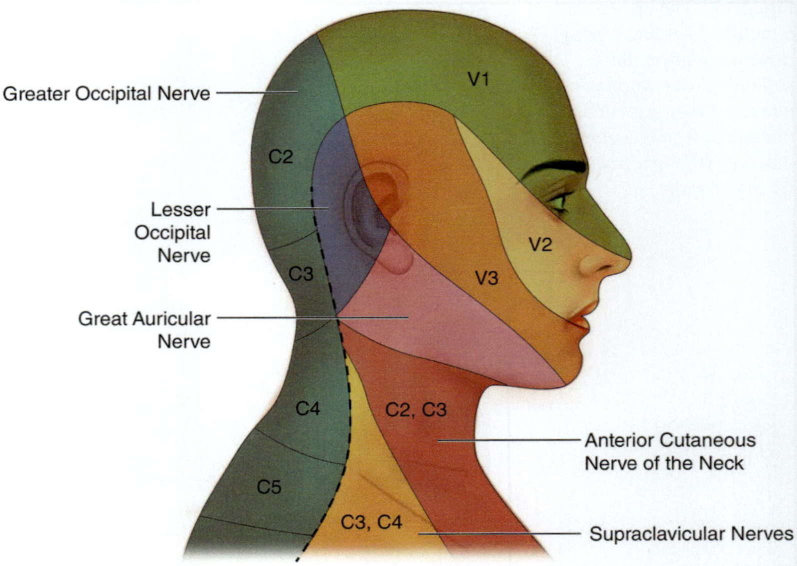

Fig. 2.21 The dermatomal mark out is the guide for the location of the random perforators coming through the fascia

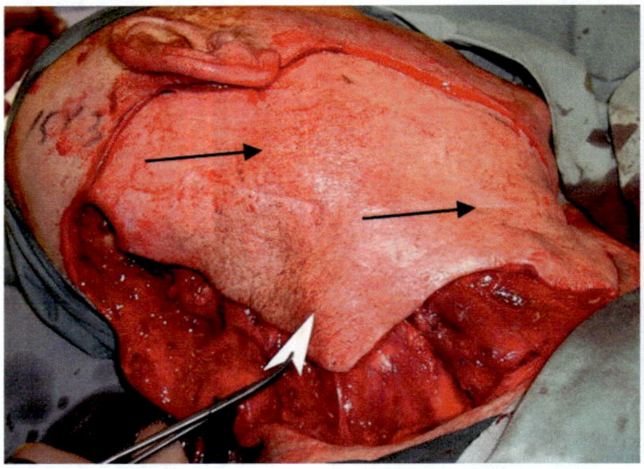

Fig. 2.22 The Keystone principle using a quadrilateral design in this case is evident. The island design anteriorly only penetrates the dermal epidermal line into the subcutaneous tissues only. Hypervascularisation becomes evident in a 10–15 min timeframe. It is hypothesised this is a sympathectomy effect at the epidermal level to increase flow. If this island is not created, flap necrosis would occur

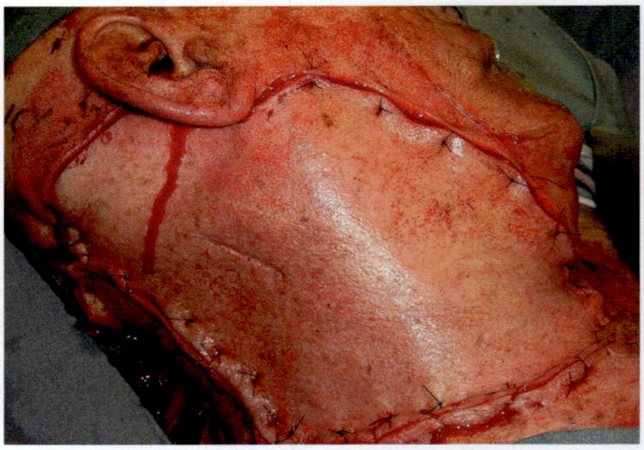

Fig. 2.23 Staged closure using the 3-phase suture technique of locking mattress sutures at the points of maximum tension to achieve cover. These stay in 21 days. The remaining wound is closed by interrupted mattress sutures, these stay in 14 days. Then a continuous nylon to achieve wound seal stays in 7–10 days. The vascular hyperaemia is evident

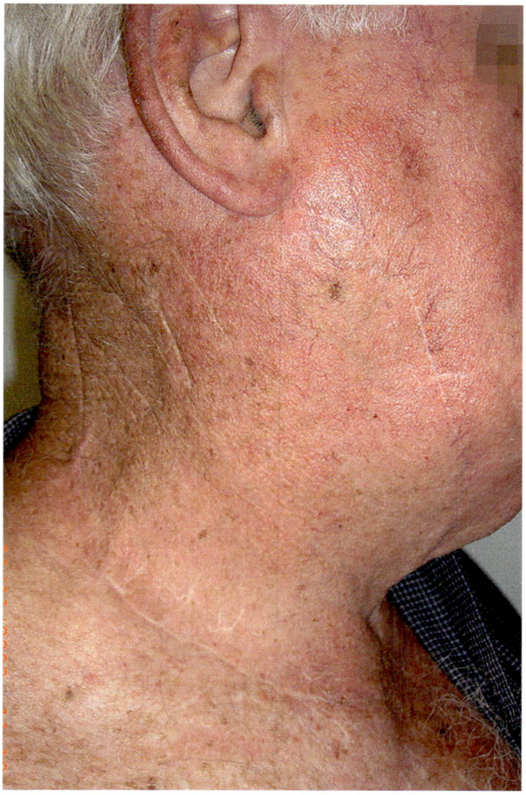

Fig. 2.24 The postoeprative healed wound appearance at 6 months. No evidence of necrosis throughout

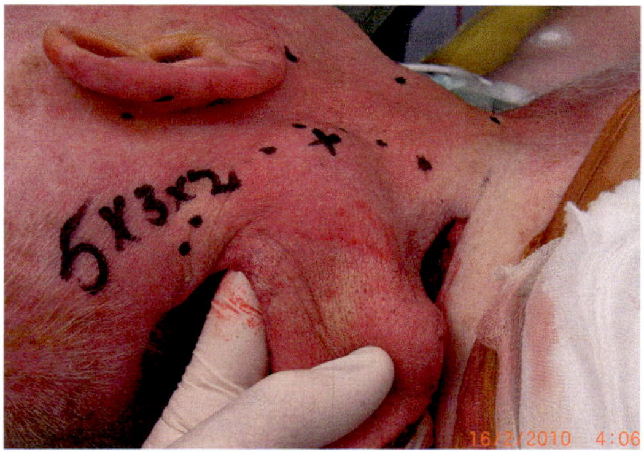

Fig. 2.25 The melanoma mass measured 5 × 3 × 2 cm in the hands of the operator before detachment and neck gland clearance

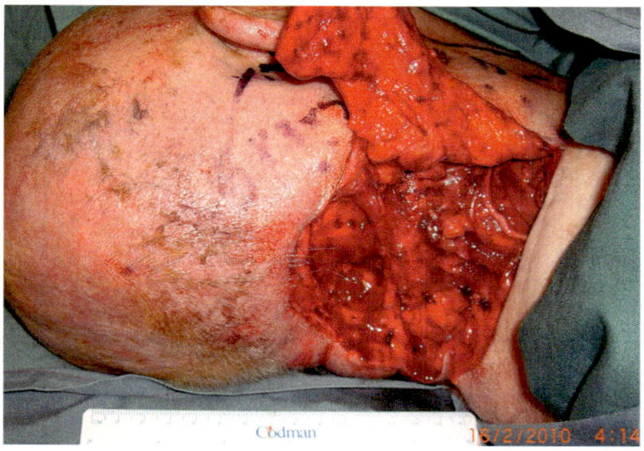

Fig. 2.26 Level cervical nodes in the R posterior triangle for clearance. Surgical defect with undermined anterior neck flaps for closure leaving one third deep attachment. The pyramidal-shaped Keystone is goverened by the surgical defect but leaving one third deep attachment below the R ear

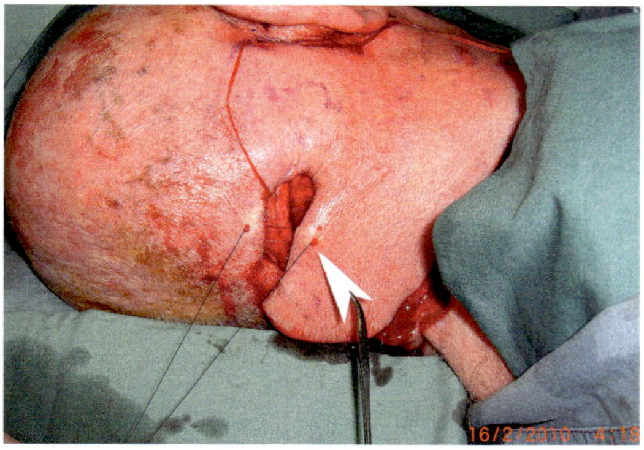

Fig. 2.27 For neck flap closure, the neck flaps are islanded in the region of the sternomastoid at the dermal epidermal level. This Keystone variant fits in with the oncological defect and requirements. The white arrow indicates the hyperaemia and the Red Dot Sign – all Keystone characteristics

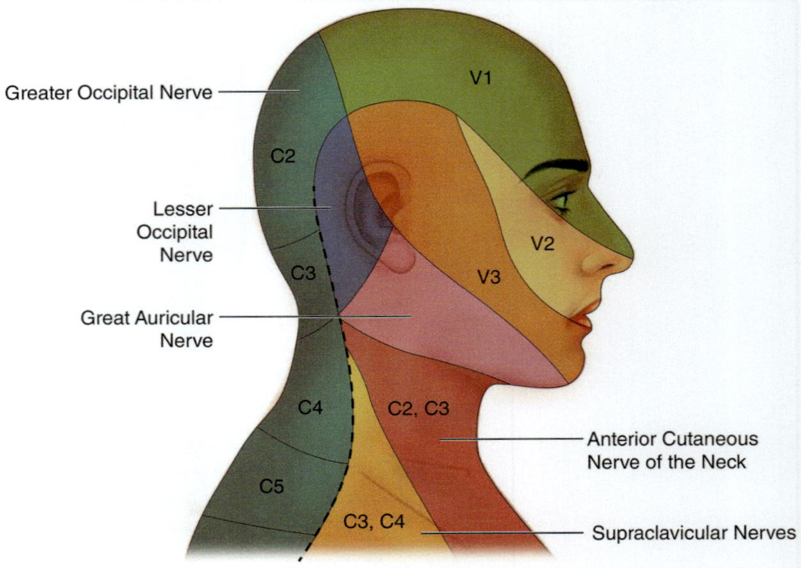

Fig. 2.28 The dermatomal mark out is the guide for the location of the random perforators coming through the fascia

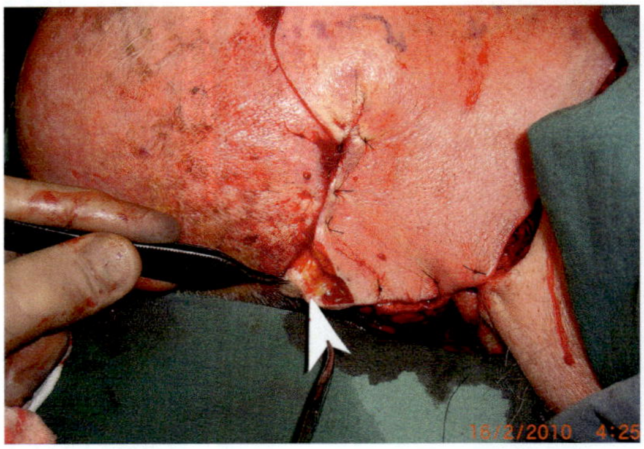

Fig. 2.29 Trimming out redundant tissue and the arrow indicates the generous subdermal flow to ensure healing without necrosis

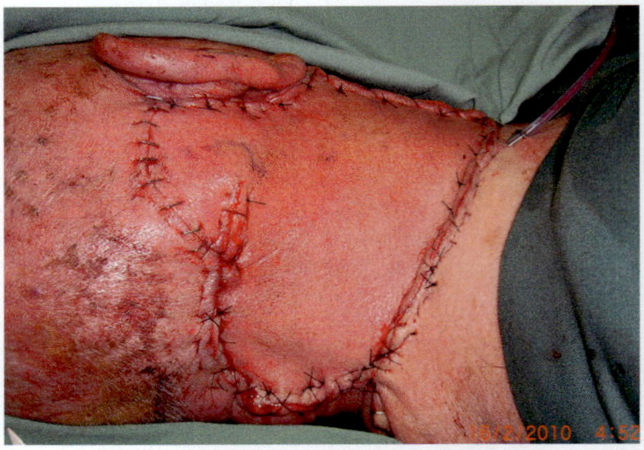

Fig. 2.30 The time taken from the timestamped images is 45 min. The 3-phase suture technique of locking mattress at tension points, ordinary mattress sutures and a continuous nylon for epidermal closure as is routinely used. RediVac drainage is mandatory

2.1.3 Forehead

The Keystones in the forehead are based on the main vessels including supratrochlear, supraorbital and superficial temporal artery neurovascular structures. The associated sensory supply, when included in the Keystone, this provides contact and protective sensation in the vicinity of the repair. One must be aware of the facial nerve innervation of the frontalis muscle and caution in reconstruction of such defects. However, the relative inelasticity of the tissue [13] is a well-recognised restriction in reconstruction in this region. Simple techniques of A-to-T flaps are part of the reconstructive options, the Bezier neurovascular island flap [14] which is an ellipsoidal design but using V-Y principles as originally documented [15]. Using local tissue for local tissue has the advantage of an aesthetic outcome with the surrounding tissues. Various locational sites will be part of the presentation.

Free tissue transfer is reserved for larger defects but the Keystone has a remarkable proclivity of spreading tension throughout the distribution of the delineated fascial island flap which seems to make closure, based on the dermatomes, a reasonable alternative. I offer you the appearance of a free flap reconstruction compared with the Keystone and the likes of latissimus dorsi and radial forearm fail abysmally from a tissue match point of view, let alone the bulky protuberance (see Figs. 2.31, 2.32, and 2.33).

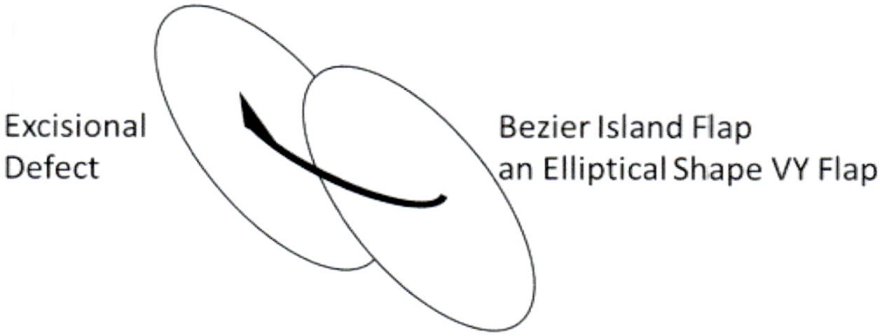

Fig. 2.31 Excisional defect with the Bezier markout

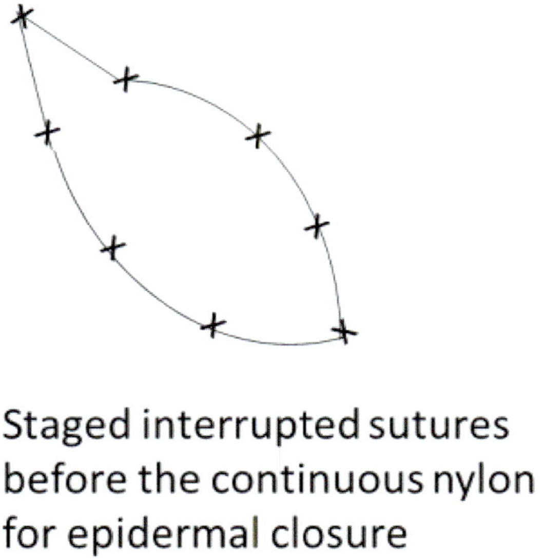

Fig. 2.32 Surgical closure with VY apposition

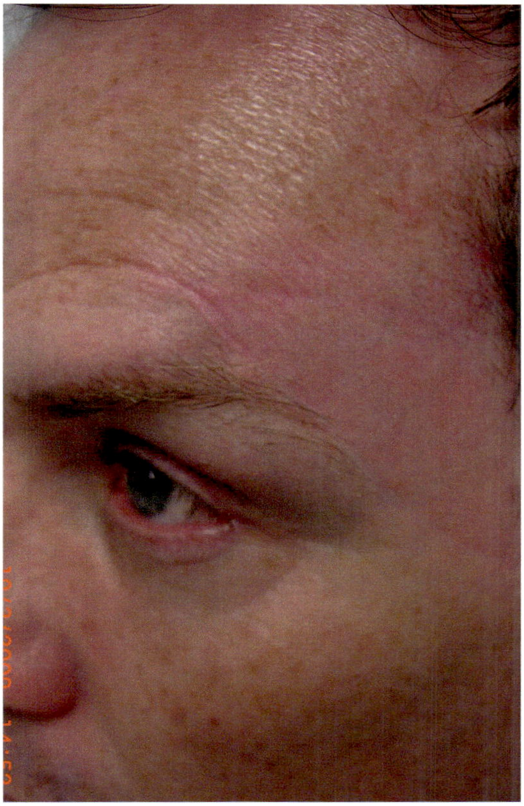

Fig. 2.33 A clinical exmaple of the Bezier curvilinear V-Y island flap – appearance at 6 months

2.1.3.1 Case 5: Bezier Flap [14] for a Mitotic Lesion of the R Temple

See Figs. 2.34, 2.35, 2.36, 2.37, 2.38, 2.39, 2.40, and 2.41

In summary, all the P.A.C.E.S. characteristics of the Keystone were evident throughout the procedure.

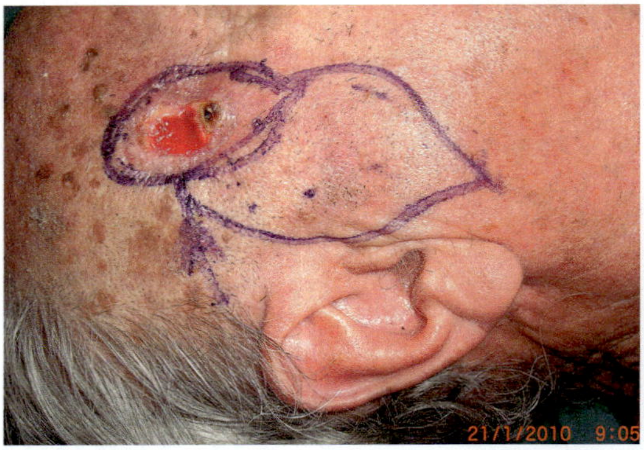

Fig. 2.34 The 6 × 4 cm excisional defect is closed by the curvilinear Bezier flap employing the same V-Y principles. Blunt dissection allows the tissue to be realigned into the surgical defect

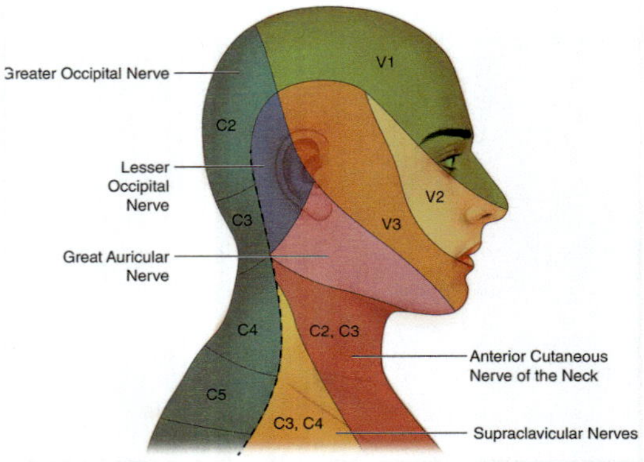

Fig. 2.35 The dermatomal mark out is the guide for the location of the random perforators coming through the fascia

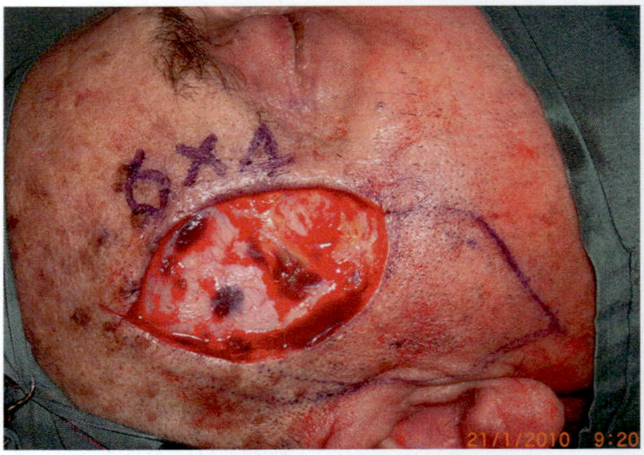

Fig. 2.36 The size of the excisional defect 6 × 4 cm

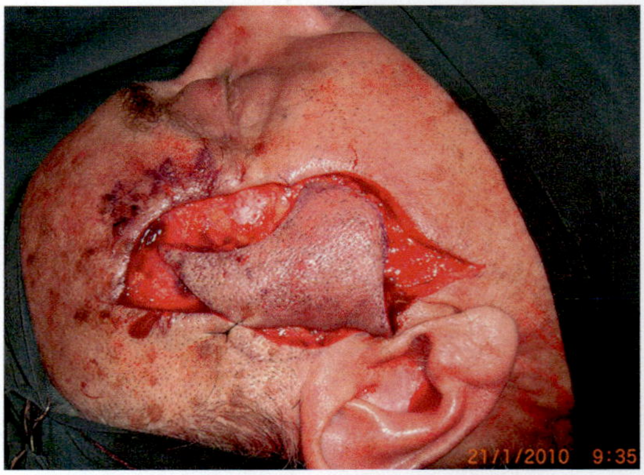

Fig. 2.37 Blunt dissection around the periphery of the flap preserves the integrity of the facial nerve branches without defining them individually leaving one third deep attachment on the deep surface

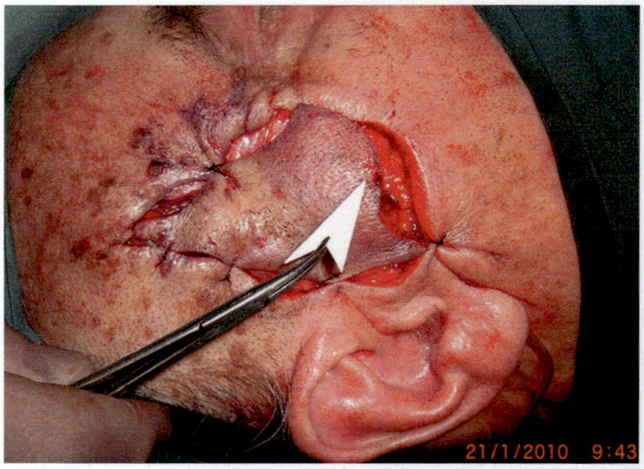

Fig. 2.38 The arrow sits on a Red Dot Sign indicating it is in the hyperaemic phase, verifying Keystone principles

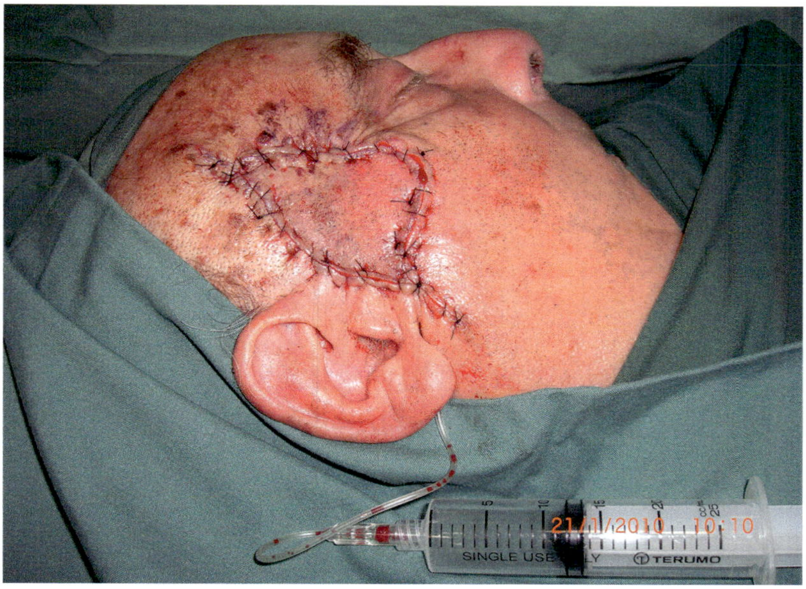

Fig. 2.39 Completed closure. Note the hyperaemia consistent with the Keystone principles, without undue lines of tension at the outer canthus. Drainage technique using a 20-ml syringe: fenestrated plastic tubing attached to a 20-ml syringe, held out to length by the needle protector sheath, volume of drainage is measured then suction reapplied

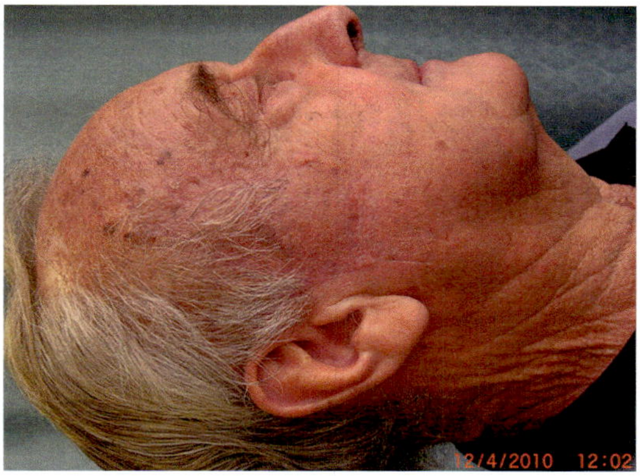

Fig. 2.40 Appearance at 3 months

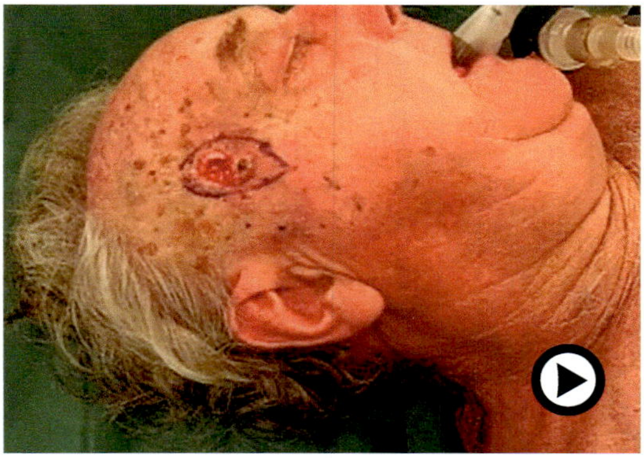

Fig. 2.41 Operative sequence (▶ https://doi.org/10.1007/000-b4n)

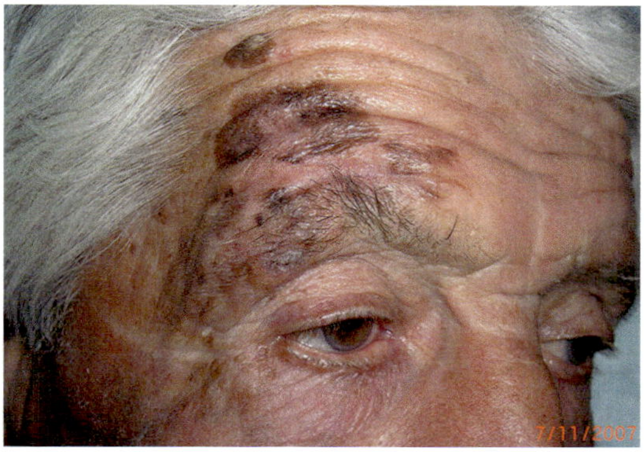

Fig. 2.42 Level II melanoma in an Hutchinson's melanotic freckle. The Hutchinson's melanotic freckle extended over a distance 6 × 6 cm of the R supraorbital region

2.1.3.2 Case 6: Level II Melanoma in a Hutchinson's Melanotic Freckle of the R Supraorbital Region

This 75-year-old male farmer had an HMF of the R forehead.

Surgically excised and delayed reconstruction awaiting pathology (the DRAPE [16] procedure).

Further surgical excision confirmed clearance histologically (see Figs. 2.42, 2.43, 2.44, 2.45, 2.46, 2.47, 2.48, 2.49, 2.50, and 2.51).

In summary, all the P.A.C.E.S. characteristics of the Keystone were evident throughout these

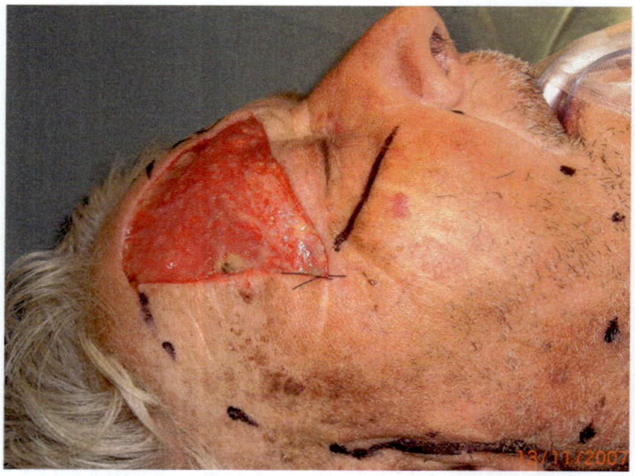

Fig. 2.43 The surgical defect 6 × 6 cm is revealed including supraorbital nerves to avoid any perineural dissemination. The Keystone flap mark out is dotted around the R cheek from the infraorbital region to the nasolabial line and up the preauricular groove. The oblique incision along the lower eyelid region is done to avoid ectropion. The skin island incision from the nasolabial region around to the angle of the jaw is not part of the flap advancement or rotation. This nasolabial incision creating the island is closed directly. It is an absolute necessity to create the hyperaemic phase in the island flap to avoid necrosis and lying within the V2 and V3 dermatomes

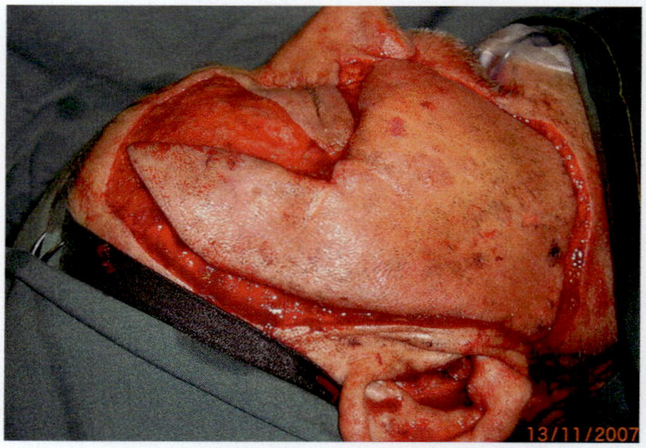

Fig. 2.45 This quadrangular shape Keystone is advanced towards the midline of the forehead with blunt dissection around the posterior and superior limits of the flap. The inferior (neck) and the anterior limits (nasolabial) are just closed directly. Islanding of a flap creates hyperaemia – an observational finding. It takes 10–15 min to show this vascular change as long as there is deep attachment throughout

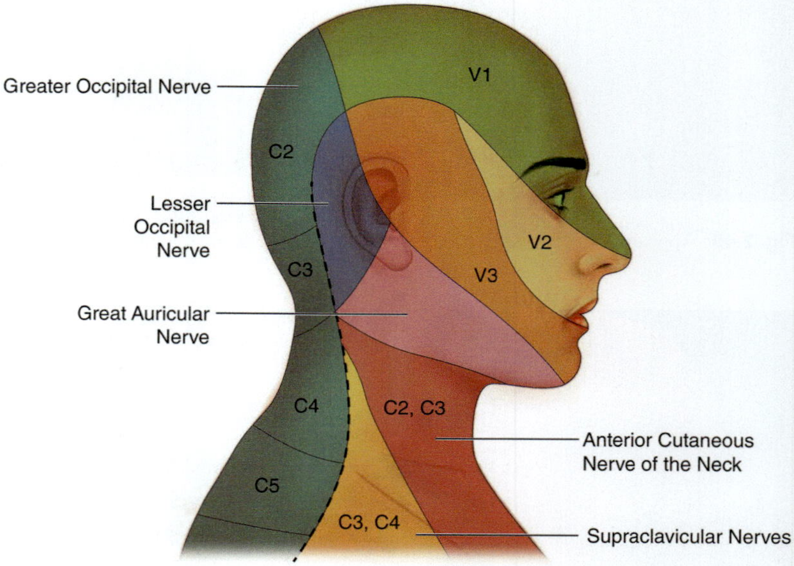

Fig. 2.44 The V2, V3 dermatomal mark out is the guide for the location of the random perforators coming through the fascia

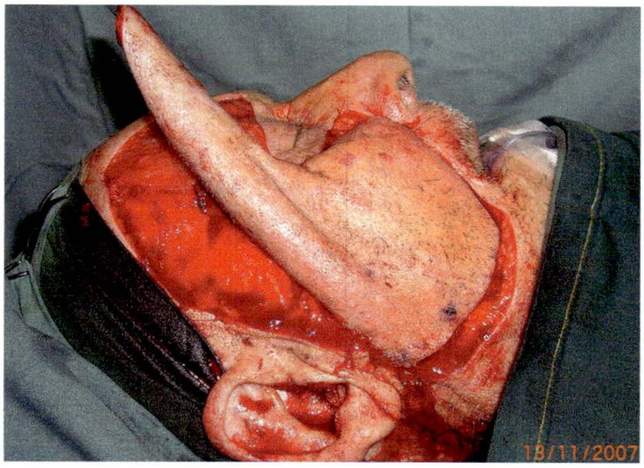

Fig. 2.46 The posterosuperior margins of the flap are undermined leaving approximately one third attached in the region of the infraorbital nerve and the neurovascular bundle on the V2 dermatome. As long as there is at least one third deep attachment in the infraorbital and nasolabial regions, this ensures the viability of the flap

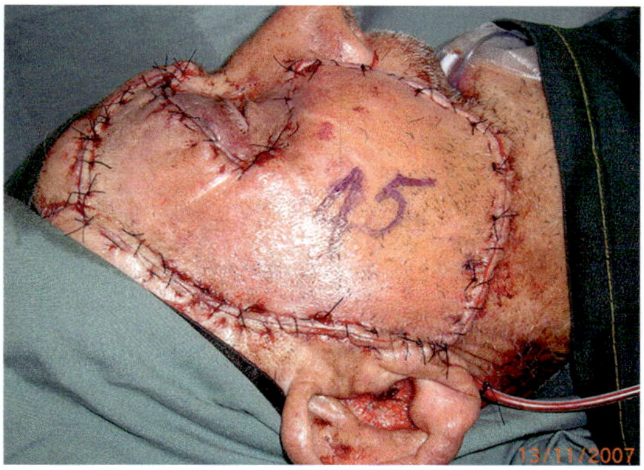

Fig. 2.47 Three-phase closure technique is repeated: locking mattress sutures at the points of maximum tension, ordinary mattress sutures to create tissue alignment and a continuous nylon suture to get epidermal seal. Suture removal comes out at 1 week, 2 weeks and 3 week intervals

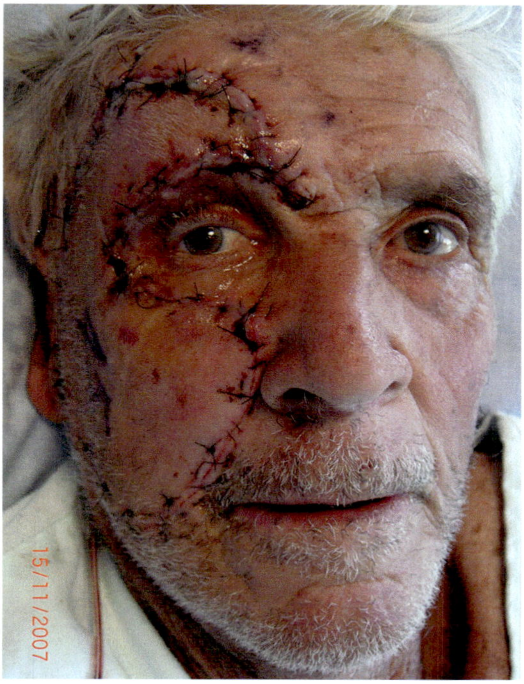

Fig. 2.48 Appearance at 2 days with no evidence of impending flap necrosis with the Redi-Vac still in situ

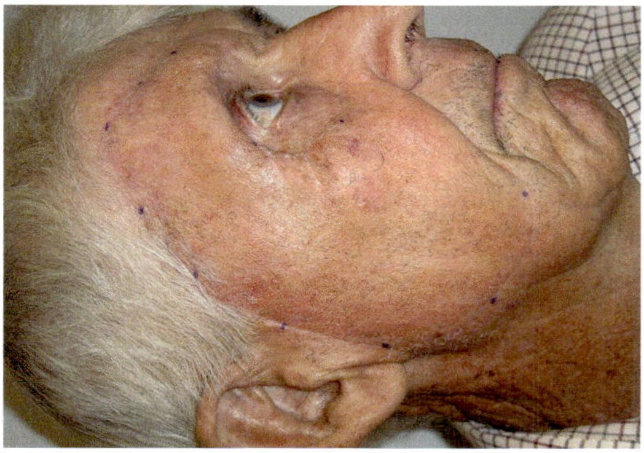

Fig. 2.49 Appearance at 6 months and to show the quality of the wound healing the suture outline has been dotted to confirm the refinement of this simple single layered closure

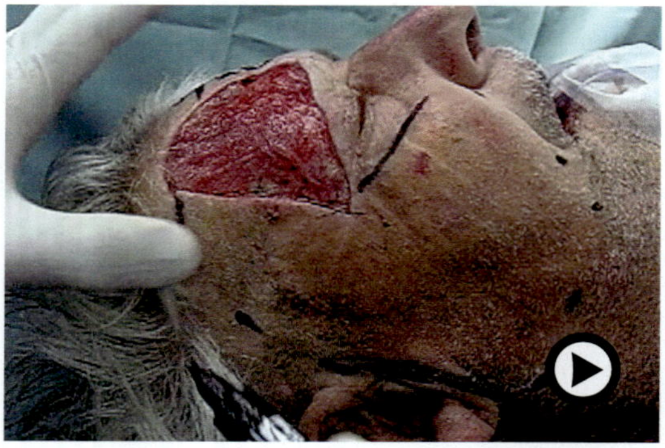

Fig. 2.50 Operative sequence (▶ https://doi.org/10.1007/000-b4p)

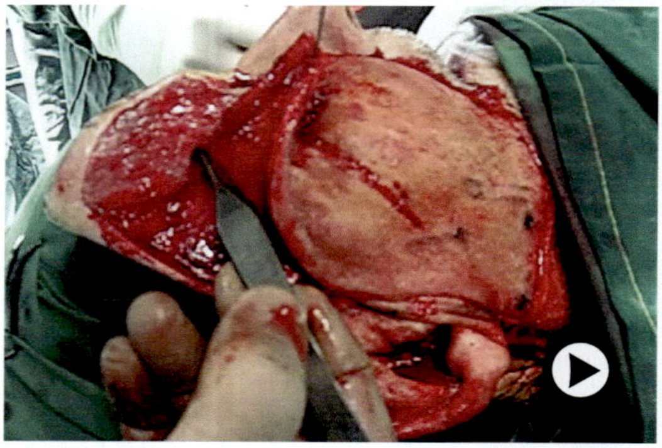

Fig. 2.51 Operative sequence (▶ https://doi.org/10.1007/000-b4q)

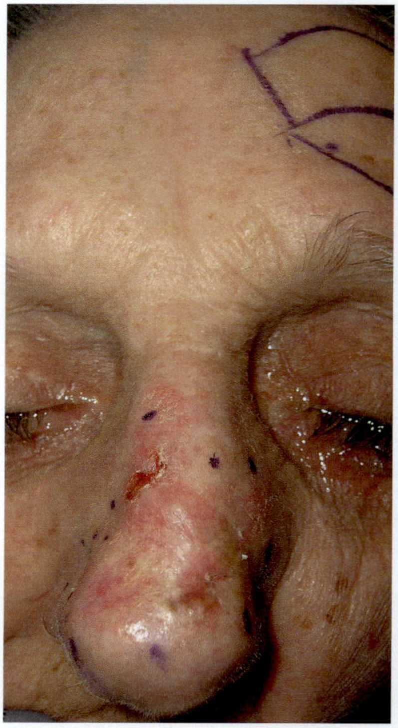

Fig. 2.52 Keystone repair of the forehead defect. The excision of the L supraorbital region is followed by a superior supraorbital Keystone and the blunt dissection is part of the technique as illustrated in Fig. 7.3

procedures. Done as a DUET procedure with Professor Andrew Sizeland at the Peter McCallum Cancer Institute.

2.1.3.3 Case 7: Forehead Reconstruction Using the Keystone

Multifocal mitotic skin lesions of the L forehead. The supraorbital Keystone design, preserving the integrity of the supraorbital vascular complex, is achieved by blunt dissection using the scissor technique, stretching the tissue, visualizing the nerve and closing in the routine Keystone manner (see Figs. 2.52, 2.53, 2.54, 2.55, 2.56, and 2.57).

2.1.4 Ear

The anatomical breakdown of the ear with its skin and cartilaginous components is easily repaired when wedge excisions and the like are necessary for melanoma. However, the Keystone has particular reference for conchal fossa reconstructions. The postauricular design using random mastoidal and postauricular neurovascular structures can be channeled from the postauricular groove into the conchal defect, attaching it to the epidermal lining of the external canal and the helix rim can be aligned back over the Keystone, which is de-epithelialised over the helical mark out, sewn together to give anatomical and aesthetic continuity.

2.1.4.1 Case 8: 3 × 3 cm Defect Conchal Fossa Involving the Mastoid Bone

A mitotic lesion of the conchal fossa with excision and closure technique using the Keystone principle along the C2, C3 dermatomes of the neck with an incontinuity neck dissection. The helical rim closure fits into the de-epithelialised

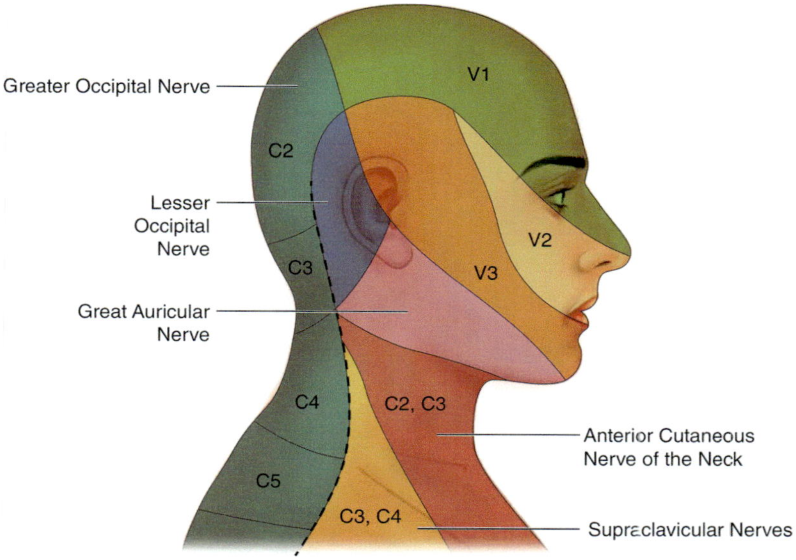

Fig. 2.53 The dermatomal mark out is the guide for the location of the random perforators coming through the fascia

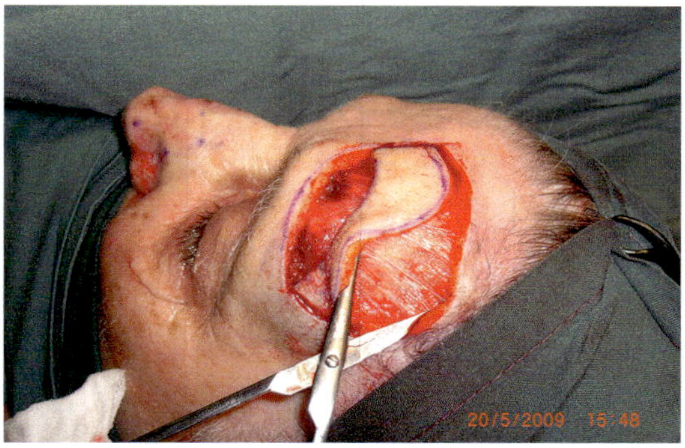

Fig. 2.54 The tissue displacement with surgical scissors preserves the integrity of the supraorbital nerve

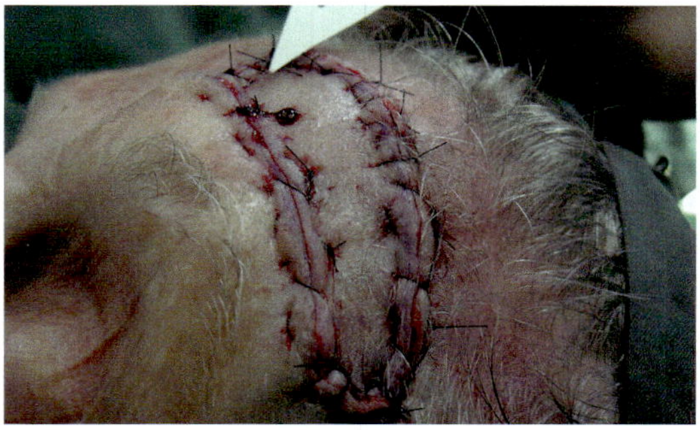

Fig. 2.55 The completion of the Keystone reconstruction. Note the Red Dot Sign on the arrow confirming its vascular integrity

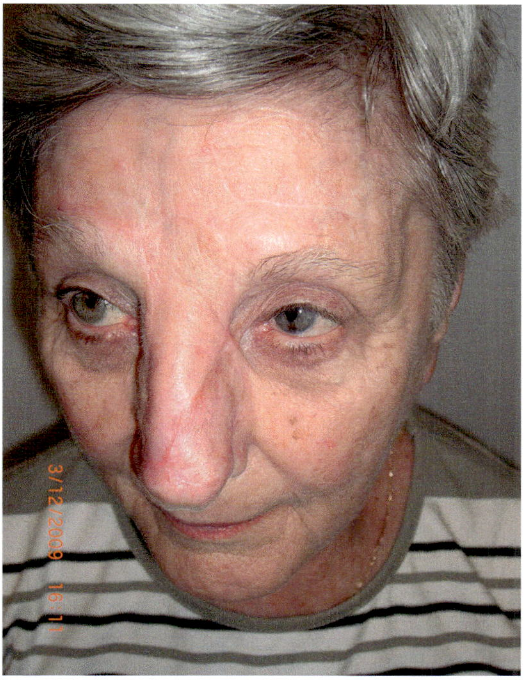

Fig. 2.56 Postoperative appearance at 6 months

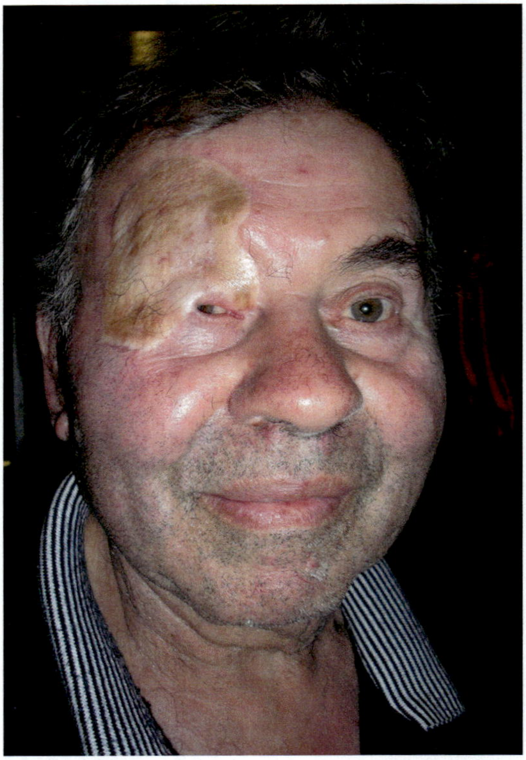

Fig. 2.57 A microsurgical reconstruction done by another unit illustrating the lack of aesthetic refinement and visual restrictions and epiphora for repair of a similar defect

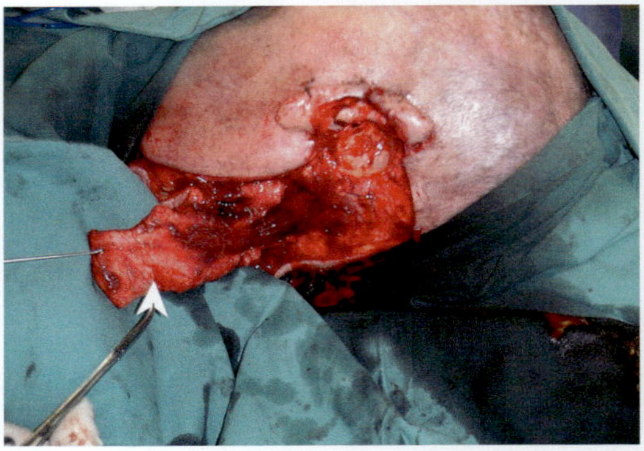

Fig. 2.58 Excision of a mitotic lesion of the L conchal fossa mastoid tip including Levels II, III and IV neck dissection

section in distal third of the cervical Keystone and closure is completed. The neck wounds, following Levels II, III and IV for the neck dissection, are also closed directly including the helical bridge. This technique has universal applications for conchal fossa and helical reconstructions (see Figs. 2.58, 2.59, 2.60, 2.61, 2.62, 2.63, and 2.64).

In summary, all the P.A.C.E.S. characteristics were evident throughout these procedures. Done as a DUET procedure with Professor Andrew Sizeland at the Peter McCallum Cancer Institute.

Fig. 2.59 The dermatomal mark out is the guide for the location of the random perforators coming through the fascia

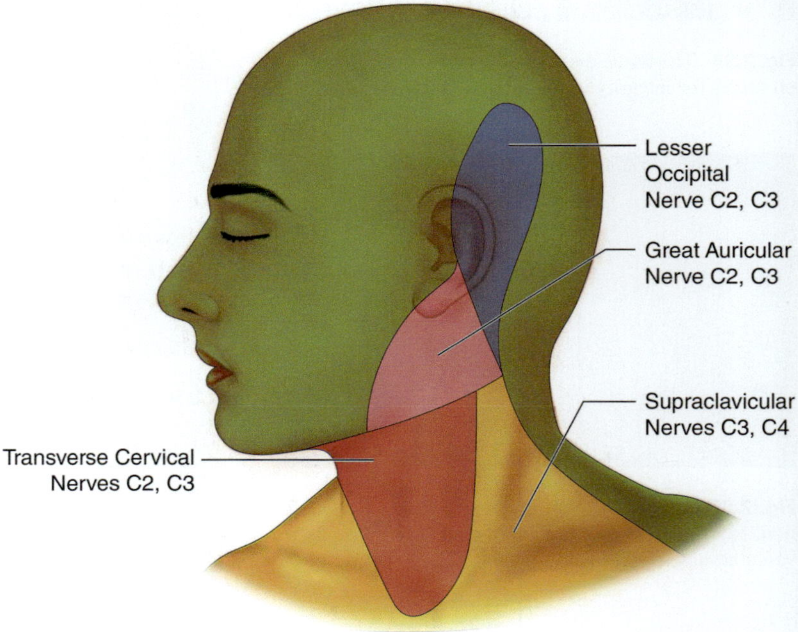

2.1.4.2 Case 9: 8 × 5 cm Defect Near Total Amputation of an Ear

Recurrent melanoma of the ear Level II melanoma in a 68-year-old male (see Figs. 2.65, 2.66, 2.67, 2.68, 2.69, and 2.70).

In summary, all the P.A.C.E.S. characteristics were exemplified.

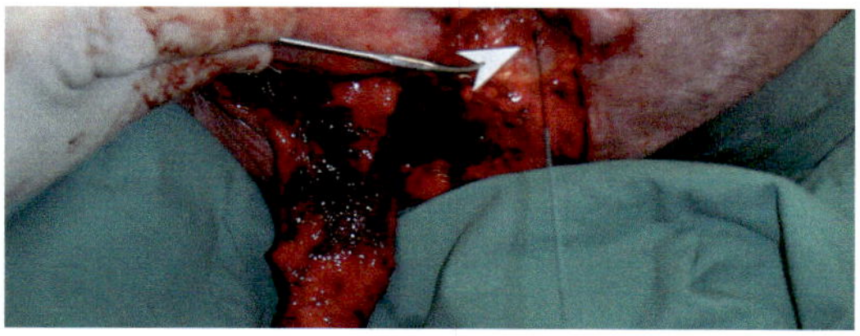

Fig. 2.60 The size of the mitotic defect including mastoid bone 3 × 3 cm

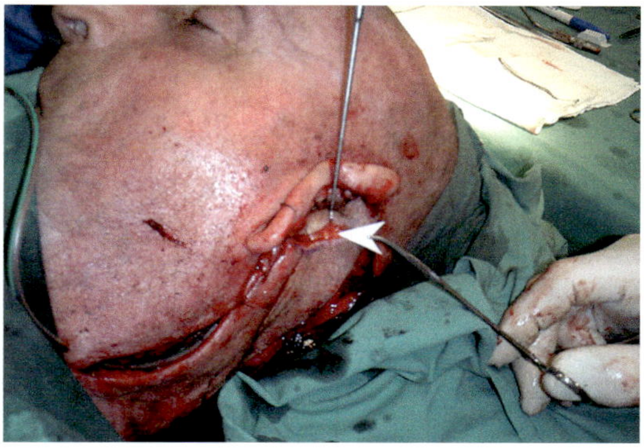

Fig. 2.61 The C2, C3 cervical Keystone closes the defect but for the helix of the ear to be reattached a de-epithelialised section allows this to be sutured in situ. This completes the ear reconstruction

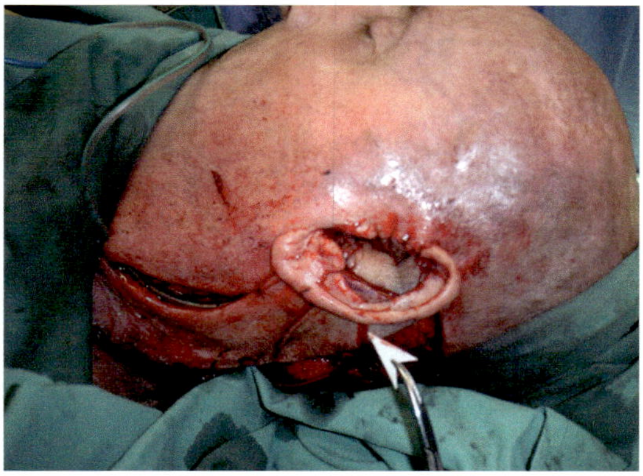

Fig. 2.62 Wound closure of the conchal fossa including the cervical Keystone flap donor site. Note the hyperaemic phase of the Keystone inspite of having a de-epitherialised section along which the helical rim is inserted

2.1.4.3 Case 10: Partial Ear Amputation – the Omega Variant of the Keystone

See Figs. 2.71, 2.72, 2.73, 2.74, 2.75, 2.76, 2.77, 2.78, 2.79, 2.80, and 2.81

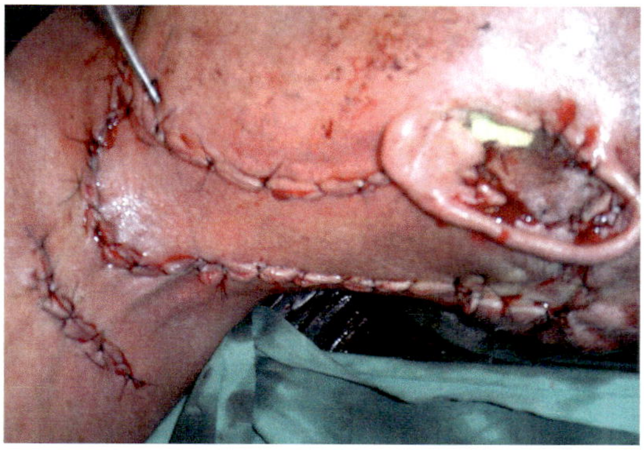

Fig. 2.63 On completion with the viable flap in the conchal fossa and the neck wound closed completely under Redi-vac seal using this standard 3-phase suture technique

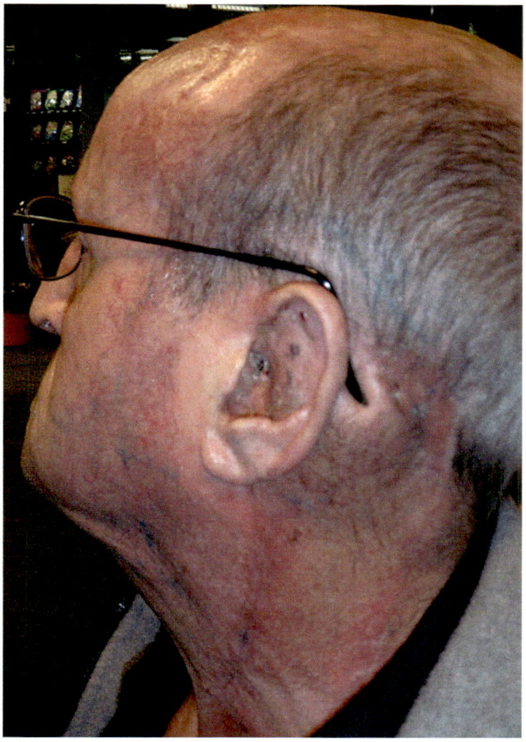

Fig. 2.64 Postoperative appearance at 6 months with no evidence of recurrence

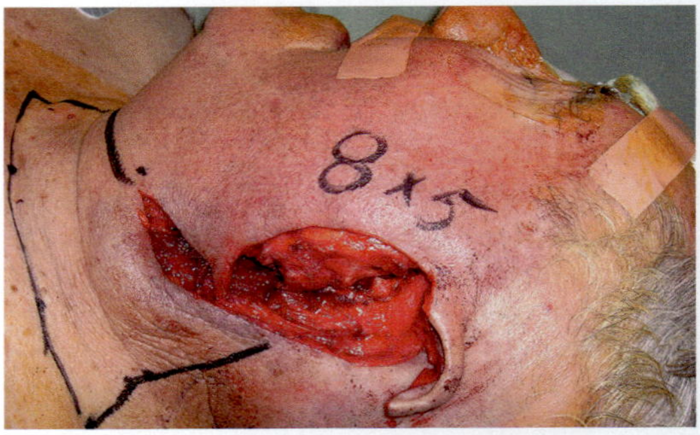

Fig. 2.65 The surgical defect 8 × 5 cm, a result of the near total ear amputation and the incontinuity neck clearance. The L ear apex is retained leaving a superior helix remnant for spectacles
The Keystone flap is outlined (transverse cervical nerves C2, C3 are used in this dermatomal alignment with the cervical fascial lined Keystone flap is the basis for the reconstruction)

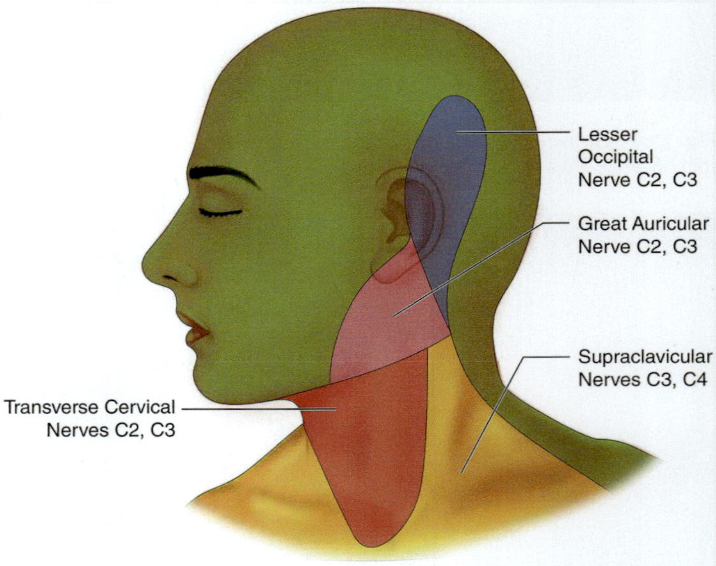

Fig. 2.66 The dermatomal mark out of the C2, C3 distribution is the guide for the location of the random perforators coming through the fascia

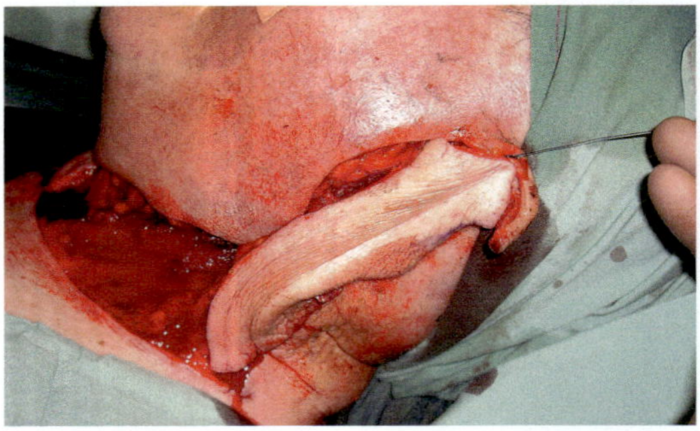

Fig. 2.67 The flap is rotated at 90°. The deep attachment is in the proximal one third sitting over the sternomastoid muscle perforators. These do not require individual dissection but are left as a random group with the deep muscle attachment

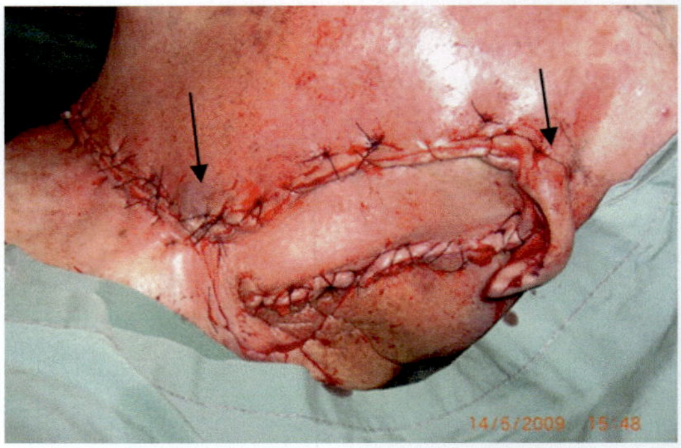

Fig. 2.68 The neck is closed directly at the V-Y point. The Keystone is inserted into the conchal fossa and its design is based on the cervico submental C2, C3 dermatomes. The arrowed points of maximum tension are the only sites where complications may arise from premature removal of the sutures. Thus, this locking mattress suture must stay in over three weeks to prevent wound rupture

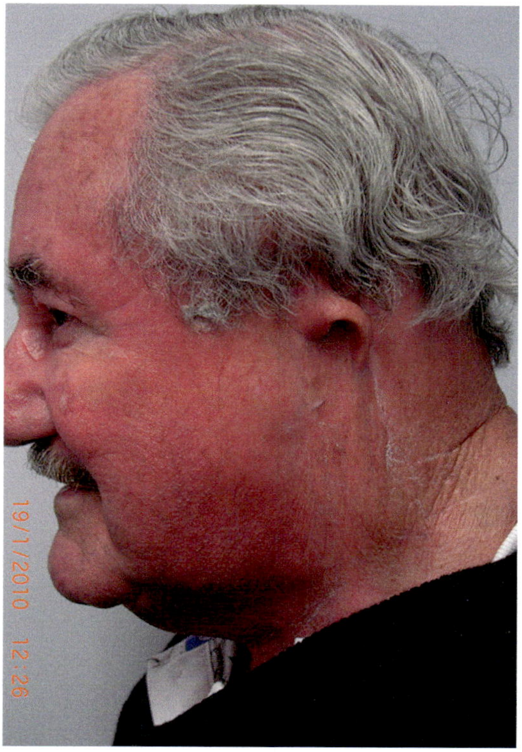

Fig. 2.69 The postoperative view of a satisfied patient. The superior remnant of the ear is for his spectacles

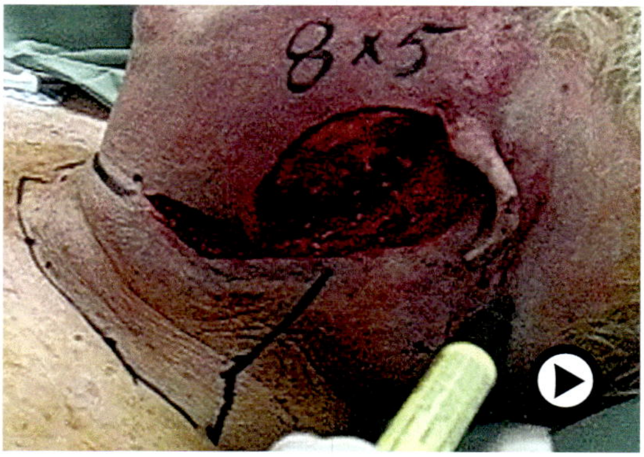

Fig. 2.70 Operative sequence (▶ https://doi.org/10.1007/000-b4r)

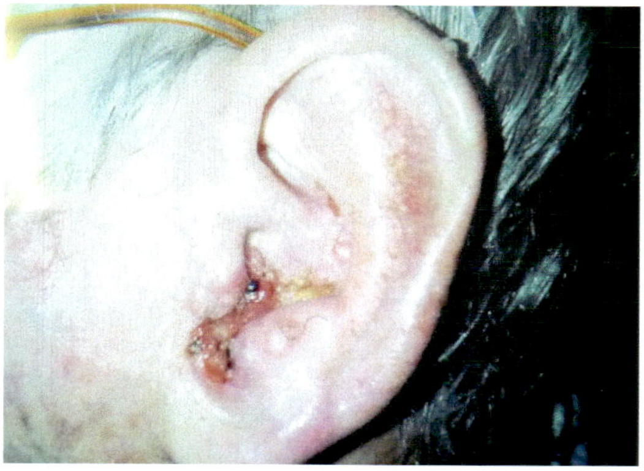

Fig. 2.71 The malignancy of the conchal fossa of the L ear involving the external auditory bony canal

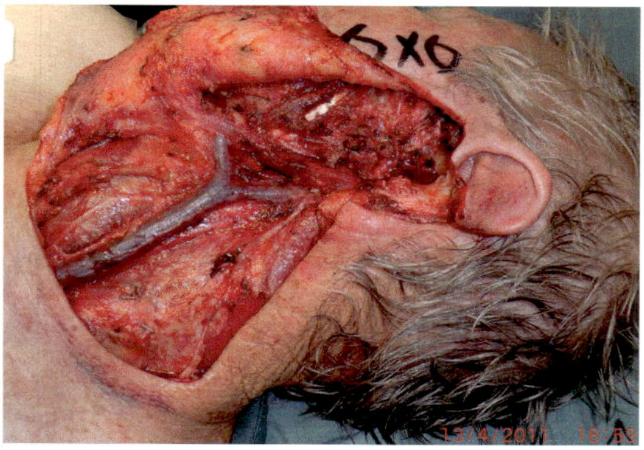

Fig. 2.72 The oncological defect is 6 × 6 cm involving a partial amputation of the ear leaving the upper helix as the only remnant. The oncological clearance of neck glands Levels II, II and IV and the external jugular vein is retained to optimise venous drainage avoiding necrosis

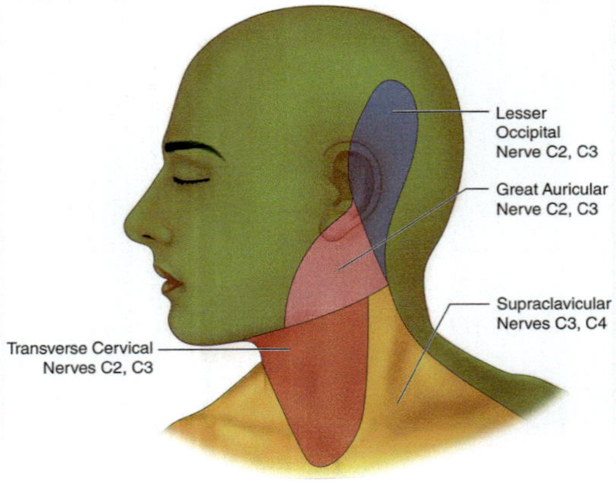

Fig. 2.73 The dermatomal mark out is the guide for the location of the random perforators coming through the fascia

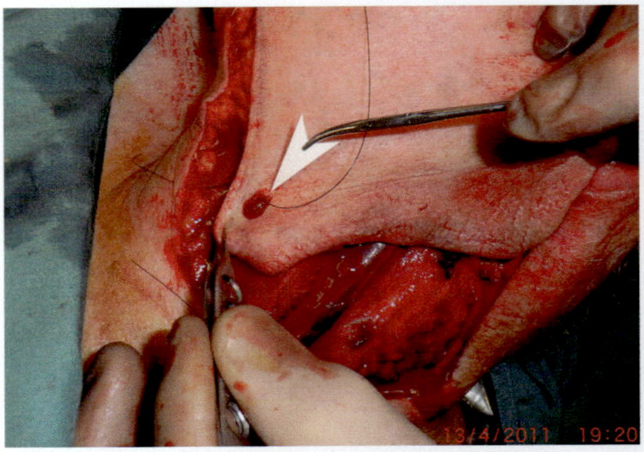

Fig. 2.75 The arrow shows the hyperaemic phase at the apex of the flap. The suture creates the Red Dot Sign bleeding more on the flap side than on the receiving site. The site of potential necrosis at the apex is overcome by this islanding technique

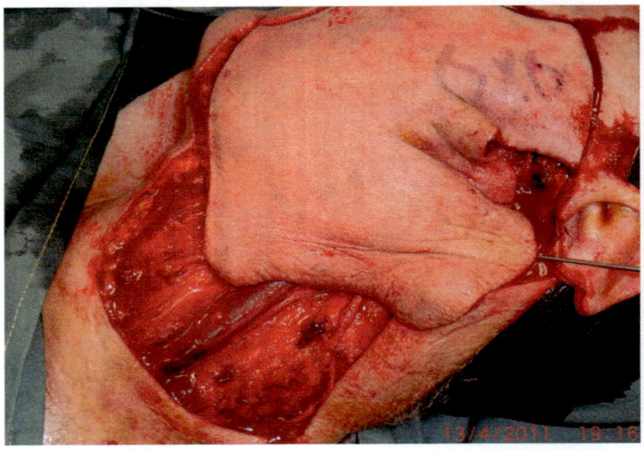

Fig. 2.74 The lower cervial tissues are part of the neck flap rotated into the defect creating the Omega variant Keystone. Islanding is an essential requirement of the technique. It is designed along the nasolabial line to ensure the hyperaemic phase, part of the Keystone concept

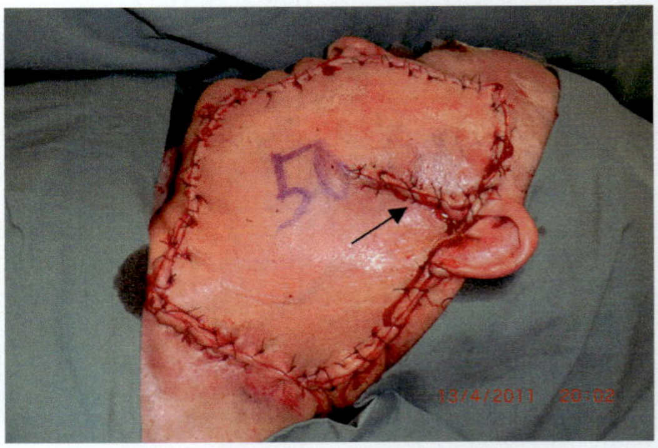

Fig. 2.76 Finally the U-shaped Omega variant Keystone allows direct closure using the 3-phase suture technique. Such is the reliabilty of the hyperaemia, any dog ears (arrowed) of redundent tissue can be trimmed with impunity at the epidermal level

2.1.5 Parotid

Melanomas in the vicinity of the parotid are usually associated with the excision of lesion and the underlying parotid mass as an oncological principle, with or without neck dissection as indicated usually in Levels II, III and IV.

The case series here ranges in age from 35 to 83 years averaging 62 years but the Keystone reconstructive principle can embrace all age groups and the speed and efficiency of reconstruction is welcomed always by the anaesthetic team, i.e. a rapid exit off the operating table for age and morbidity reasons.

This case series covers simple and complex reconstructions depending on the location and whether or not there is recurrent pathology. However, all the Keystone clinical characteristics are evident and have been recorded from the patient's response as summarised in P.A.C.E.S.

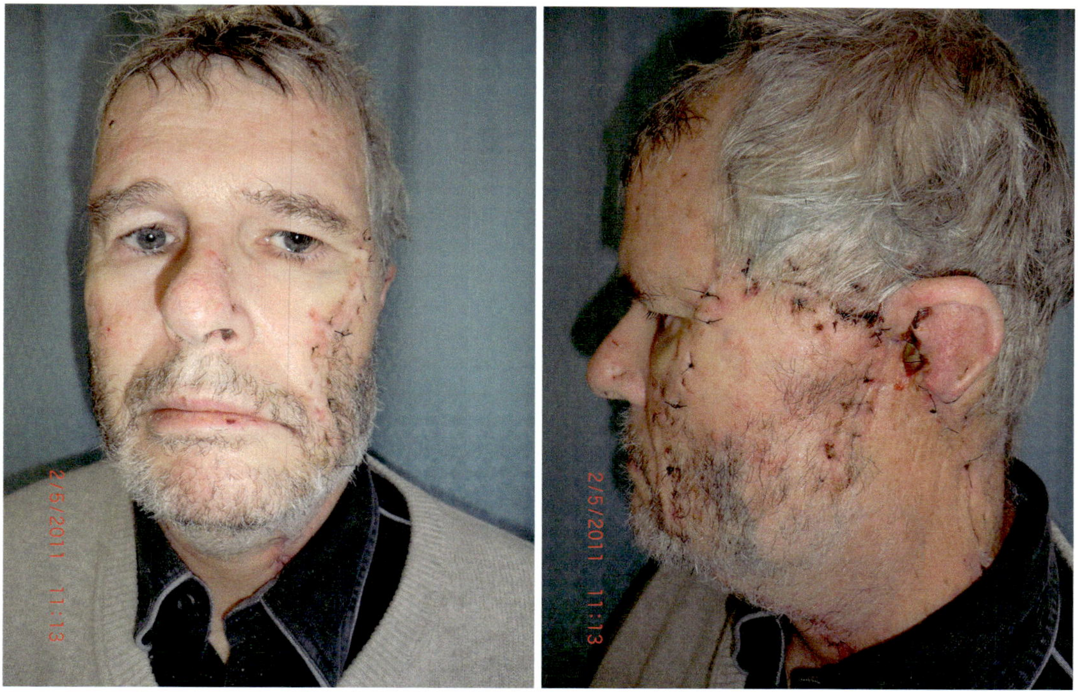

Fig. 2.77 Postoperative appearance at 2 weeks in between staged removal of sutures

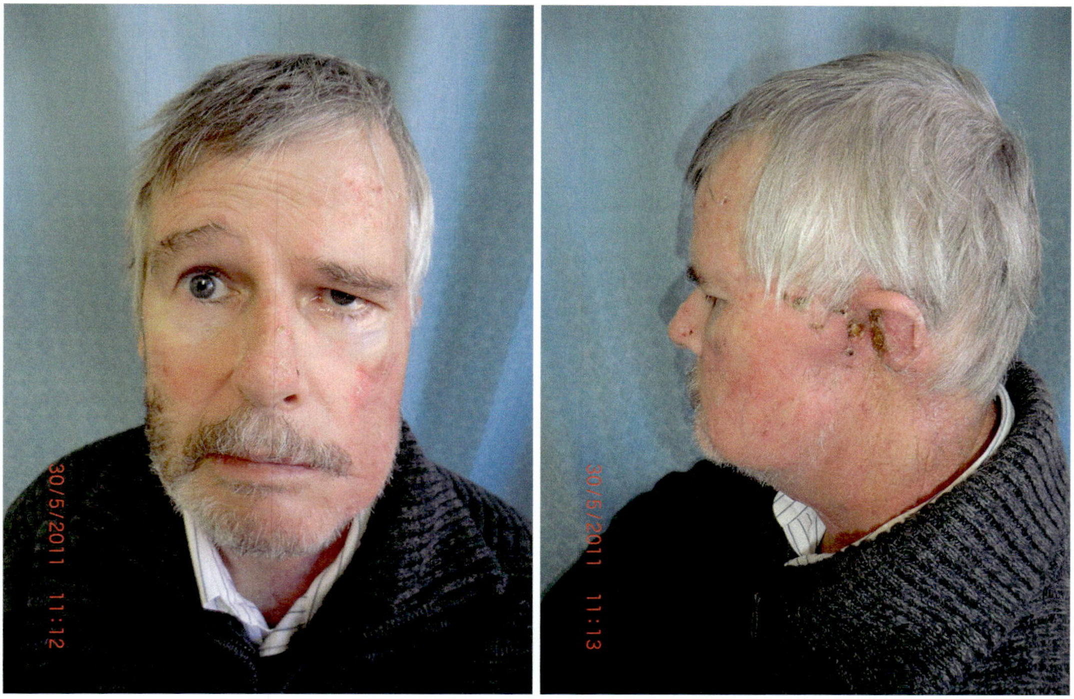

Fig. 2.78 Postoperative appearance at 6 weeks with removal of sutures. Note how the islanding of the neck flaps eliminates necrosis

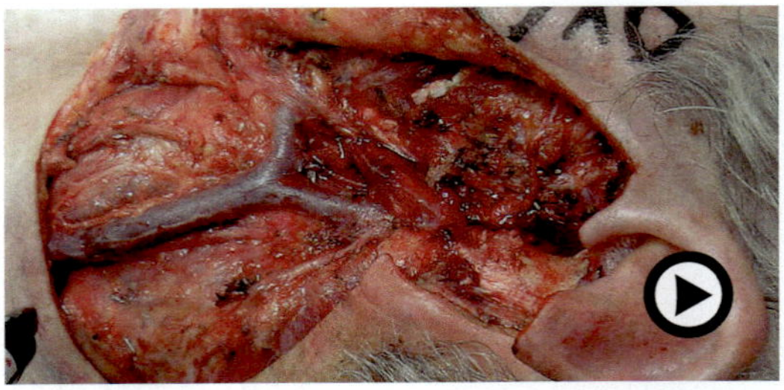

Fig. 2.79 Operative sequence (▶ https://doi.org/10.1007/000-b4s)

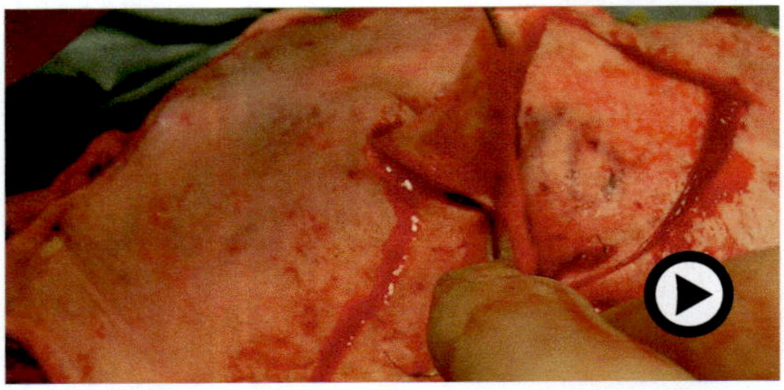

Fig. 2.80 Operative sequence (▶ https://doi.org/10.1007/000-b4t)

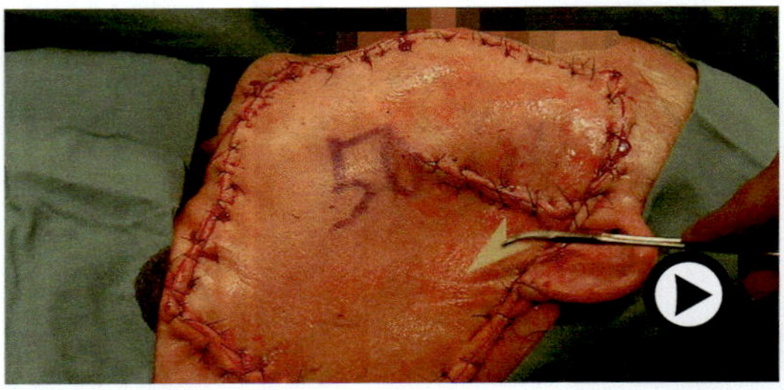

Fig. 2.81 Operative sequence – dog ear excision (▶ https://doi.org/10.1007/000-b4v)

Size of the oncological defect is not a contraindication of the Keystone application as in Case 13. Closing under tension while not impeding the hypervascularisation without impeding healing.

Recurrent melanoma as in Case 15 is reconstructed using a loco-regional flap but delineated in the V2 dermatome at the skin epidermal level to create the island and its hyperaemic perfusion – the regular characteristic of the Keystone. This has the advantage of increasing vascular flow to the limits of the loco-regional flap, which otherwise would necrose if this Keystone manoeuvre (islanding) had not been employed.

2.1.5.1 Case 11: Melanoma Overlying the Parotid – Cheek Keystone Embracing the V2/V3 Aspect of the Trigeminal Nerve – Involving Infraorbital Cheek Tissue as an Island

Melanoma overlying the R parotid in a 39-year-old female of New Zealand origin. The operation consisted of a parotidectomy in association with excision of tumour, a fairly uncomplicated procedure (see Figs. 2.82, 2.83, 2.84, 2.85, 2.86, and 2.87).

The P.A.C.E.S. characteristics were all evident. The patient returned to New Zealand; no follow-up images are available.

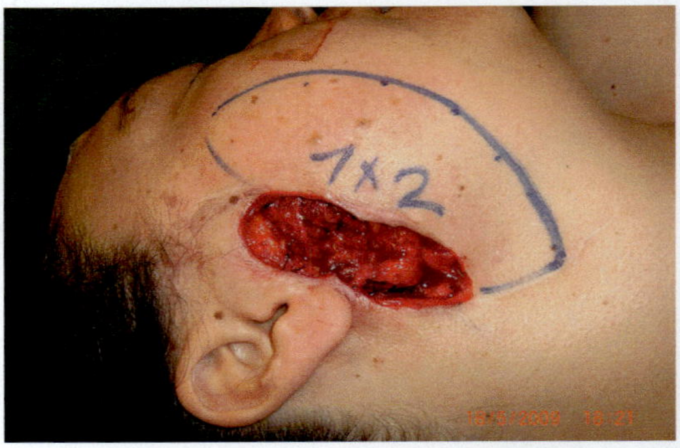

Fig. 2.82 The 7 × 2 cm excisional defect over the R parotid region was closed by a standard Keystone cheek flap. The arc of the Keystone in the V2/V3 dermatome which spreads the tension like an umbrella of tissue over four sites anterior, posterior, superior and inferior sliding on the SMAS layer with no undermining beneath the Keystone

Fig. 2.83 The V2, V3 dermatome of the trigeminal template completely covers the area of excision and Keystone flap closure, ensuring wound healing with hypervascularity evident

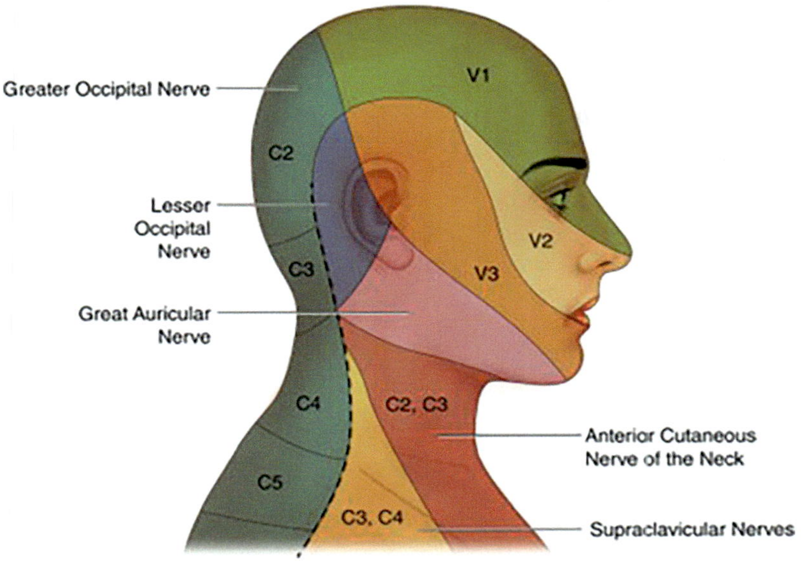

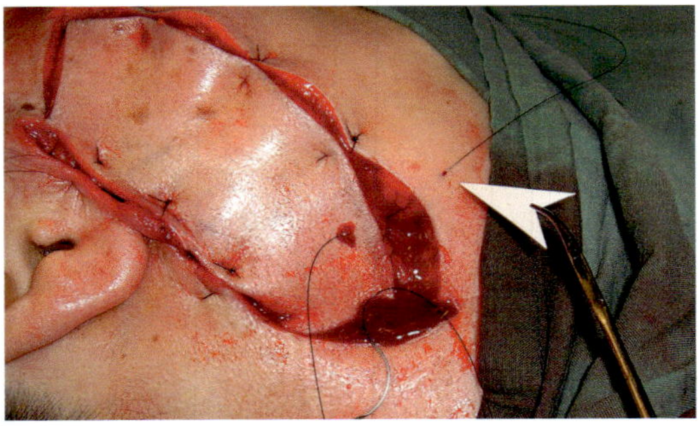

Fig. 2.84 Note the 15-min timeframe for the Red Dot presentation reflecting the reactive hyperaemia. This is an excellent example of the comparison of the Red Dot on the flap and the insignificant dot on the receiving side of the flap (arrowed)
Staged insertion, the superior V-Y closes directly followed by the inferior V-Y and the arrow indicated the suture entry and exit line. I repeat the Red Dot Sign sits on the Keystone confirming its hyperaemia – a constant observation in Keystone reconstructions

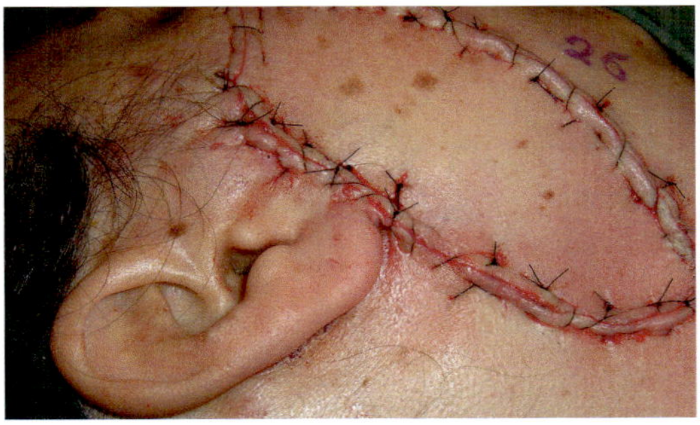

Fig. 2.85 The closure in 25 min with the 3-phase single layer suture technique. Note in the lower third of the Keystone the hyperaemia sitting over the branch of the facial artery (not defined)

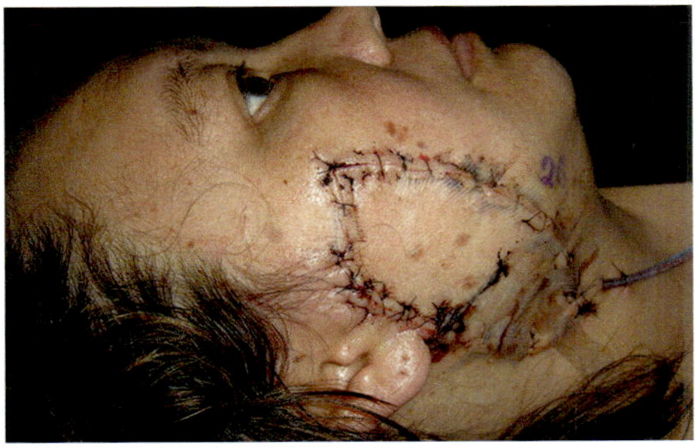

Fig. 2.86 The 3 day postoperative appearance without any evidence of facial nerve dysfunction

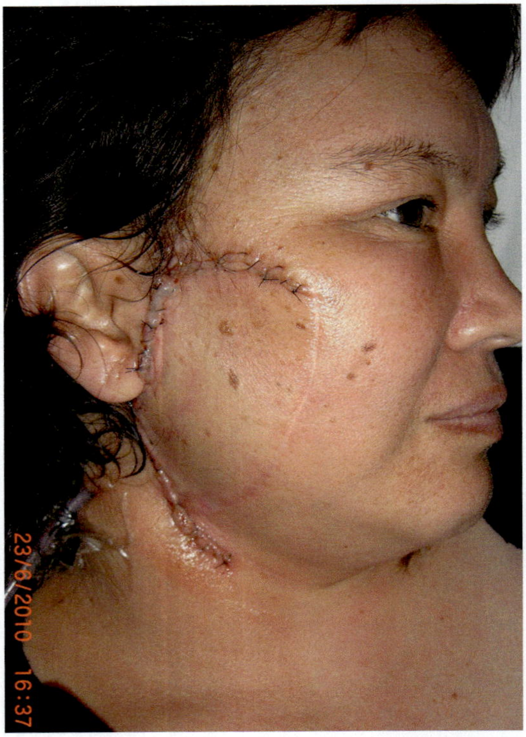

Fig. 2.87 Five day postoperative appearance

2.1.5.2 Case 12: Level II Melanoma over the R Parotid and the Keystone Cheek Repair Overlying the V2 Region

This 63-year-old female with a level II melanoma overlying the R parotid excised in continuity (see Figs. 2.88, 2.89, 2.90, 2.91, 2.92, 2.93, 2.94, 2.95, 2.96, and 2.97).

In summary, all the P.A.C.E.S. characteristics have been exemplified to the patient's satisfaction.

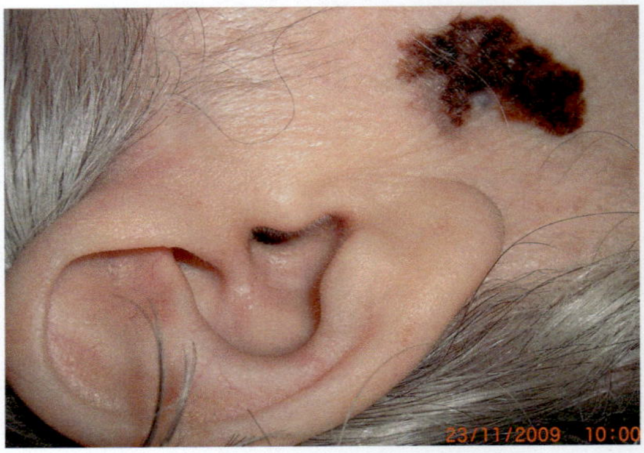

Fig. 2.88 Level II in a Hutchinson's melanotic freckle confirmed by the variations in colour at the margins

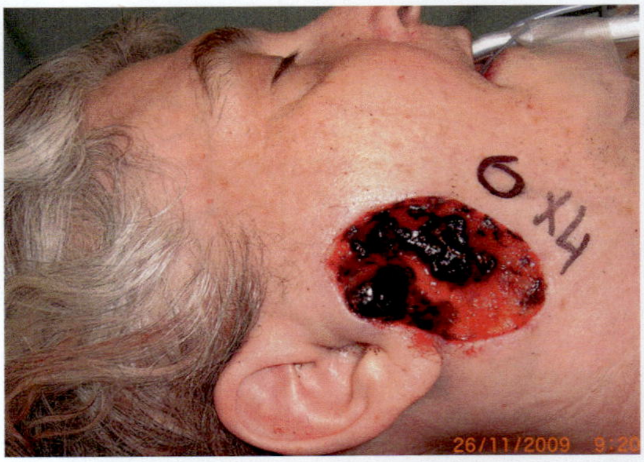

Fig. 2.89 The surgical defect 6 × 4 cm with a parotidectomy

2.1.5.3 Case 13: Parotid Melanoma in an 83 Year Old and a V2 Cheek Keystone for Closure

Level II/III melanoma R cheek in this 83-year-old patient over the angle of the mandible (see Figs. 2.98, 2.99, 2.100, 2.101, 2.102, and 2.103).

In summary, all the P.A.C.E.S. characteristics have been exemplified.

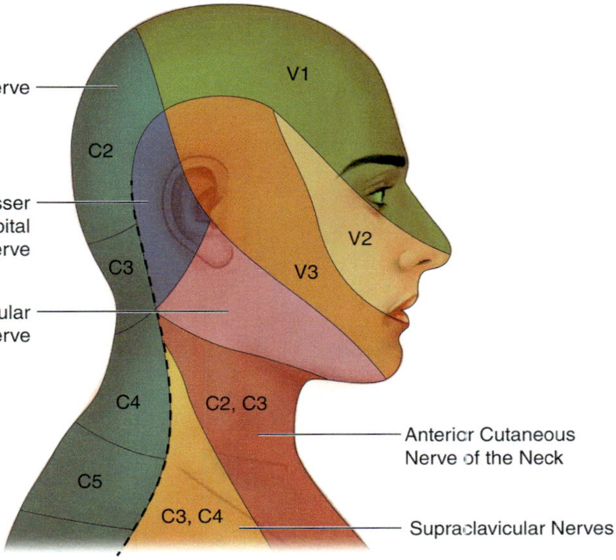

Fig. 2.90 The Keystone design anteriorly is totally within the V2/V3 dermatomes overlying the facial artery. The facial artery supplies the integument of the face but its branches network throughout this V2 distribution

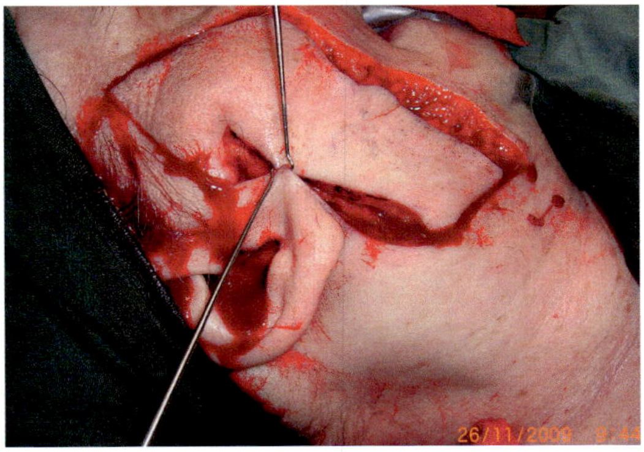

Fig. 2.91 The Keystone closure under tension where the hyperaemia ensures flap viability. The anterior arc of the Keystone sits along the nasolabial line incised at the skin epidermal dermal level only without undermining and the skin hooks reveal the approximation of the closure of the 6 × 4 cm defect. Without undermining, this is the basis of the Keystone principle to produce the hyperaemic reflex based on random perforators from the major arterial supply of the face

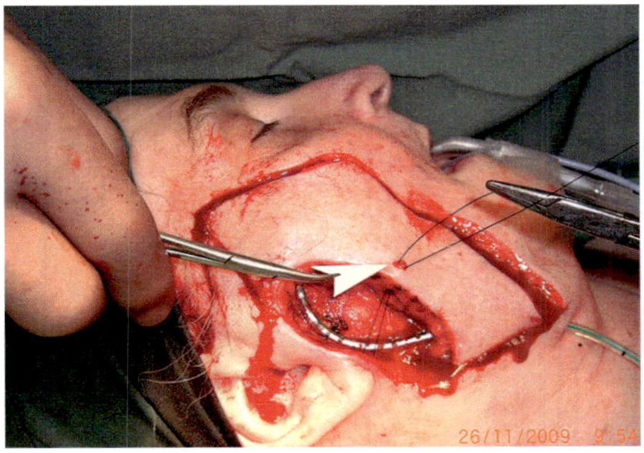

Fig. 2.92 The arc shape of the Keystone allows it to fill the oncological site. Note the inferior hyperaemia in the lower half of the flap adjacent to a branch of the facial artery. Then this transition of flow, presumably along facial artery branches before spreading upwards, creating complete hyperaemia in the flap. This confirms the facial artery perforators are predominant in the inferior aspect of the Keystone. A network of vessels must exist to allow this complete perfusion within the limits of the V3 dermatome mark out. Note the arrow on the Red Dot Sign which ensures flap viability and reliable healing. The Redi-Vac drainage is bent in a u-shape manner underneath the flap so the anterior section and the posterior section can be drained by a single unit

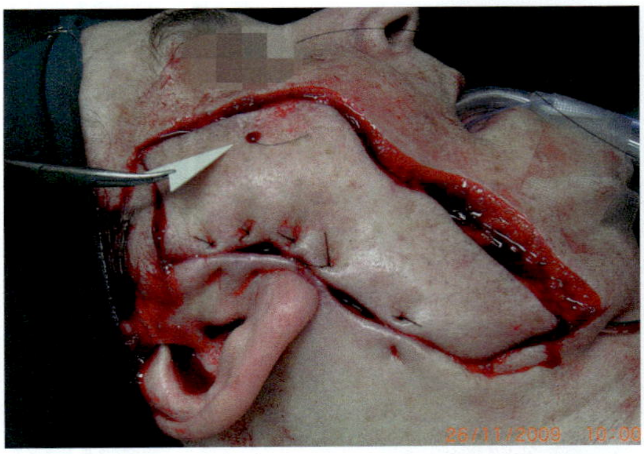

Fig. 2.93 The Red Dot Sign (arrowed) confirms increased vascular perfusion at the apex. The Keystone arc has now been distorted governed by the anatomical site. Lines of tension transversely cause temporary embarrassment to the vascular supply but this vascular impendence disappears thanks to the fascial vascular support. The hyperaemic phase becomes evident usually after 15 min and eliminates lines of tension (timestamped images)

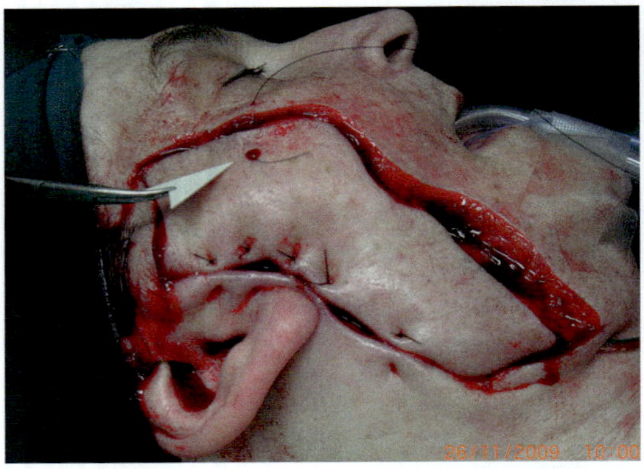

Fig. 2.94 The single layer 3-phase suture technique is used. The Red Dot Sign, in spite of this tensional alignment, confirms the increased vascular flow at the subdermal plexus before epidermal pinkness confirms its reliability

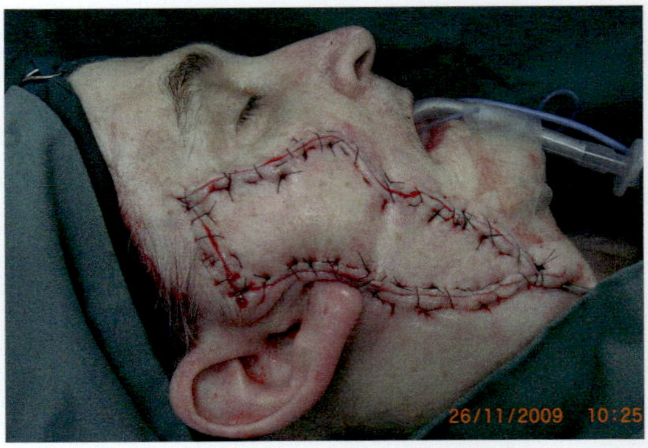

Fig. 2.95 The wound closure at 55 min completes the procedure. Note there is no external pull at the R outer canthus because of the upwards angulation of the Keystone

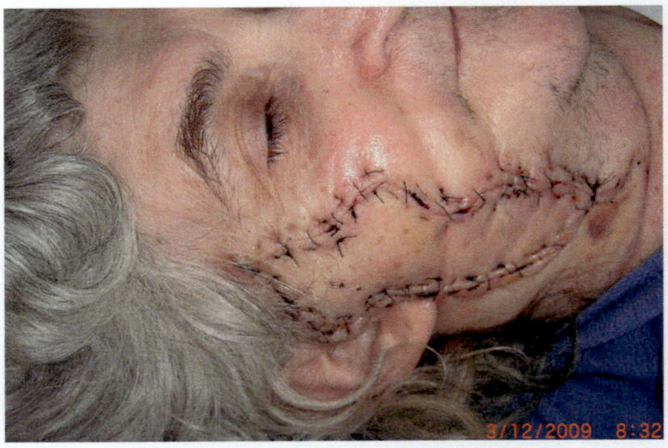

Fig. 2.96 Appearance at 8 days before the initial standard wound dressing technique is commenced

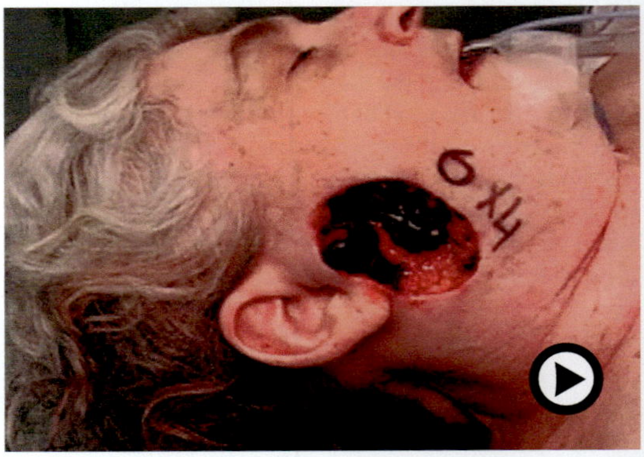

Fig. 2.97 Wound closure (▶ https://doi.org/10.1007/000-b4w)

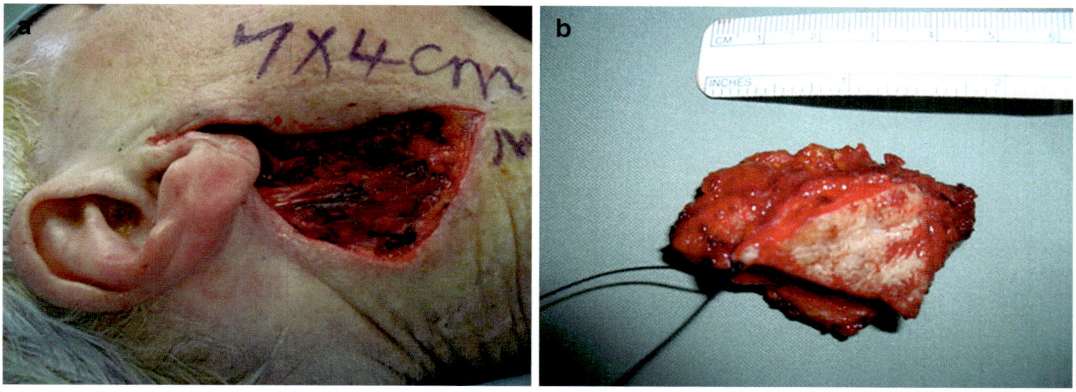

Fig. 2.98 (**b**) Pathology specimen. Note the cyanotic changes in the undermined cheek flap following the parotidectomy – a sign of potential necrosis if closed directly. The hyperaemic phase of the Keystone salvages this tissue problem

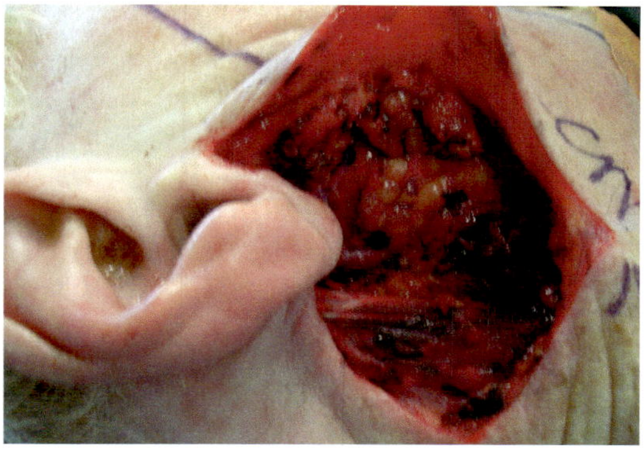

Fig. 2.99 The excisional parotid defect measuring 7 × 4 cm with preservation of the facial nerve

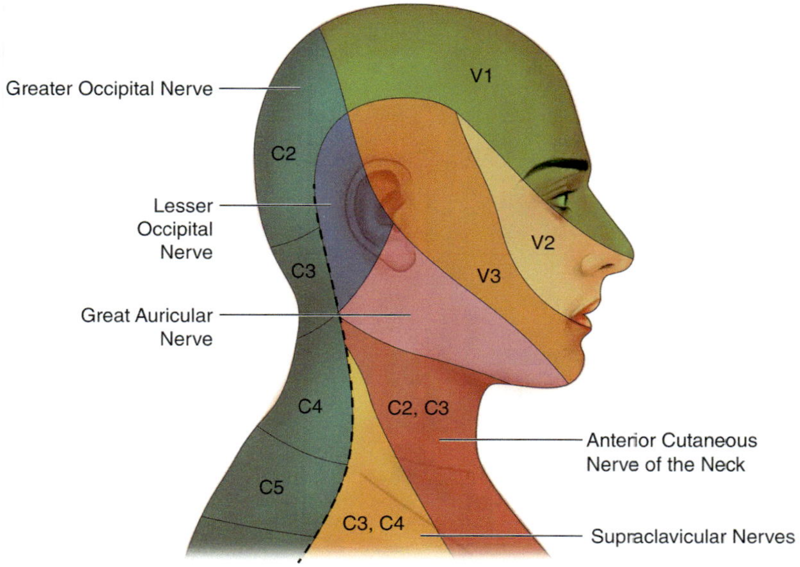

Fig. 2.100 The V2, V3 dermatome of the R cheek outlined. The island mark out in the V2 dermatome involving the whole cheek is the basis for the Keystone repair. Extending from the nasolabial incision along the line of the mandible inferiorly and extending up along the preauricular groove creates a triangulate island flap overlying the V2 dermatome. This is not quite a Keystone design but repeats the Keystone principles of vascularity and reliability

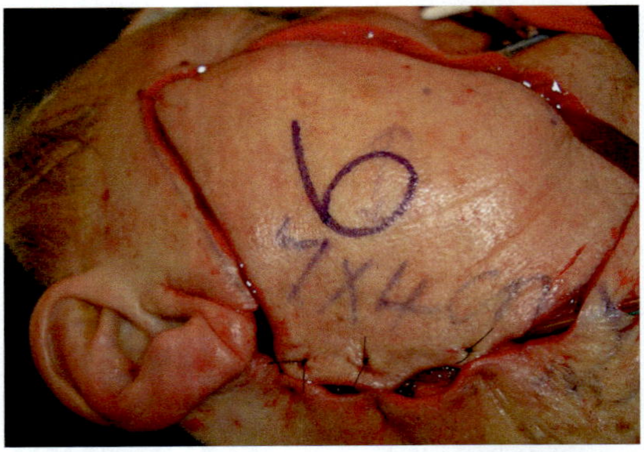

Fig. 2.101 Staged closure for the parotidectomy defect. Note the cyanotic phase has disappeared (Fig. 13.1a). This triangulate Keystone flap is outlined on the R cheek from the nasolabial line across the submandibular region and up the preauricular groove. The timeframe to raise that flap is only 6 min. The 3-phase single layer wound closure suture technique is utilised

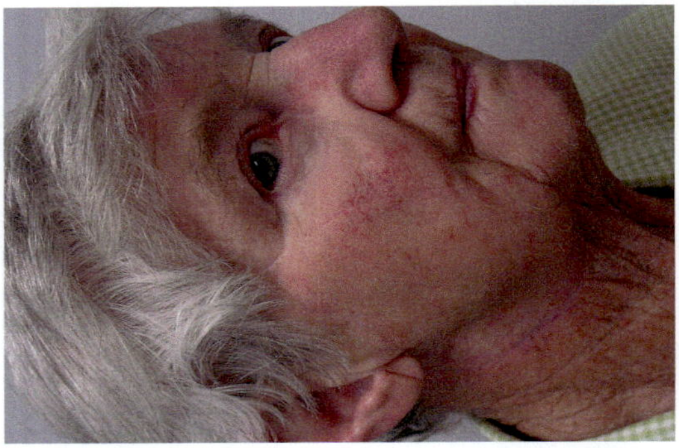

Fig. 2.102 Postoperative appearance 12–18 months after procedure

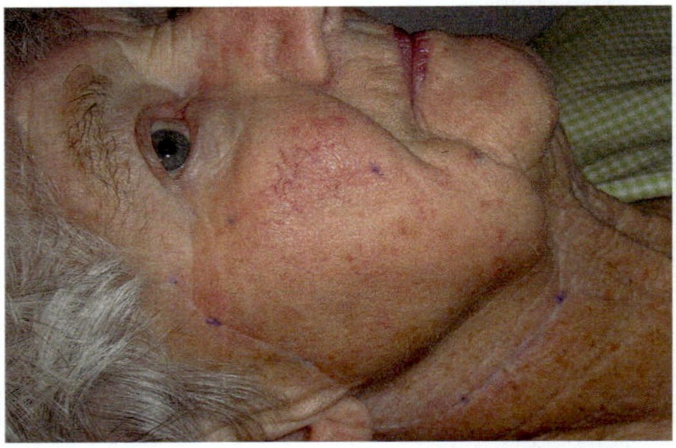

Fig. 2.103 Postoperative appearance 12–18 months after procedure and the dots are there to outline the margins of the flap which are almost indiscernible

2.1.5.4 Case 14: Massive Parotid Defect 10 × 9 cm with a Neck Dissection Levels II, III and IV Closure with a Cervical Keystone

Level III melanoma over the R parotid with secondary dissemination into the R neck.

Clearance of the tumour including levels II, III and IV neck dissection with venous preservation.

Cervical undermining is indicated by the digital elevation of the cervical skin and fascia and neck tissue in this 70-year-old female (see Figs. 2.104, 2.105, 2.106, 2.107, 2.108, 2.109, 2.110, 2.111, 2.112 and 2.113).

In summary, all the P.A.C.E.S. characteristics of the Keystone are once more exempliflied.

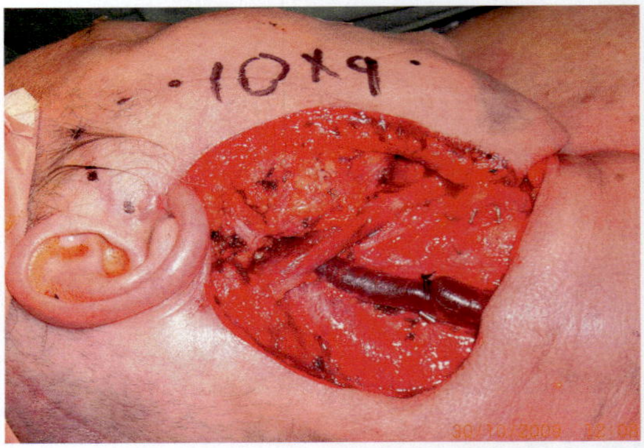

Fig. 2.104 The defect size 10 × 9 cm. Facial nerve preserved. External jugular vein preserved to ensure adequate venous drainage from the random perforator vascular supply in the Keystone. As McGregor [17] said never forget, flap necrosis usually is a consequence of venoustasis and not arterial insufficiency

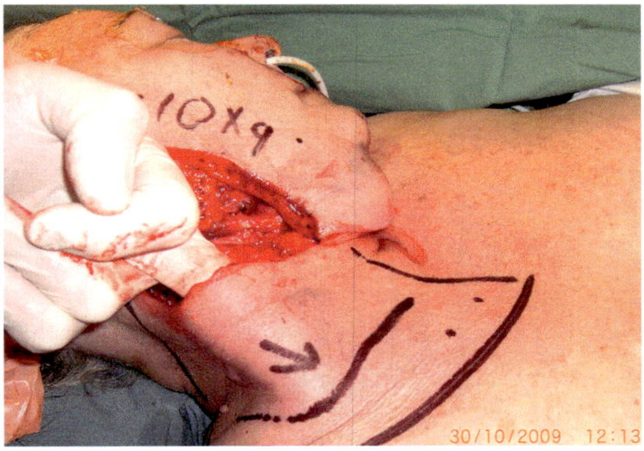

Fig. 2.105 The extent of undermining of neck tissue for cervical nodal clearance levels II and III from the neck dissection. The working rule for the design of the infra-supraclavicular circulatory perforator support is as long as there is one third of deep flap attachment distal to the undermined section, circulatory healing is achieved. The dots are a guide to the random supraclavicular perforators, randomly located and not specifically sited

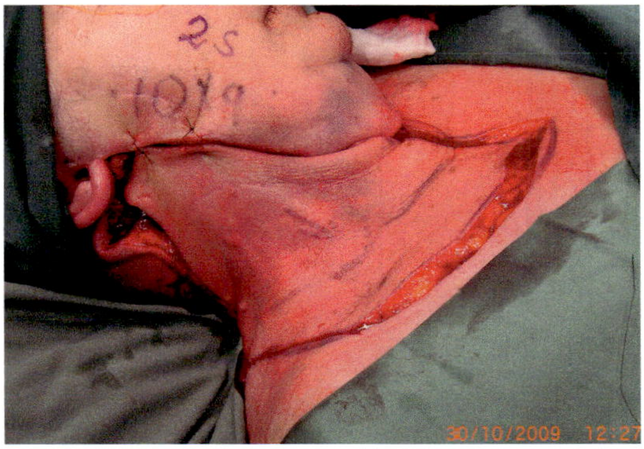

Fig. 2.107 Islanding creates hyperaemia ensuring flap viability. The closure is achieved with a neck tilt with some tension at the apical 3-phase standard locking mattress suture technique. The island flap mark out ensures Keystone hyperaemia to guarantee successful repair under tension and also pain free in the postoperative phase

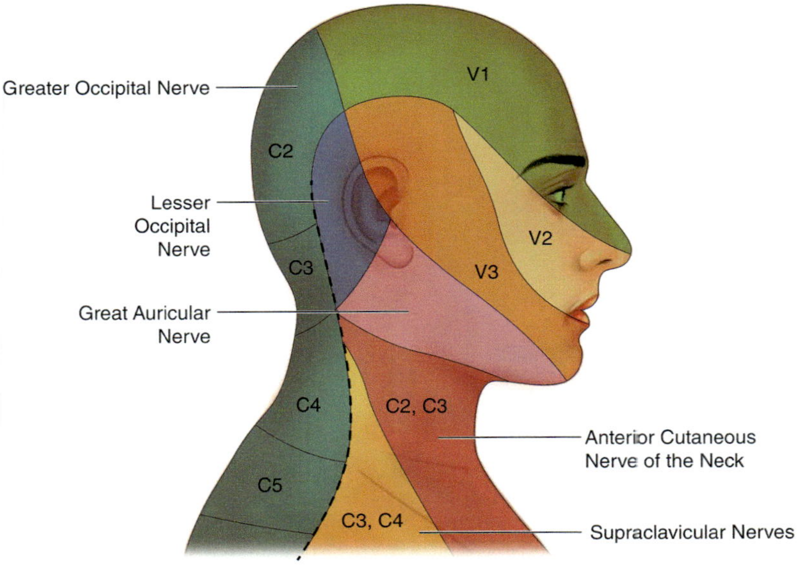

Fig. 2.106 The dermatomal mark outs of the anterior cutaneous nerve of the neck C2, C3 and the supraclavicular nerves C3, C4 is the compass alignment for the random perforator support for this neck flap

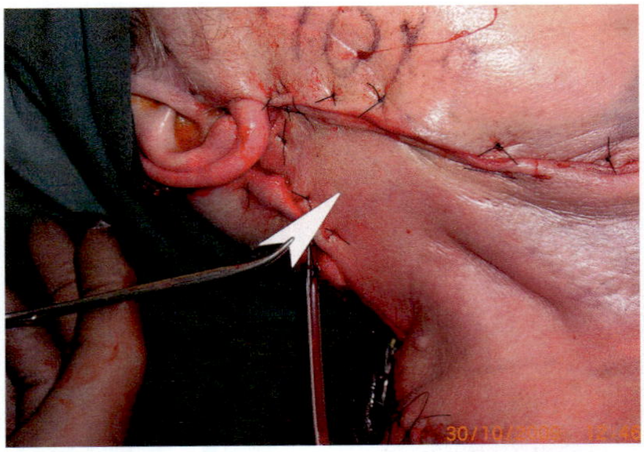

Fig. 2.108 Staged closure of the wound and the apex of the flap (arrowed) shows no sign of vascular impedence confirming the Keystone characteristic. The standard 3-phase single layer suture technique is employed: 1. Locking mattress sutures at the tension points. 2. Interrupted mattress aligns the wound. 3. Continuous nylon closes the epidermal level

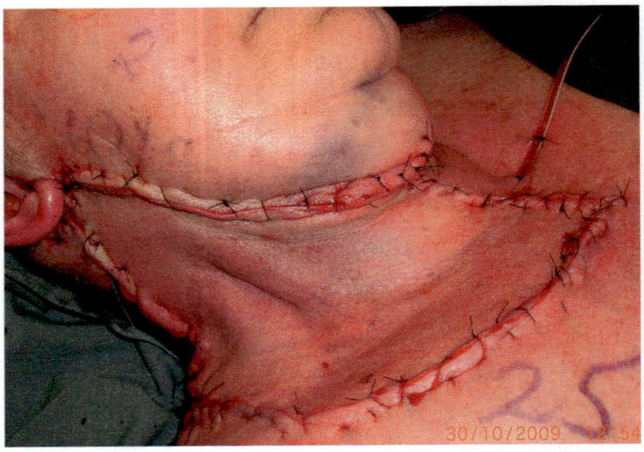

Fig. 2.109 On completion the timeframe of 25 min relates to the second part of the closure where the total time was 50 min. All under Redi-Vac drainage

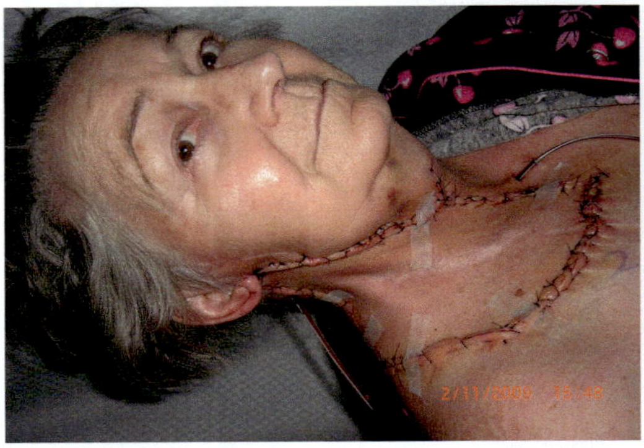

Fig. 2.110 The postoperative ward appearance at 3 days from the timestamped images and the patient has a satisfied appearance confirming that Keystone characteristic of being pain free

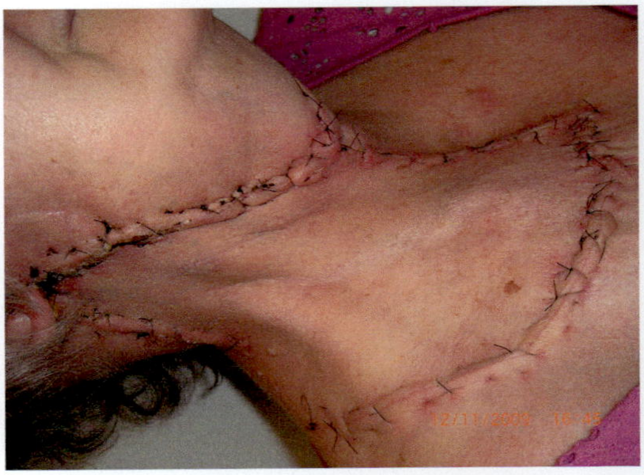

Fig. 2.111 Wound dressing at 10 days. No necrosis evident. The continuous epidermal nylon is released to remove cross hatch marks. The standard mattress sutures are then removed at 2 weeks and locking mattress sutures at 3 weeks

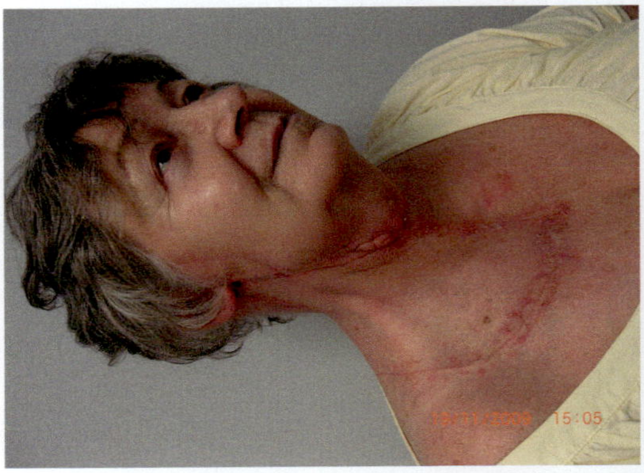

Fig. 2.112 At 3 weeks and note the patient's satisfied appearance

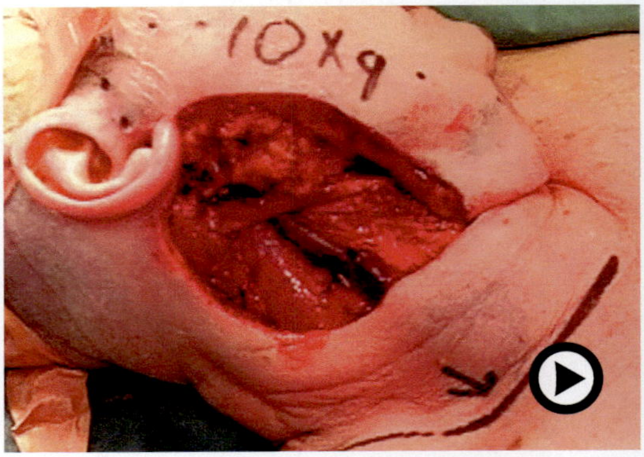

Fig. 2.113 Operative sequence (▶ https://doi.org/10.1007/000-b4x)

2.1.5.5 Case 15: Recurrent Melanoma of the L Ear Tragus

Level II/III melanoma of the L preauricular region in this 68-year-old male farmer. Recurrence following initial management (see Figs. 2.114, 2.115, 2.116, 2.117, 2.118, 2.119, 2.120, 2.121, 2.122, 2.123, 2.124, 2.125, and 2.126).

In summary, islanding of the V2 dermatome ensures hyperaemic perfusion to the distal limits of the L cheek rotation flap to cover the L TMJ site.

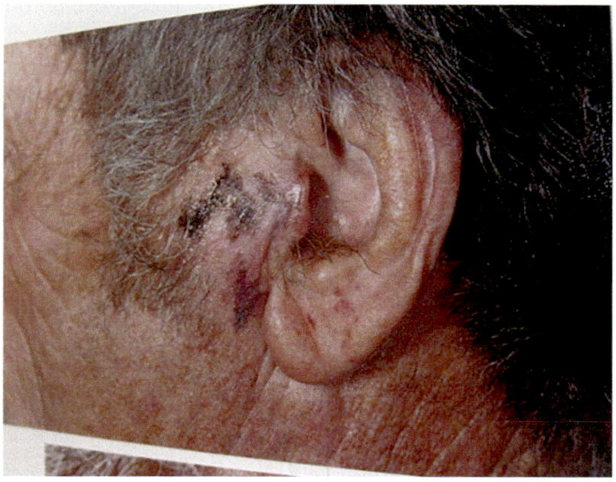

Fig. 2.114 Initial presentation of the level II/III melanoma. Three years after initial management before presenting with the recurrence involving the temporomandibular joint

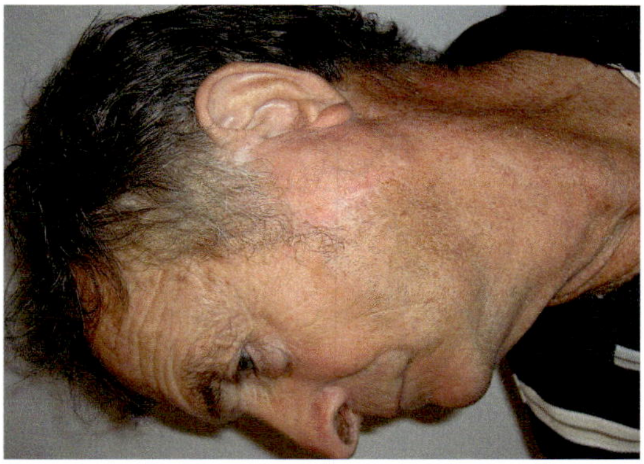

Fig. 2.115 Recurrent melanoma mass at 3 years over the preauricular site and parotid

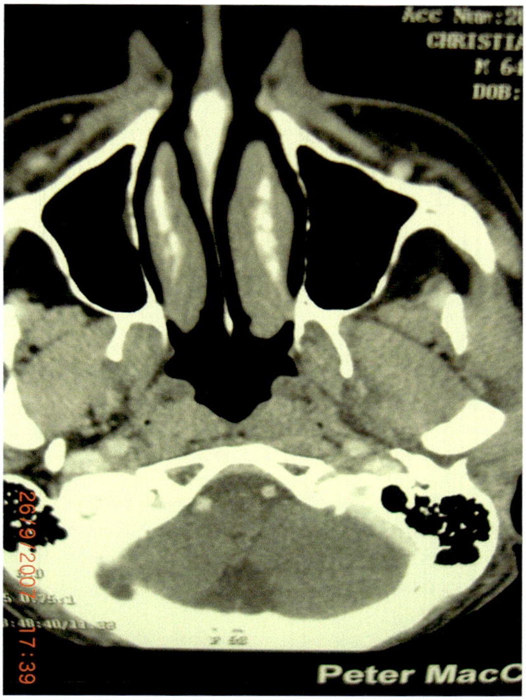

Fig. 2.116 CT X-ray image showing involvement of the tumour above the parotid and adjacent to the (L) temperomandibular joint

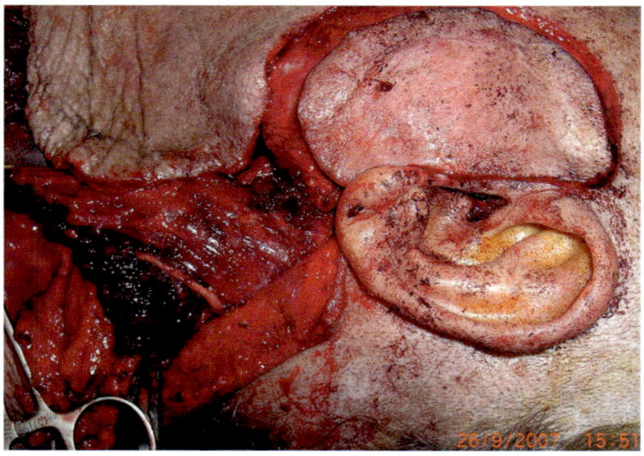

Fig. 2.117 The staged surgical excision and neck dissection including the TMJ. Note the cyanosis following undermining of the cervical exposure flap. Note how the Keystone concept can eliminate this potential apical necrosis

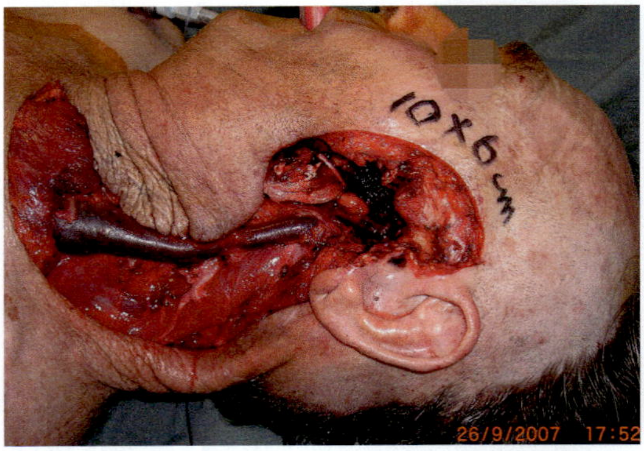

Fig. 2.118 The 10 × 6 cm defect. The surgical excision included parotidectomy and facial nerve and temporomandibular joint (TMJ) including neck dissection of levels II, III and IV. Note the cervical cyanosis in the cervical flap which normally would be a contraindication for use but the Keystone islanding principle can salvage this problem. All venous drainage sites are retained to minimise any possible venoustasis hence necrosis

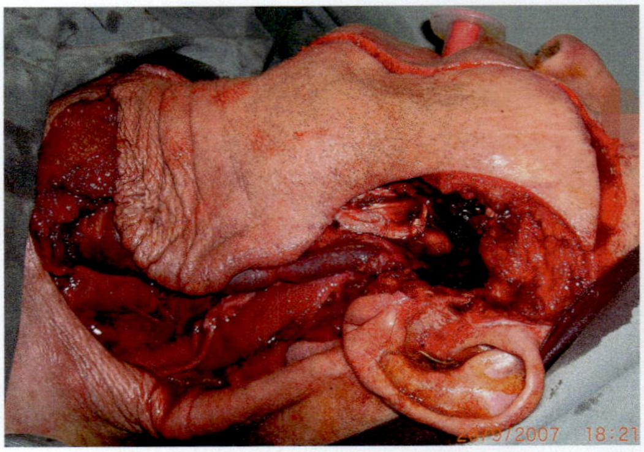

Fig. 2.119 The incision down the nasolabial line over the point of the chin creates the island flap of the C2, C3 dermatomes. The island flap of cheek and neck tissue has gone into its hyperaemic phase eliminating the cyanotic tip. Thus, the neck flap can be advanced and rotated to close the defect of the TMJ. This technique ensures hypervascularity and note how the cyanotic cervical flap now has a normal perfusional appearance

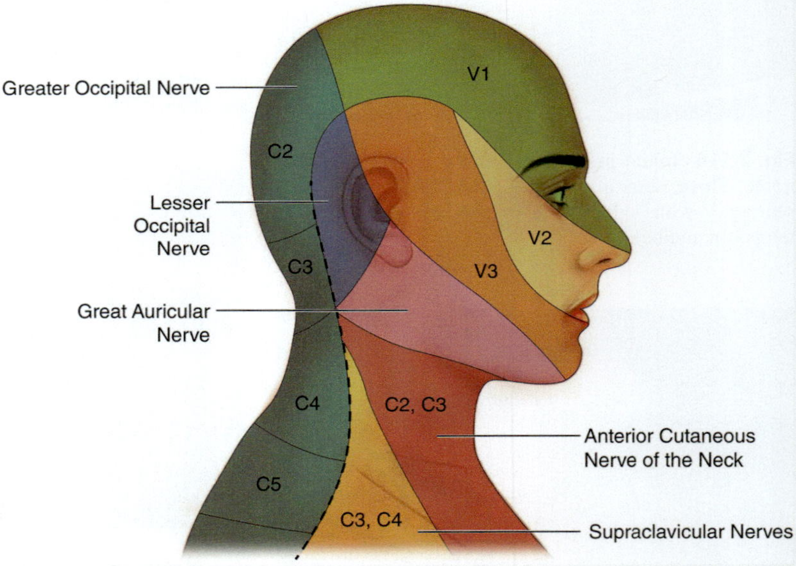

Fig. 2.120 In this case here, the Keystone mark out moves over three territories from the V2 infraorbital area, V3 preauricular area and the C2, C3 anterior cervical area

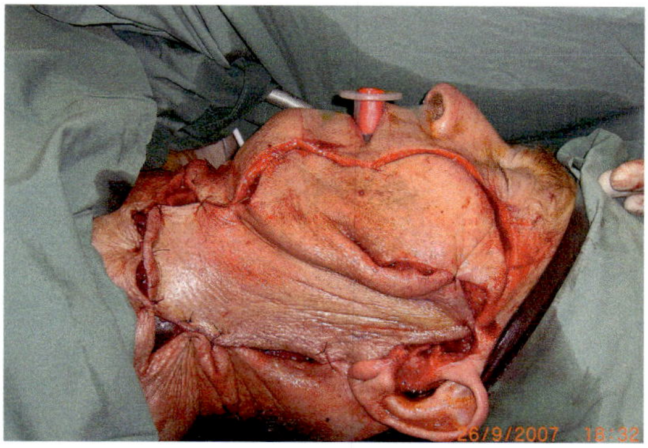

Fig. 2.121 The inferior limit of the flap closes into the preauricular defect and the cyanotic lines of tension are subsequently overcome by the hyperaemic phase. Any dog ear or redundant tissue can be excised at the epidermal level and is not a contraindication for immediate surgical excision because the cervical fascial base ensures circulation

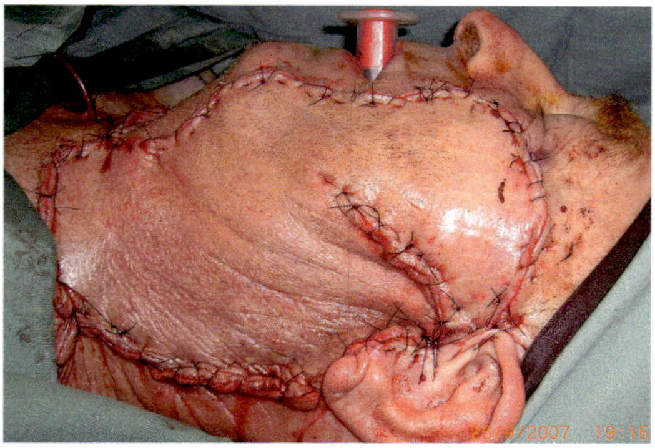

Fig. 2.122 The reliability of the circulation allows one to trim the dog ear in the acute phase and the surgical delineation of the island is closed directly down the nasolabial line. Some clinical points from this image: 1. The L infraorbital wound closure is angled upwards to minimise any ectropion. 2. The flap closure under tension allows tightness of the L cheek and is a form of static facial nerve reconstruction. No microsurgical nerve grafting was done. 3. The 'dog ear' excision is completed at the time of the initial closure because of the hyperaemia developed in the tissues with the Keystone Island principle. 4. The tensional closure and the static facial nerve manoeuvre eliminates any need for an initial tarsorrhaphy

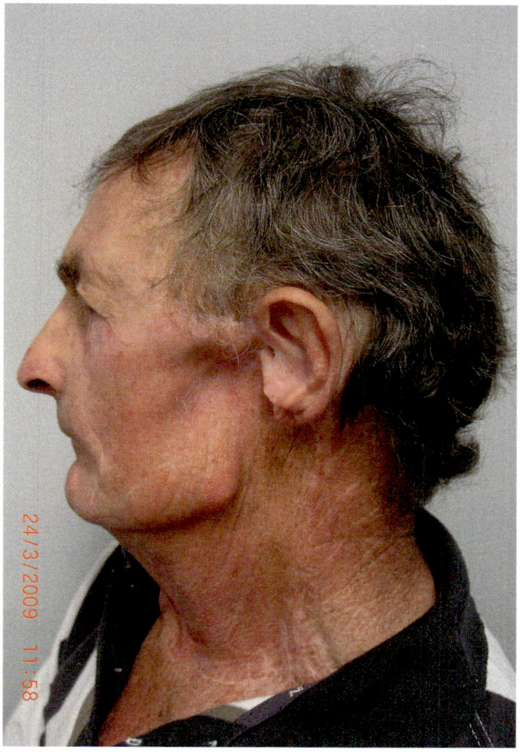

Fig. 2.123 The appearance at 2 years following radiation. There is no element of any ectropion evident at this early stage. However, subsequently the weight of the tissue caused some element of droop and for comfort; a tarsorrhaphy was performed only after 3 years

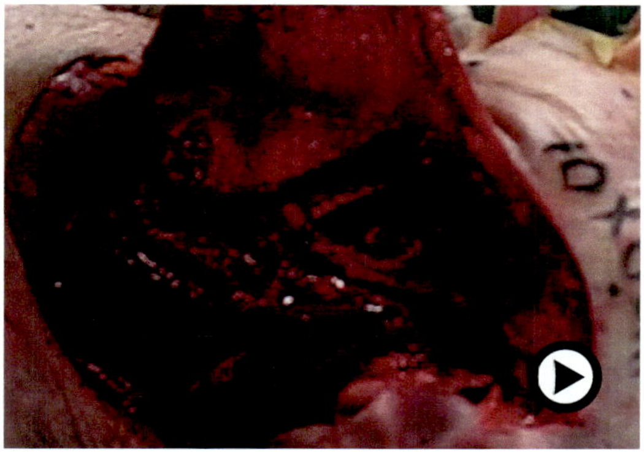

Fig. 2.124 Operative sequence (▶ https://doi.org/10.1007/000-b4y)

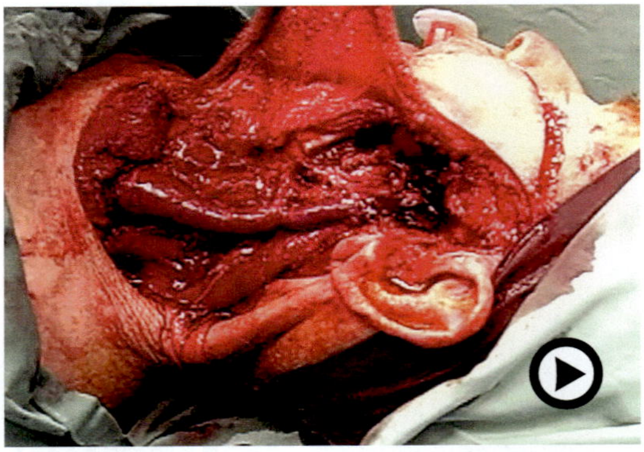

Fig. 2.125 Operative sequence (▶ https://doi.org/10.1007/000-b4z)

2.1.5.6 Case 16: Anterior Cervical Submental Keystone for a Large Parotid Defect in a 75 Year Old

Melanoma level III, IV over the parotid with R neck clearance with sentinel node (negative). A DRAPE procedure was performed, i.e. Delayed Reconstruction Awaiting Pathology Evaluation (see Figs. 2.127, 2.128, 2.129, 2.130, 2.131, and 2.132).

In summary, the P.A.C.E.S. charactristics of the Keystone were all exemplified.

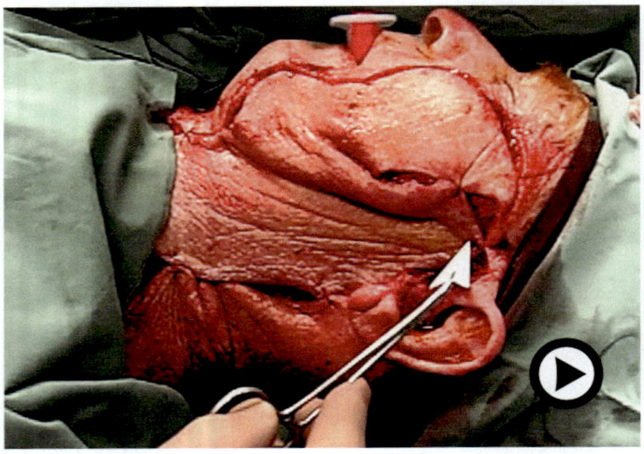

Fig. 2.126 Operative sequence (▶ https://doi.org/10.1007/000-b50)

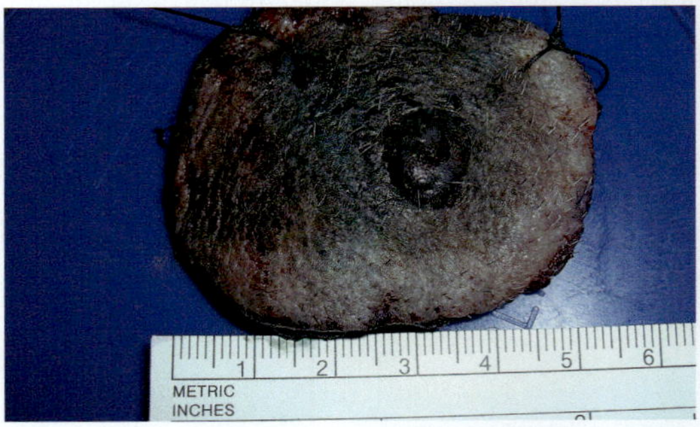

Fig. 2.127 The surgical specimen 5 × 5 cm with the sentinel node staining

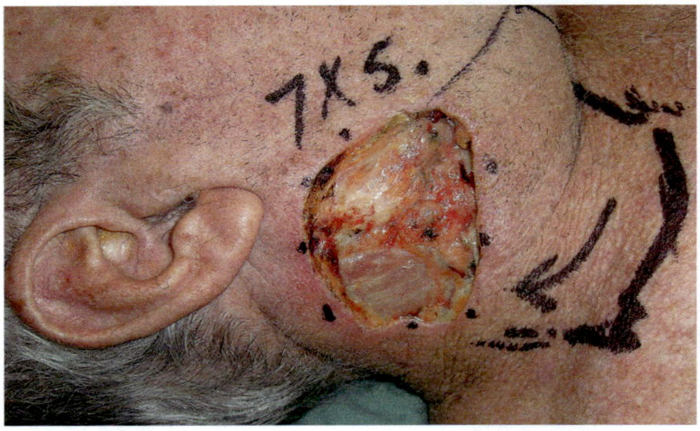

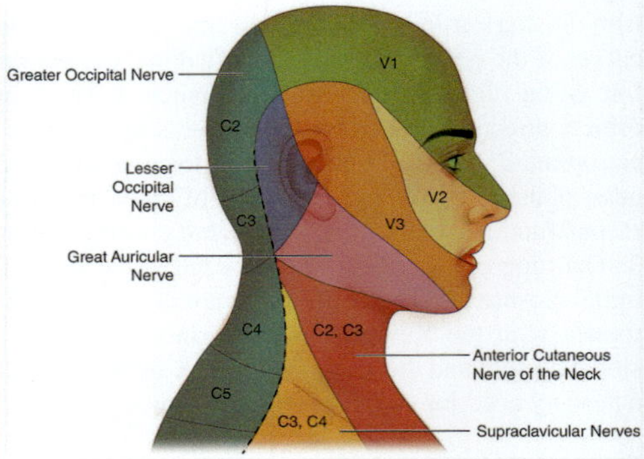

Fig. 2.128 The 7 × 5 cm defect sitting over the angle of the mandible. The cervico-submental Keystone (arrowed) for closure of the defect. The excisional defect after tumour removal was closed. The cervico-submental flap from the neck to the point of the chin incorporating anterior cutaneous nerves C2, C3 from the dermatomal mark out

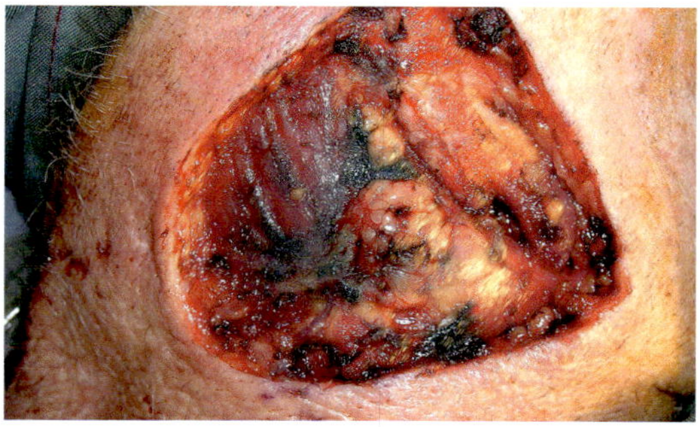

Fig. 2.129 Close-up of the excisional defect

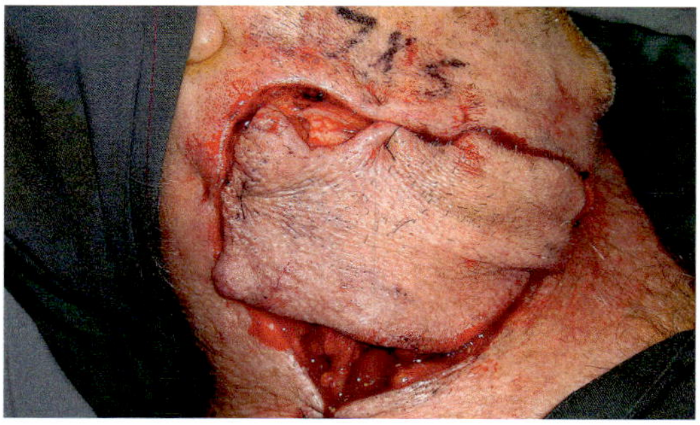

Fig. 2.130 The cervico-submental Keystone based on cervical fascia and designed within the dermatomes C2, C3 is undermined two thirds. The proximal one third attachment over sternomastoid random perforators ensures viability. The Keystone is then rotated into the defect and then the single layer 3-phase suture technique is employed using locking mattress sutures in a single layer at the points of maximum tension, ordinary mattress to close the wound and an epidermal continuous nylon to produce cutaneous seal. The 30-min timeframe (time-stamped) for the reconstruction and Keystone insertion and closure of the secondary defect

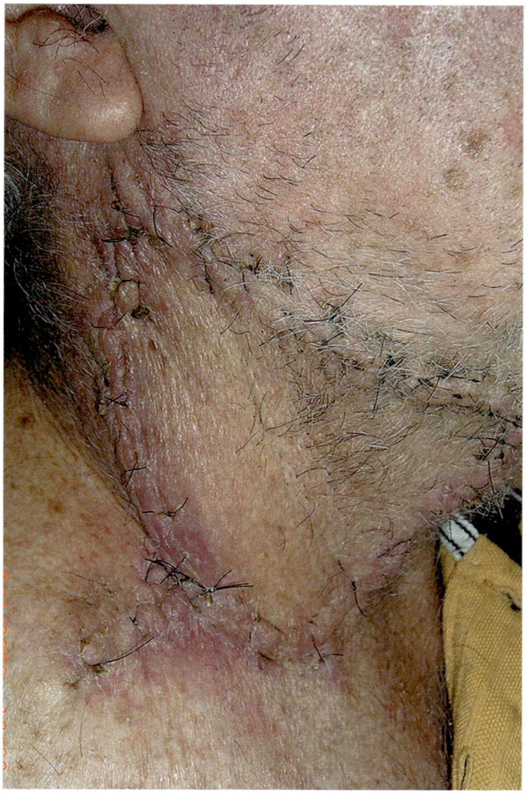

Fig. 2.131 Appearance at 14 days from timestamped image

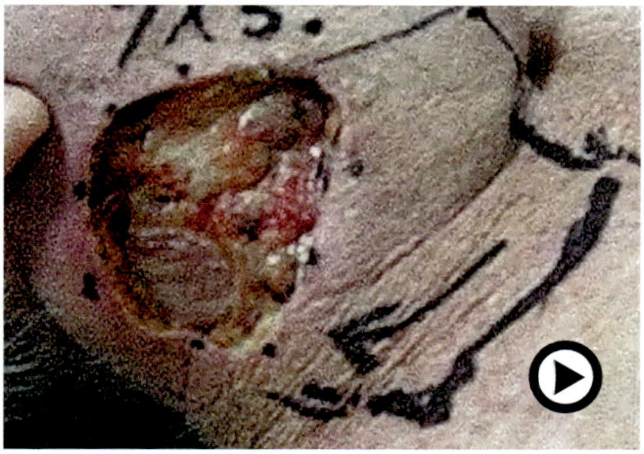

Fig. 2.132 Operative sequence (▶ https://doi.org/10.1007/000-b51)

2.1.5.7 Case 17: Posterior Cervical Orientated Keystone for a Mitotic Lesion in a 35 Year Old

See Figs. 2.133, 2.134, 2.135, 2.136, and 2.137

In summary, the P.A.C.E.S. charactristics of the Keystone were all exemplified in this young male smoker who was warned accordingly.

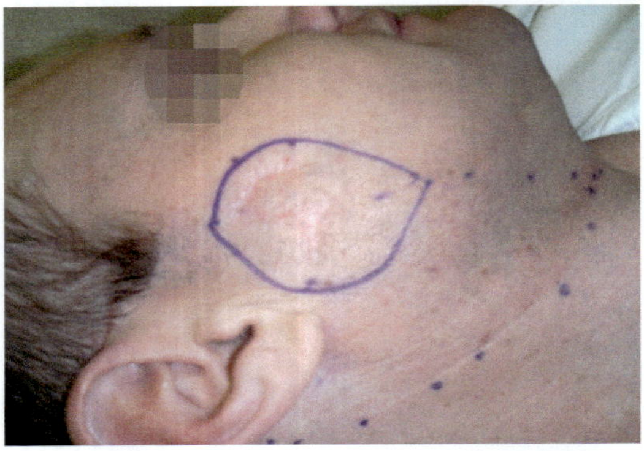

Fig. 2.133 The recurrent mitotic lesions over the parotid which was cleared including a parotidectomy and no neck dissection

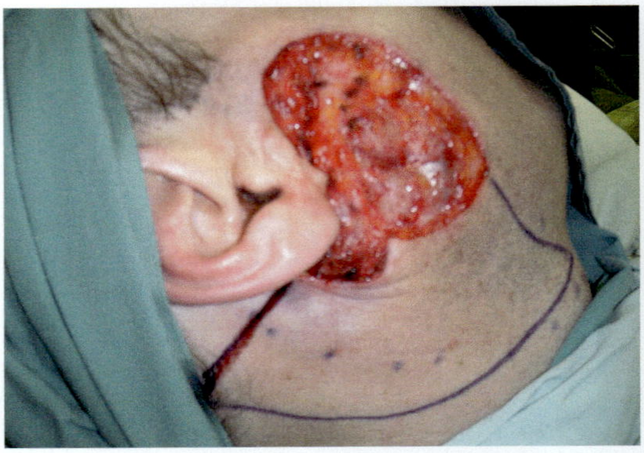

Fig. 2.135 Defect size 8 × 5 cm and the closure with a posterior orientated cervico Keystone based on sterno-mastoid perforators with the superior limits of the Keystone to close the cheek defect leaving one third deep attachment inferiorly over the random sternomastoid perforators

Fig. 2.134 The dermatome mark out

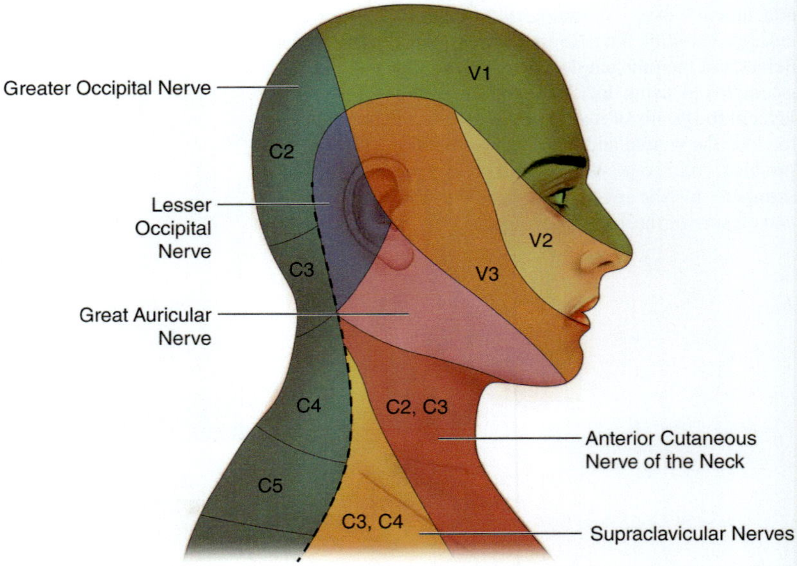

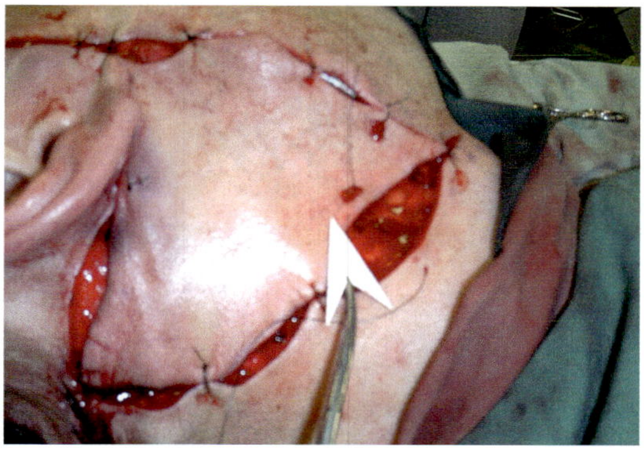

Fig. 2.136 The Red Dot Sign confirming the hyperaemic phase and therefore the increased vascularity eliminates any necrosis with the closure under tension

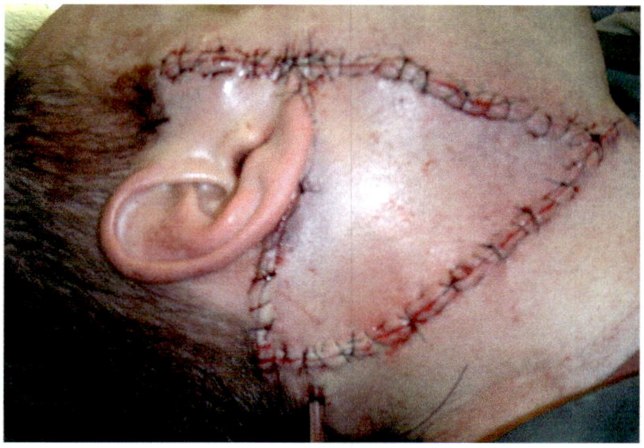

Fig. 2.137 The appearance on completion using the single layer 3-phase suture technique of locking mattress sutures, simple mattress sutures and continuous nylon for epidermal seal. Note the hyperaemia throughout the flap compared with the surrounding tissues. The wound is healed normally

2.1.6 Nose

This Keystone technique in nasal reconstruction for melanoma and other mitotic lesions has wide application. Incidentally, the multifocal skin lesions of the nasal bridge were excised and once pathology clearance was achieved [16], a forehead island flap was used for closure. The standard vertical flap rotated to 180° often leaves a secondary defect at the hairline needing grafting. This supraorbital forehead island flap overcomes that problem, in spite of closing under tension, a characteristic of the Keystone. It is noteworthy this patient wanted the secondary procedure done during the healing phase of the L forehead lesion, showing again, the reliability of the Keystone vascularity, based on anatomical norms using the dermatomal mark outs. In this case, the supratrochlear and supraorbital neurovascular structures producing an acceptable aesthetic outcome.

The principles of nasal reconstruction have a long tradition referring to Burget and Menick's work (1994). In these Melanoma cases, usually the skin cover only is required and the Keystone provides vascular foundation in the nasal reconstruction reconstructing the cutaneous envelope. Free tissue transfer has no applications in this Keystone concept and has universal application in covering all elements of this nasal envelope. The Keystone provides excellent colour match, thickness and texture in the reconstruction.

The principal melanoma excision and closure by elements of secondary intention is something that is not practiced by plastic surgeons in spite of a 1 cm defect in spite of the aesthetic drawbacks. Never forgetting, the grafting option is always a possibility.

The Keystone principle seems to universalise the collection of loco-regional flaps in nasal reconstruction – too many to list, including advancement, rotation and transposition types including Bi-lobed and the Hatchet variants [8]. Even Rohrich et al. 1999 nasal tip repair is based on traditional techniques with skin from the proximal two thirds, whereas the Keystone design seems to incorporate this reference.

The staged midline forehead flap variety [18, 19] has its drawbacks with tightness, vascular impedance and hairline secondary defects are impediments to a good aesthetic outcome, let alone subsequent repeat procedures looking for surgical scar revision.

2.1.6.1 Case 18: Side of the Nose

The nasolabial line of reconstruction based on random branches of the facial artery (see Figs. 2.138, 2.139, 2.140, 2.141, 2.142, 2.143, 2.144, 2.145, and 2.146).

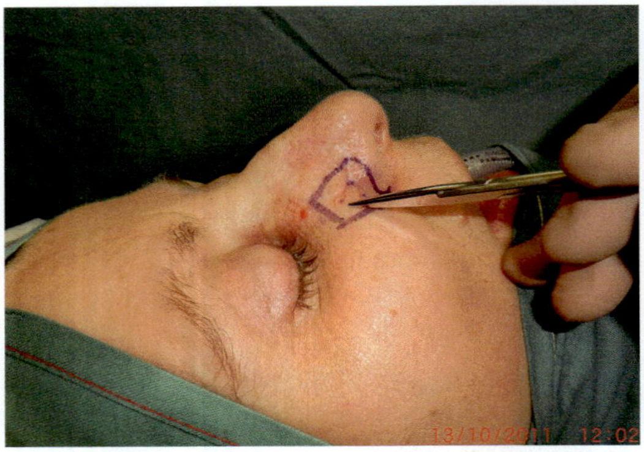

Fig. 2.138 Recurrent mitotic lesion of the R side of the nose 6 months following initial surgery

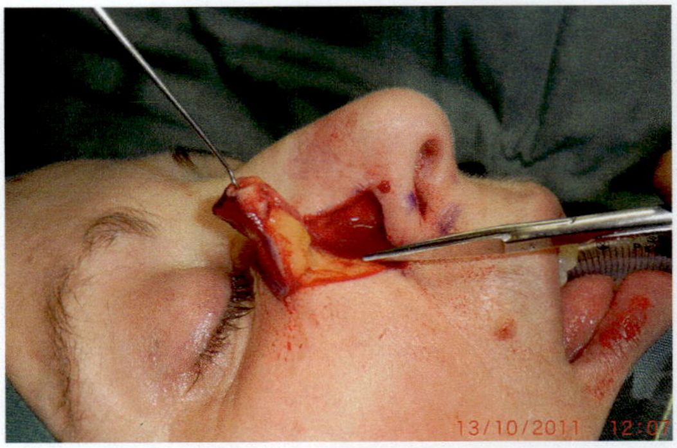

Fig. 2.140 Removal of the tumour. The underlying neurovascular axis (with the nasal branch of the facial artery) is evident but not skeletonised or stripped. The DRAPE procedure applied again. Following pathology clearance, the Keystone repair was completed

Fig. 2.139 The dermatome mark out – the basis for the Keystone island flap design

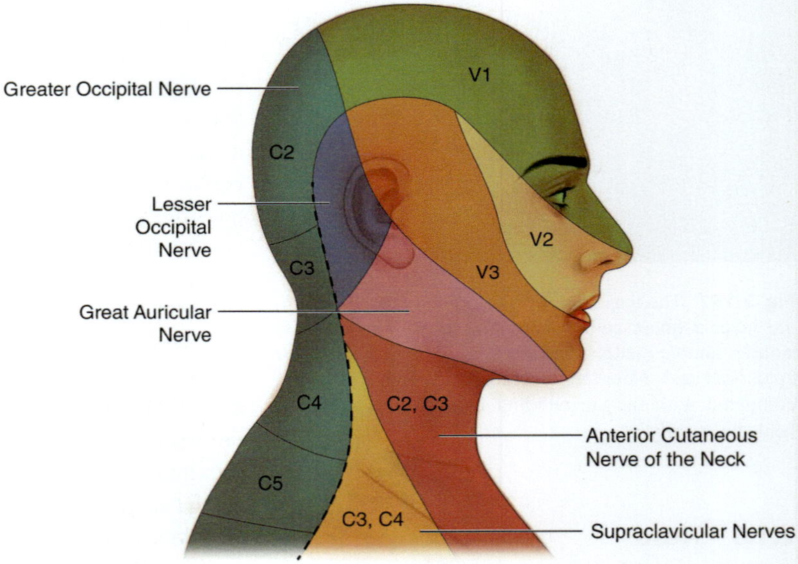

In summary, an aesthetically acceptable outcome using the V-Y Dieffenbach flap based on random neurovascular perforators from the nasal branch of the facial artery. The tissues are teased with blunt dissection to facilitate advancement of the flap into the defect.

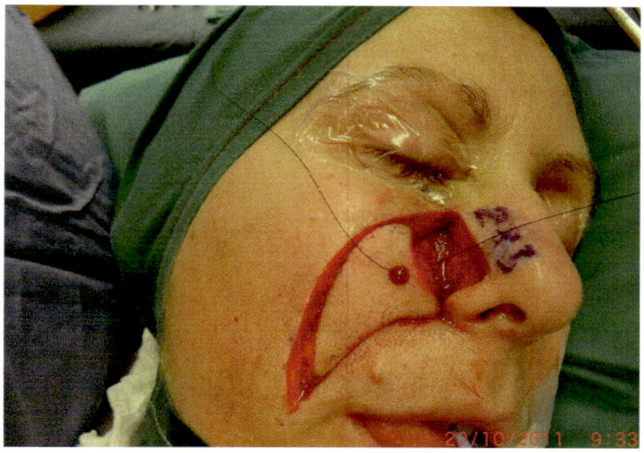

Fig. 2.141 The Red Dot Sign at the suture point, indicating the reflex hyperaemia evident in this V-Y island flap as happens in the Keystone. The flap is supported by random perforators from the nasal branch of the facial artery to explain the hyperaemia. All vessels are not skeletonised as this unnecessary manoeuvre may strip autonomic fibres along the vessel

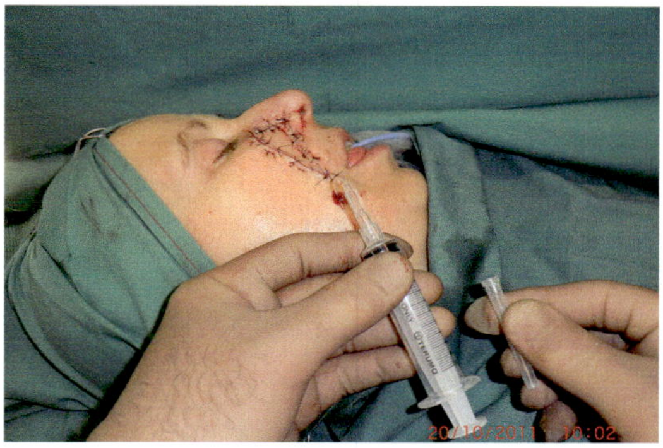

Fig. 2.142 Drainage technique using a 10-ml syringe with perforated plastic tubing attached. It is held out to suction length and secured using the plastic sleeve of the hypodermic needle

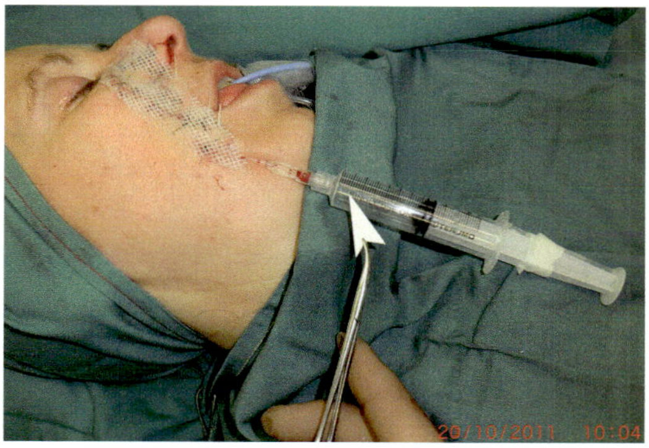

Fig. 2.143 Reinstating suction after release. The volume contained in the syringe is a measure of blood loss in mls. Reinstating the suction and reattaching the tubing allows ongoing drainage to be monitored and measured until it ceases

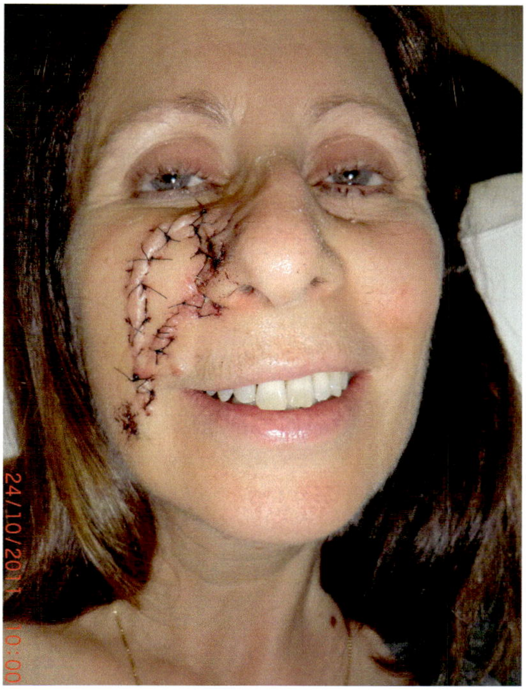

Fig. 2.144 Appearance at 24 h. The wound is closed with the standard single layered 3-phase suture technique and the nylon suture on the epidermis creates eversion to produce an excellent scar line as in the Keystone the P.A.C.E.S. factors also apply (because this is comparable to a hemi-Keystone in design)

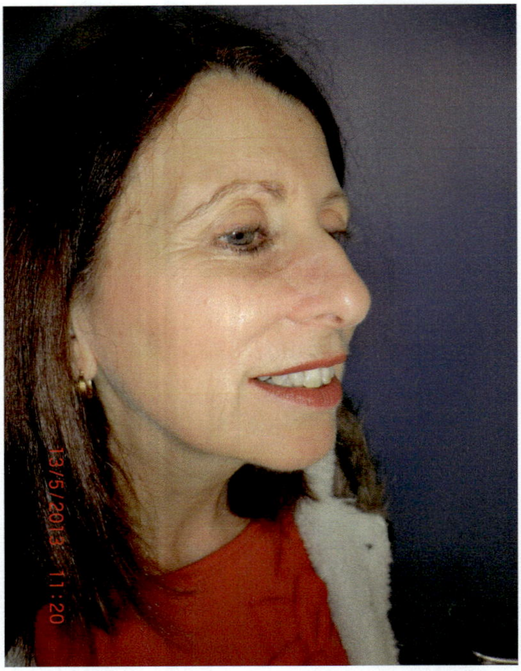

Fig. 2.145 Postoperative appearance at 2 years and the P.A.C.E.S acronym have all been exemplified. This anxious patient appreciated the outcome of the modified Keystone which is really a conjoined/double V-Y flap

2.1.6.2 Case 19: Total Nasal Cover Reconstruction Using a Transverse Keystone Design Variant from the Forehead

Multifocal mitotic skin lesions of the nasal bridge are the background pathology. The lesion over the L frontal eminence has successfully healed (Case 7) (see Figs. 2.147, 2.148, 2.149, 2.150, 2.151, 2.152, 2.153, and 2.154).

In summary, each reconstruction exemplified the P.A.C.E.S. characteristics of the Keystone as applied to this variation of a forehead island flap. It is simpler to execute with upward closure over the R frontal eminence and no doubt sitting along the supraorbital and supratrochlear angiotome supply – V 1.

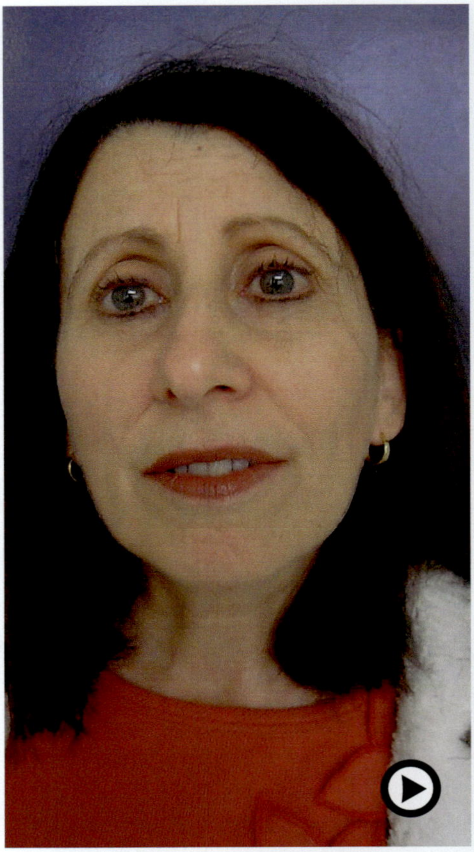

Fig. 2.146 Postoperative 6 years – patient perspective (▶ https://doi.org/10.1007/000-b52)

2.1.6.3 Case 20: Nasal Tip Reconstruction

A 63-year-old female nasal tip melanoma in association with an adjacent BCC component creating a defect 3 × 2 cm with 7 mm clearance achieved (see Figs. 2.155, 2.156, 2.157, 2.158, 2.159, 2.160, and 2.161).

In summary, the P.A.C.E.S. charactristics of the Keystone were all exemplified in this island flap repair.

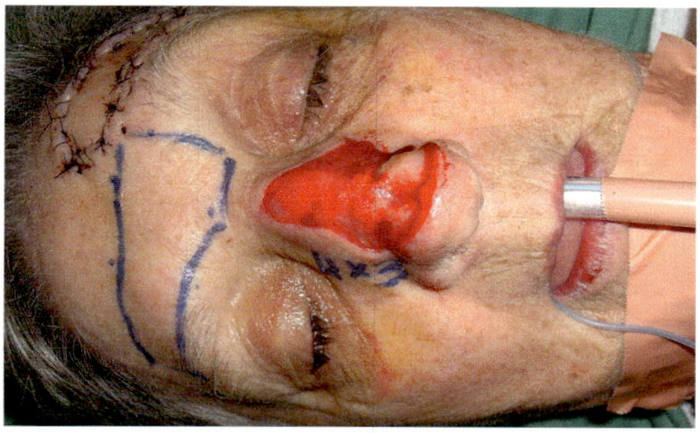

Fig. 2.147 The multifocal lesions of the nasal bridge. Defect is 4 × 3 cm awaiting pathology clearance (DRAPE). The forehead island flap mark out, based on the R supratrochlear and supraorbital neurovascular dermatome

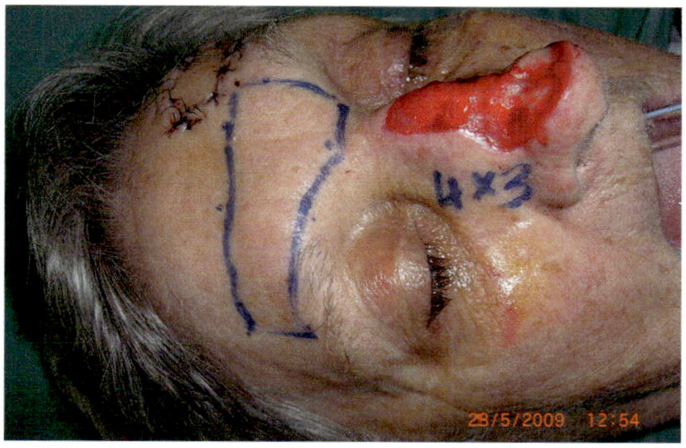

Fig. 2.148 Lateral view of the same defect in the V1 dermatome

Fig. 2.149 The dermatome mark out for the trigeminal nerve – V 1

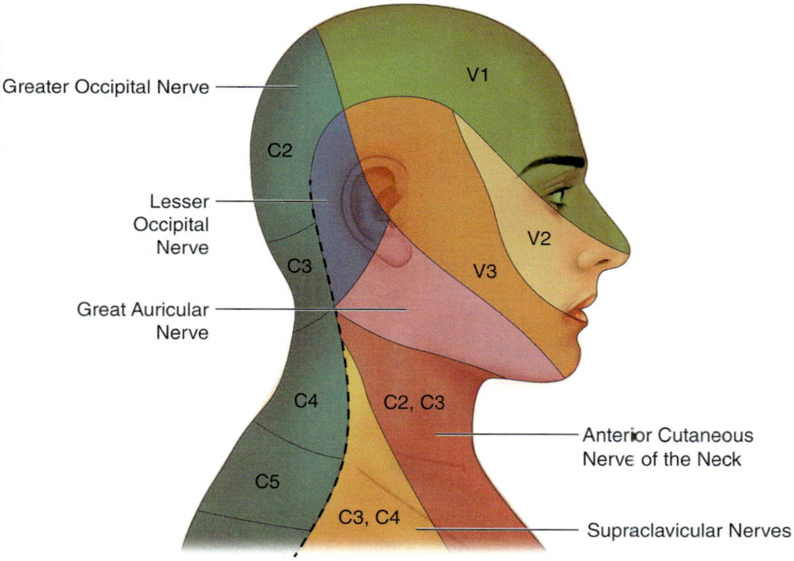

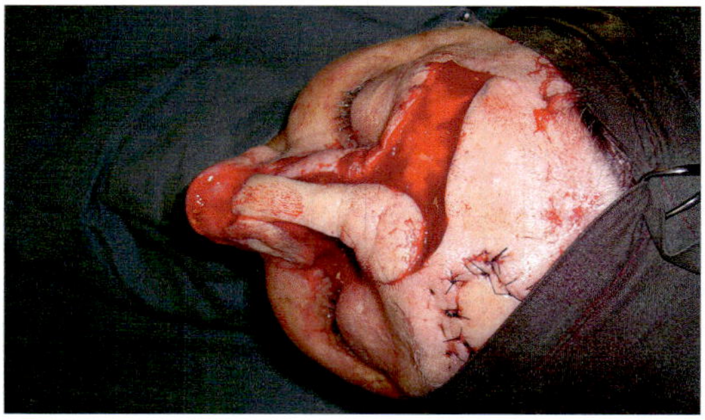

Fig. 2.150 Staged insertion of the forehead island flap to close the bridge

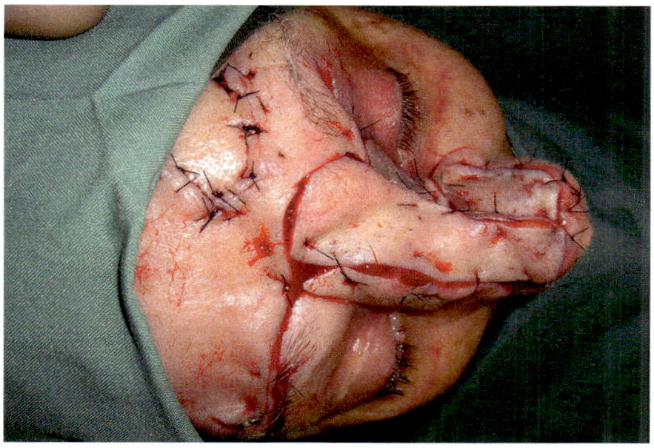

Fig. 2.151 Closing of the secondary defect under tension. Note the viability of the nasal Keystone and the upper forehead Keystone has not been compromised and the defect on the lateral side of the nose was full-thickness grafted

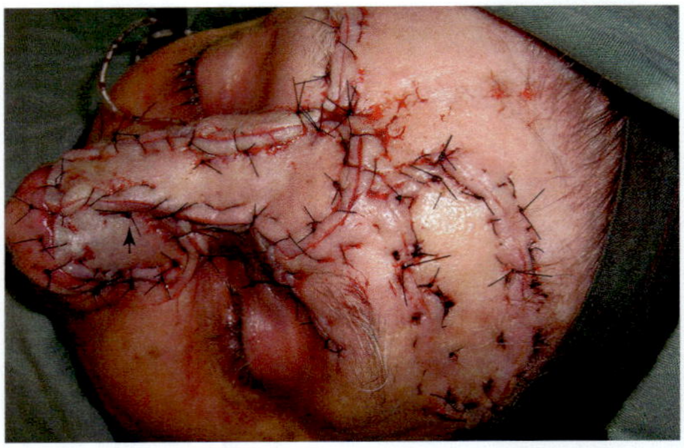

Fig. 2.152 The L forehead lesion with staged removal of sutures. The fenestrated full thickness graft on the L side of the nose (arrowed) and the forehead island flap completes the closure

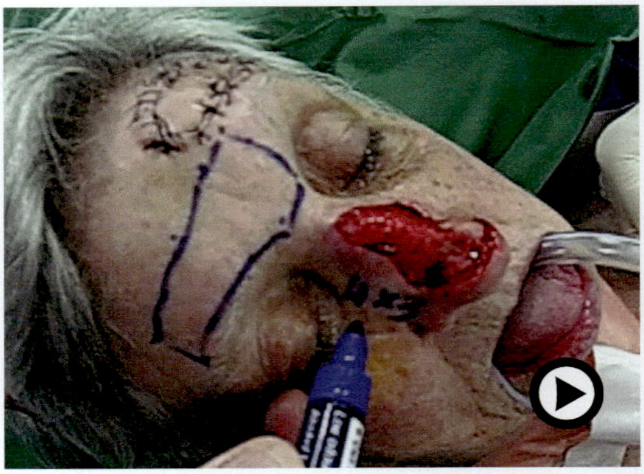

Fig. 2.154 Operative sequence (▶ https://doi.org/10.1007/000-b53)

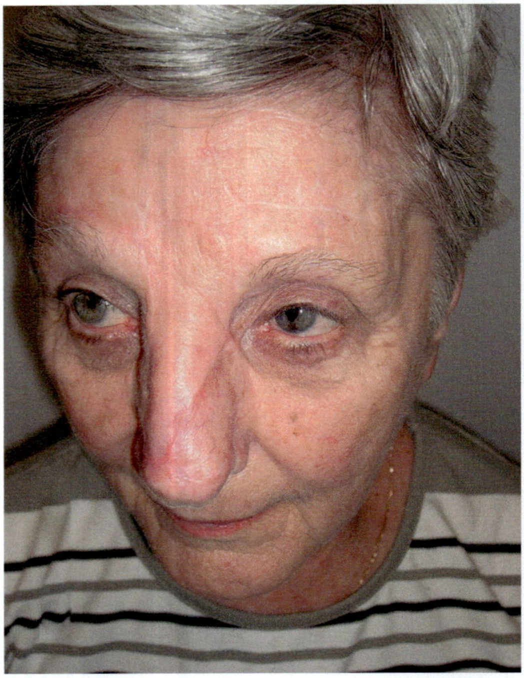

Fig. 2.153 Appearance at 6 months postoperative

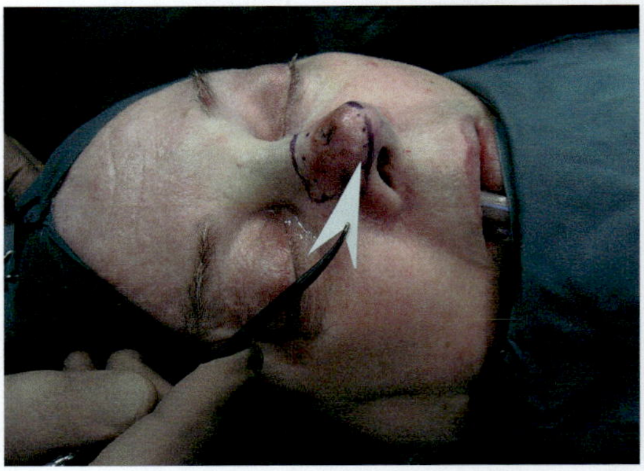

Fig. 2.155 The arrow indicates the planned tumour clearance incision

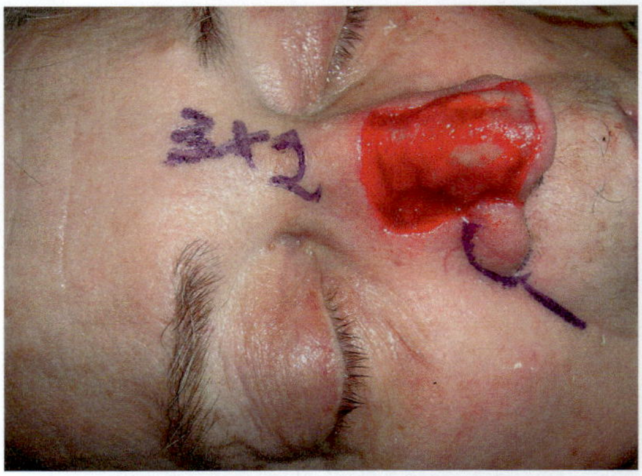

Fig. 2.156 The oncological defect 3 × 2 cm

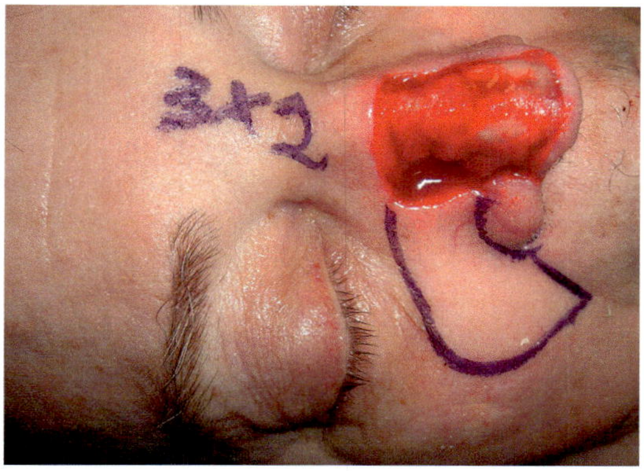

Fig. 2.157 The Keystone flap repair on the infraorbital neurovascular axes and the nasal branch of the facial artery. The Keystone is outlined and raised with blunt dissection ensuring one third deep attachment at the flap origin to reach over the nasal bridge providing soft tissue cover. Remnants from the infraorbital neurovascular axis and the nasal branch of the facial artery form a network of circulation of vascularity to allow the flaps placement at the nasal tip

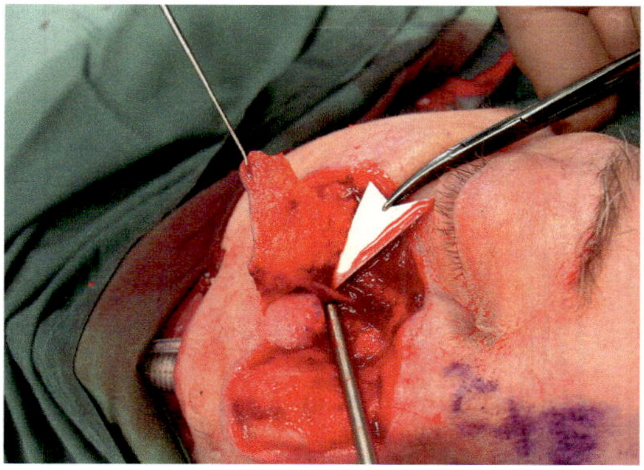

Fig. 2.159 The arrow indicates the nasal branch of the facial artery defined but not skeletonised

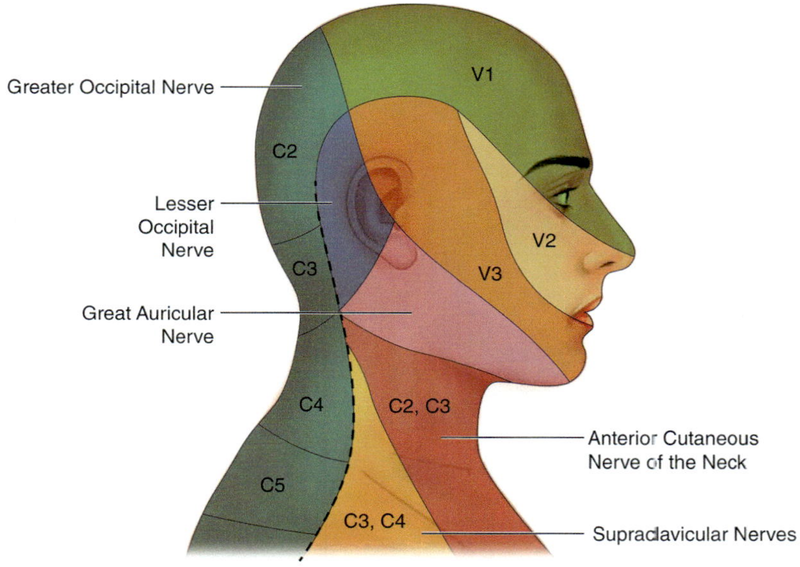

Fig. 2.158 The V2 dermatome of the trigeminal nerve is the neurovascular support for this island technique utilising nasal branches of the facial artery and nasal branches of the infraorbital neurovascular system. These are not specifically dissected

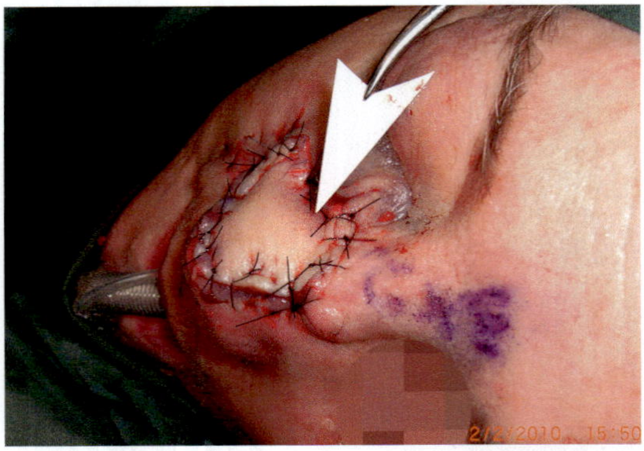

Fig. 2.160 The flap insertion using the standard 3-phase single layer suture technique

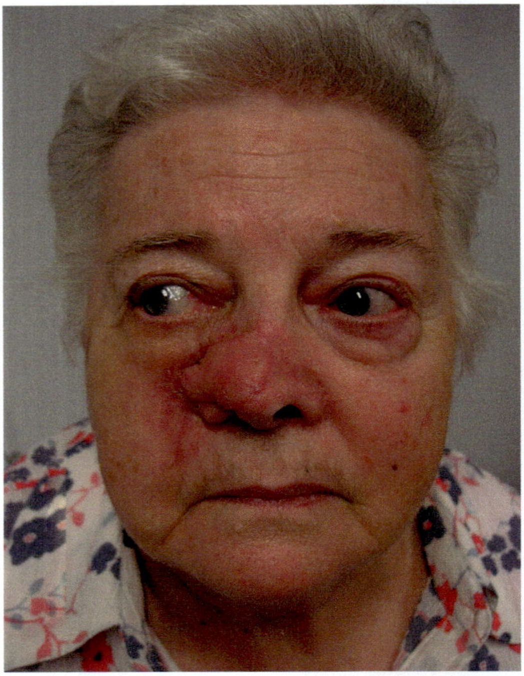

Fig. 2.161 Postoperative appearance at 2 weeks after removal of sutures

2.1.7 Cheek

The Keystone has universal applications in closure of defects from the infraorbital region, the preauricular region and the bucco-mandibular alignment. The principles of direct closure, though possible in the loose elderly skin, often give a furrow arrowing in the initial deformity – whereas the Keystone, a single island flap, bridges two surgical defects (the tumour site and the origin of the Keystone). Simplistically, we have an umbrella of tissue, the Keystone which opens to cover both sites acting in the same manner as an open umbrella. I will not list the umpteen cases of cheek rotation flaps, V-Y island flaps, Mustarde's rotation flap, even quoting Moncrief as a style of reconstruction. The Rhombic flap or Dufourmental [5] creates angular designs with V-Y closures at the apical sites. The Keystone combines a lot of these designs with random subcutaneous pedicles which are not defined. But the fact that there is an island, this apparently sympathectomises the tissues around the designs of the Keystone to increase vascularity and create the hyperaemic appearance externally visualised by the Red Dot Sign. The alignment of flaps around the dermatomes of the trigeminal design and the cervico-facial outlines is the success of this reconstructive tool. The problem of undermining to allow advancement in large wound closure is thus avoided because the tensional apposition – an edict of surgery we have all experienced and respected – is now obsolete as the hyperaemia is based on perforator circulation in this island concept and has no part with the subdermal plexus, except for input and the perforators lie in the 'stalk of the umbrella' that is used to cover the tissue defect. Microvascular free flap reconstruction, radial forearm, even parascapular almost ordain secondary procedures to improve contour and bulk and volume because these three extremes seem to characterise microvascular reconstruction. However, if it is needed it is needed, particularly covering large bony defects.

2.1.7.1 Case 21: Malar Region

This level II melanoma created an infraorbital defect 5 × 4 cm. The important aspects of the Keystone design must have a directional pull in an upward and outward alignment so there is no ectropion produced which would occur if the Keystone was placed laterally and not superiorly (see Figs. 2.162, 2.163, 2.164, 2.165, 2.166, 2.167, and 2.168).

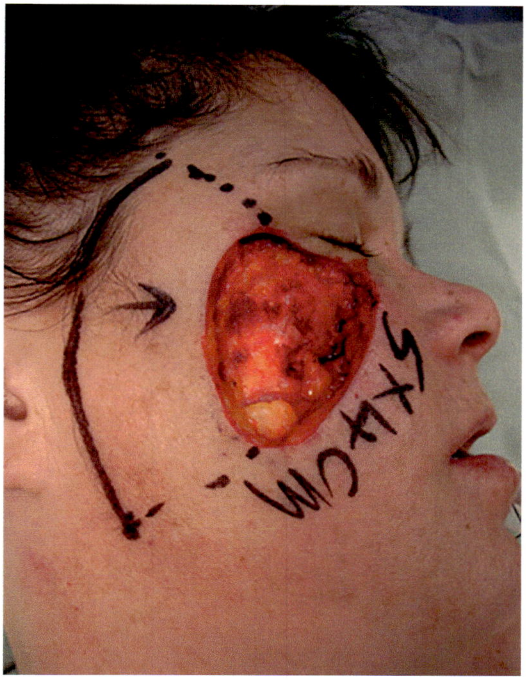

Fig. 2.162 Melanoma of the R malar eminence. Note the discreet way the defect was excised with the line of the superior excision aligned upwards and outwards to minimise subsequent ectropion development. The arrow in the Keystone flap indicates the line of pull. If it is more inferiorly placed the ectropion factor may emerge. The circulation, no doubt, is based on random perforators from the facial artery which are not specifically localised while the hyperaemic phase is still evident

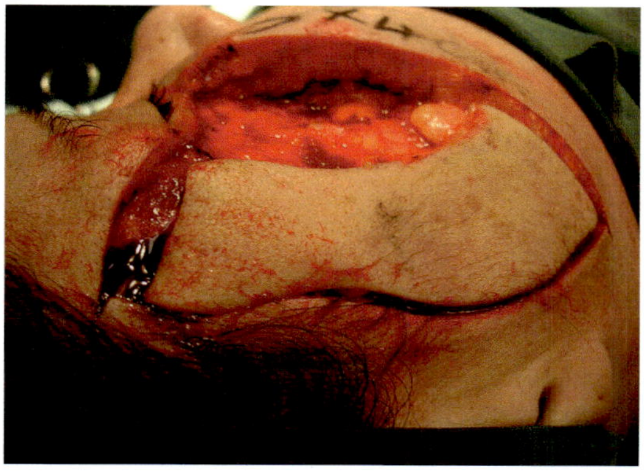

Fig. 2.164 The preauricular Keystone mark out to align with the excisional defect of the cheek with the closure in the upward and outward direction to minimise ectropion

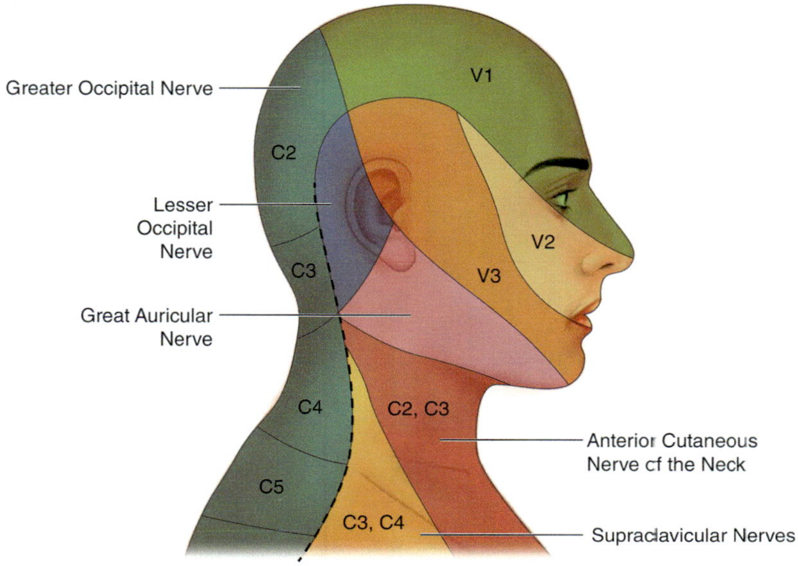

Fig. 2.163 The dermatomal mark out is the guide for the location of the random perforators coming through the fascia

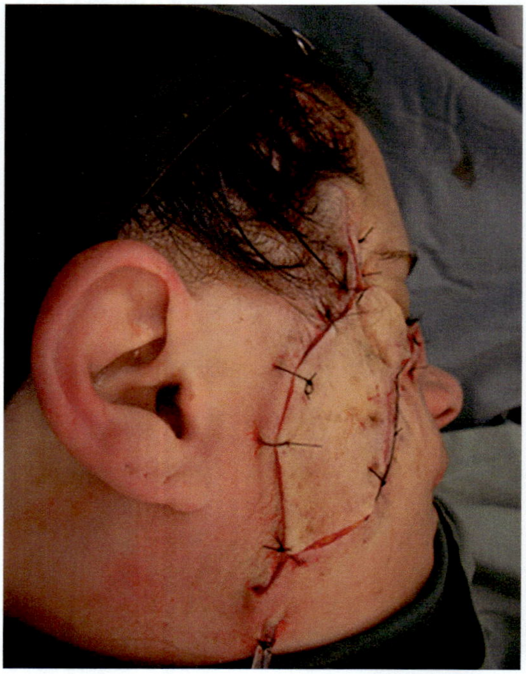

Fig. 2.165 Staged repair using the 3-phase single layer nylon suture technique (mattress locking and mattress standard sutures) and epidermal closure using a continuous 4/0 nylon suture removed at 7 days

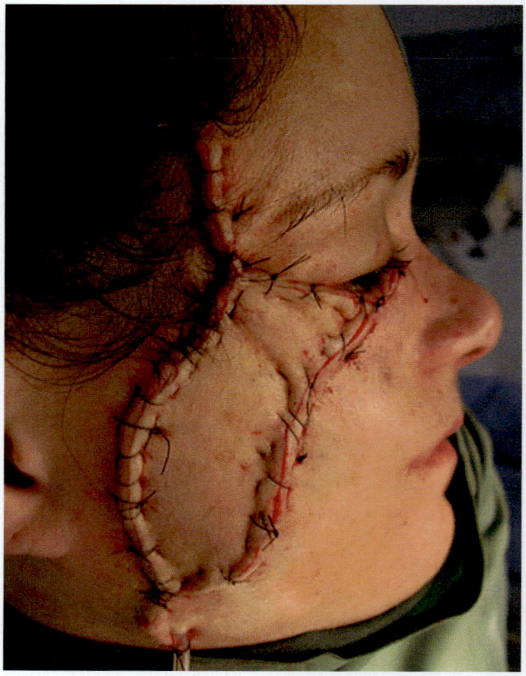

Fig. 2.166 Postoperative appearance without any ectropion. Note the hypervascularity reflex in the flap which is pinker than the surrounding flaps in the cheeks – confirming the P.A.C.E.S. characteristics of the Keystone

Fig. 2.167 Staged wound dressing on the face where the cutaneous loops are cut at 7 days, some of the mattress at 10 days and the points of maximum tension at the locking mattress sutures may stay up to 14 days. Note there is no ectropion of the R lower eyelid

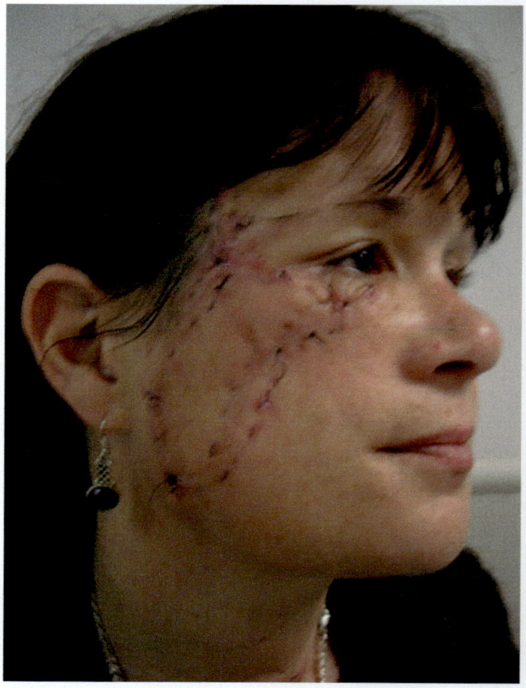

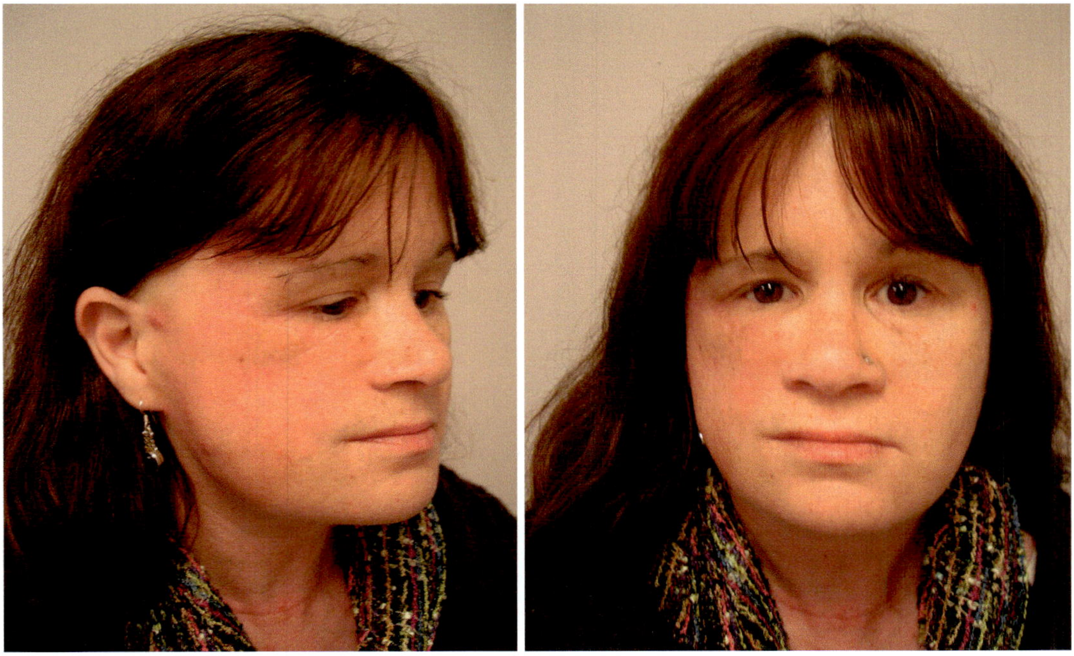

Fig. 2.168 The postoperative result showing the patient's satisfaction in this anxious young person. The only important aspect here in reconstruction is to design the Keystone so the direction of tensional closure is in an upward and outward direction to minimise the development of any ectropion on that R lower eyelid

In summary, the P.A.C.E.S. charactristics of the Keystone were all exemplified in this island flap repair.

2.1.7.2 Case 22 – Melanoma of the R Lower Cheek

Level I/II cheek melanoma in a Hutchinson's melanotic freckle overlying the R cheek in the bucco-mandibular region (see Figs. 2.169, 2.170, 2.171, 2.172, 2.173, 2.174, 2.175, 2.176, and 2.177).

In summary, the P.A.C.E.S. charactristics of the Keystone were all exemplified in this island flap repair.

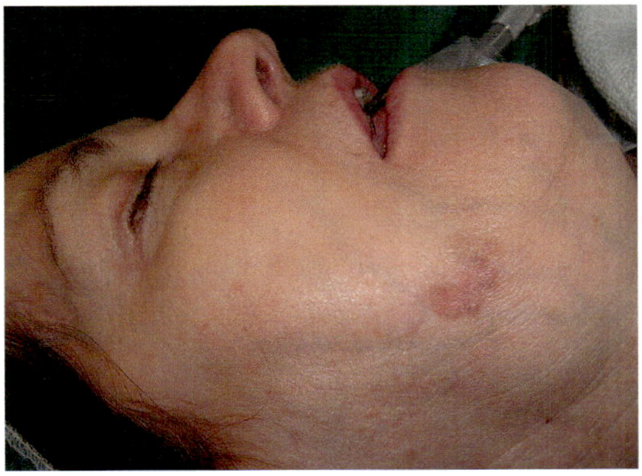

Fig. 2.169 The 3 × 2 cm melanotic lesion of the R cheek

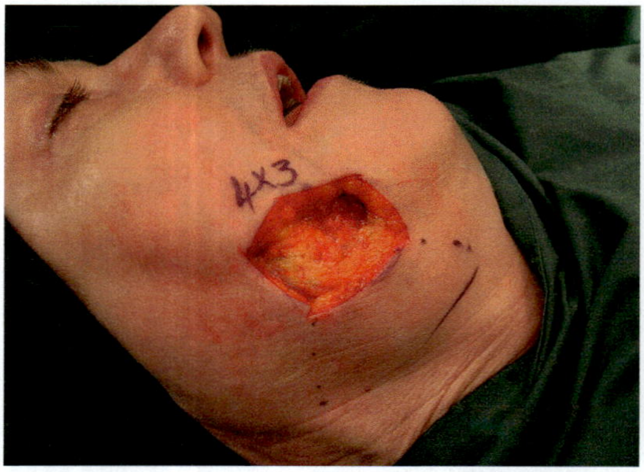

Fig. 2.170 The surgical excision defect 4 × 3 cm down to the buccal pad of the R cheek and circumventing the mandibular branch of the facial nerve

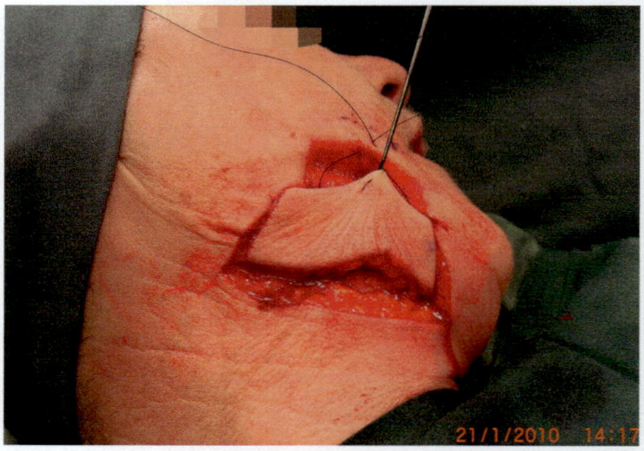

Fig. 2.172 The looseness of tissue in the submandibular region is the perfect baseline for the Keystone design leaving one third of deep attachment beneath the Keystone. The skin hook shows the alignment around the oral aperture. This is the site for the tension sutures using locking mattress techniques which produce the best aesthetic outcome, eliminating lip drag or angle of the mouth distortion

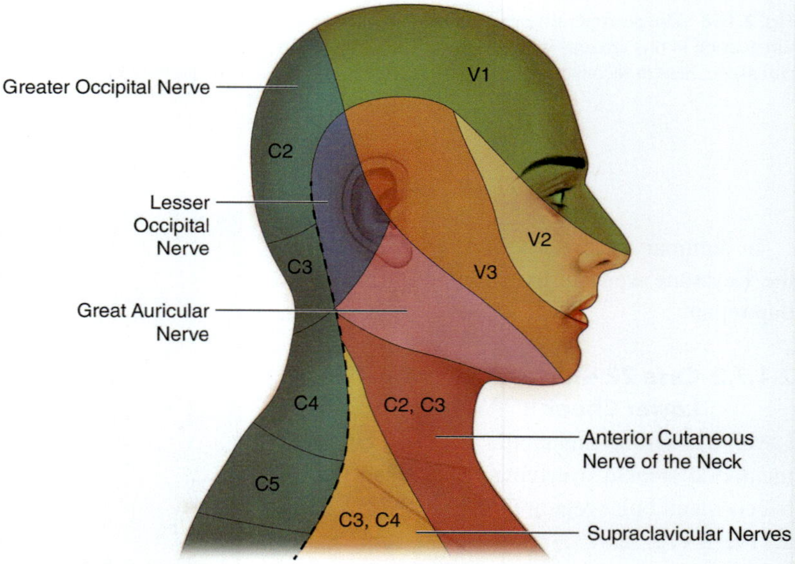

Fig. 2.171 The Keystone flap based on random perforators from the facial artery sitting in the C2, C3 dermatome posteriorly and the V3 dermatome anteriorly. However, an underlying principle of leaving one third of deep attachment of the Keystone flap guarantees vascular perfusion

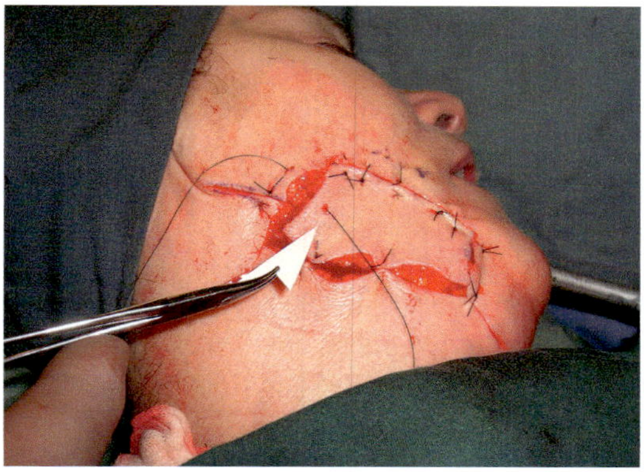

Fig. 2.173 Repair in progress. Note the arrow is indicating the Red Dot Sign which is the hyperaemic flow indicator characteristic of the Keystone island flap design. Here the suture point exit site bleeds more than the suture receiving site on the attached tissue surrounding this Keystone. This Red Dot Sign confirms the absence of any vascular impedance, in fact quite the reverse

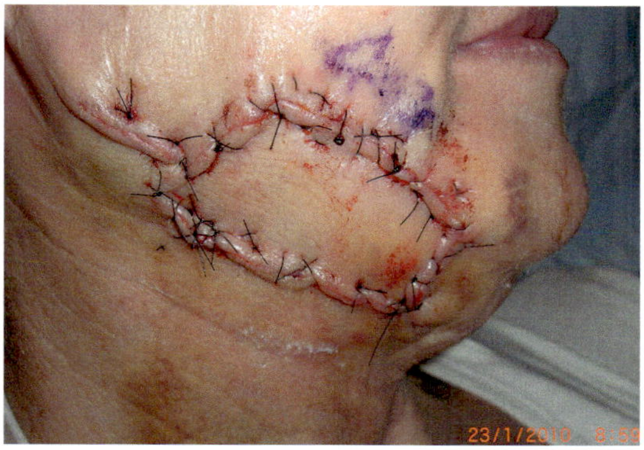

Fig. 2.174 Two days postoperative appearance with no signs of vascular necrosis

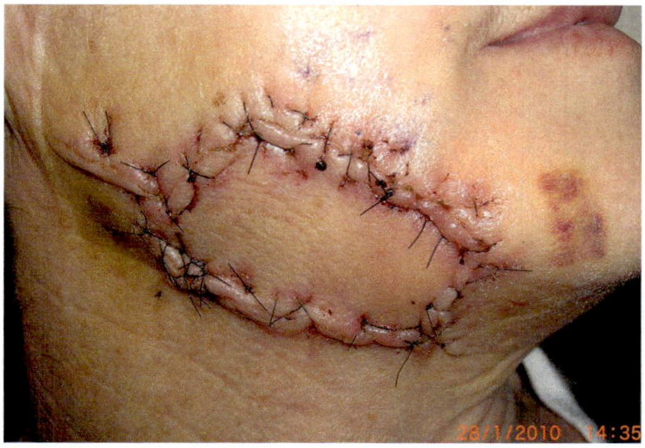

Fig. 2.175 One week postoperative appearance

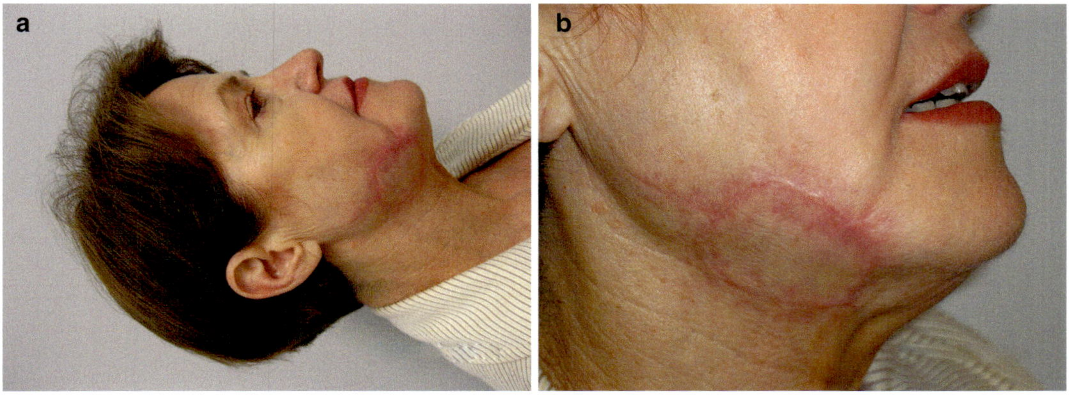

Fig. 2.176 (**a**) Appearance at 6 weeks. (**b**) Close up of same

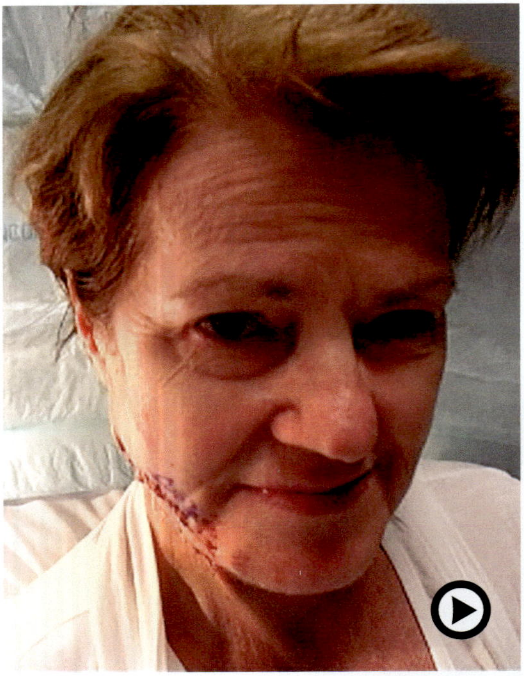

Fig. 2.177 Postoperative—patient perspective (▶ https://doi.org/10.1007/000-b54)

2.1.7.3 Case 23: Melanoma in an Irradiated Field

Melanoma in the R cheek in an irradiated field in this 62-year-old male.

He had a past history of cancer of larynx treated with radiation. His lower neck skin necrosis was treated with pectoralis-major reconstructive flap before the biopsy of the cheek lesion which confirmed melanoma (see Figs. 2.178, 2.179, 2.180, 2.181, 2.182, 2.183, and 2.184).

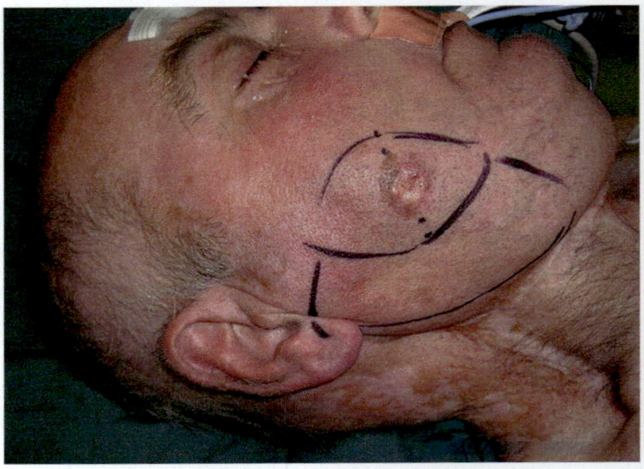

Fig. 2.178 This level II melanoma in an irradiated field doubled in size during the postoperative treatment of the lower cervical radio-necrosis treated with a pectoralis-major flap

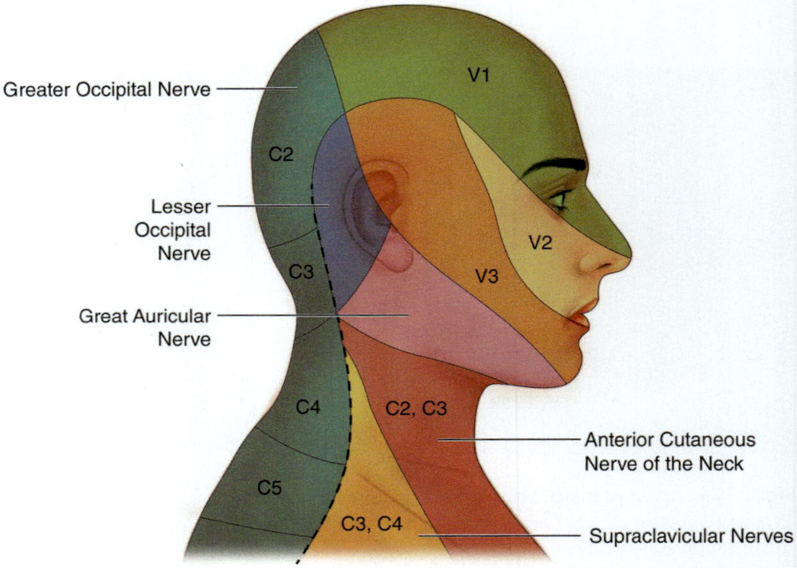

Fig. 2.179 The cheek lesion sits over the V2 dermatome – the site of the excision. The C2, C3 dermatomes are the site of the R submandibular Keystone repair using random branches of the facial artery

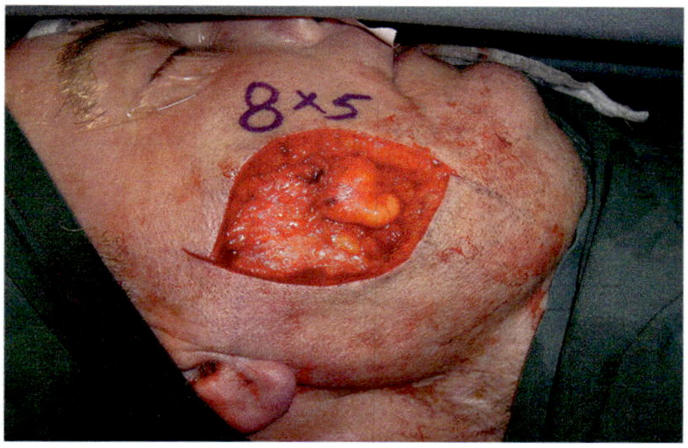

Fig. 2.180 The defect 8 × 5 cm and the buccal pad of fat is evident in the depths of the wound

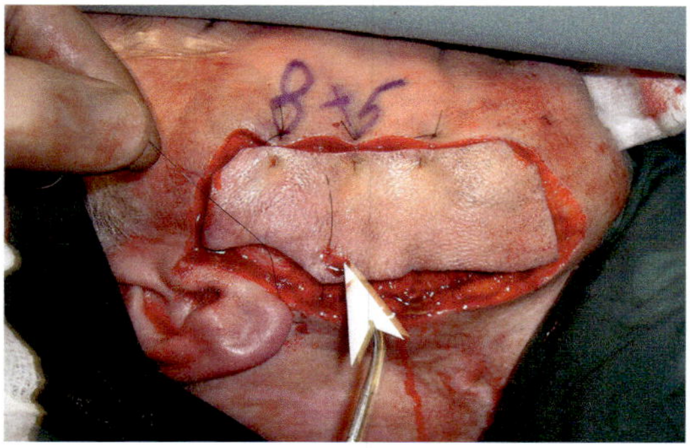

Fig. 2.181 The wound is closed under tension in this irradiated field, a Keystone characteristic reflecting the hyperaemic reflex is evident in the posterior aspect of the Keystone (closer to a branch of the facial artery). The cyanotic superior margin indicating the possible vasculitis associated with radiation. The Red Dot Sign is arrowed confirming its hypervascularity to ensure healing in this irradiated field – usually a contraindication for loco-regional reconstruction

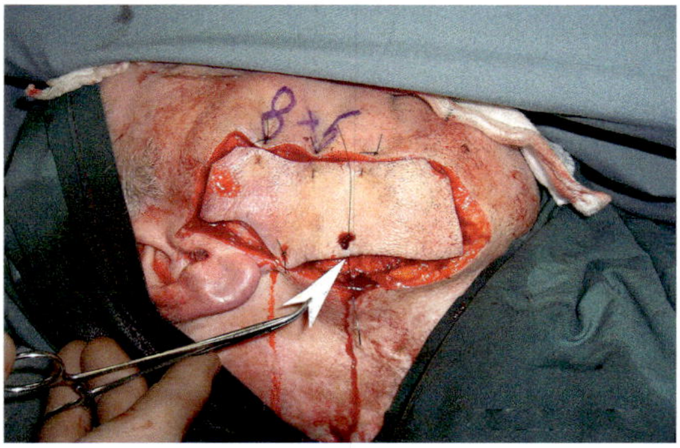

Fig. 2.182 The Red Dot Sign in an irradiated field reflecting the slight vascular impedance and it borders on the cyanotic appearance

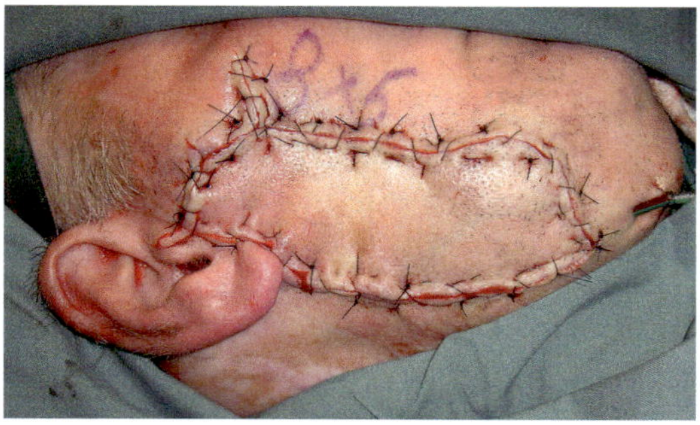

Fig. 2.183 The closure complete in a timeframe of 90 min with the standard 3-phase suture technique. The difference in vascular perfusion is evident starting inferiorly and spreading up the flap

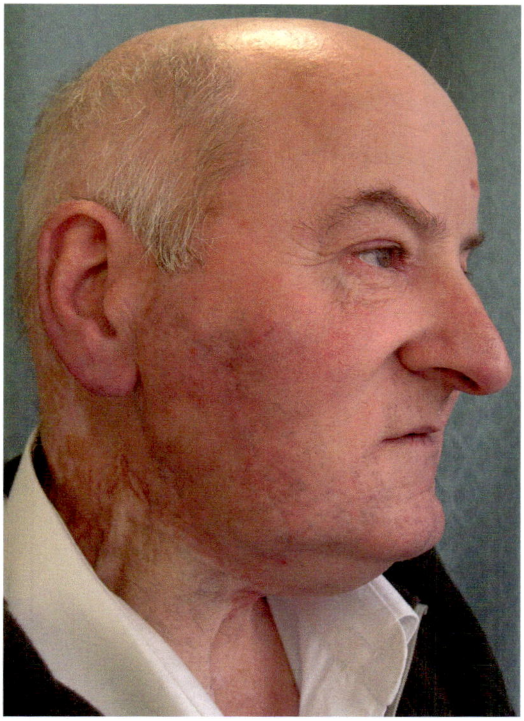

Fig. 2.184 Normal appearance at 6 weeks, meeting the patient's satisfaction in this barber. The scar is indiscernible reflecting the value of the single layered 3-phase nylon closure technique

In summary, the P.A.C.E.S. charactristics of the Keystone were all exemplified in this island flap repair. An acceptable surgical repair in irradiated tissue, not a contraindication to Keystone applications as it is for other loco-regional flaps. The islanding hypervascularises the tissue in spite of dermal and subdermal fibrous atrophy post radiation vasculitis.

2.1.7.4 Case 24: DRAPE Procedure – Referral from Another Unit

Hutchinson's melanotic freckle and melanoma of L cheek in an 80 year old. The pathology indicated incomplete removal that is why a DRAPE (Delayed Reconstruction Awaiting Pathology Evaluation) procedure was performed (see Figs. 2.185, 2.186, 2.187, 2.188, 2.189, 2.190, 2.191, 2.192, 2.193, and 2.194).

In summary, the DRAPE procedure thus delaying repair until pathology clearance is achieved is a sound clinical principle.

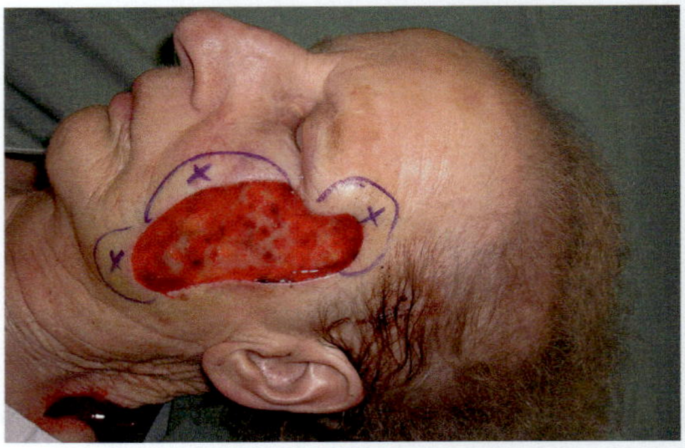

Fig. 2.185 The three curvilinear mark outs at the lateral eyebrow, the nasolabial cheek and along the line of the mandible all needed re-excision

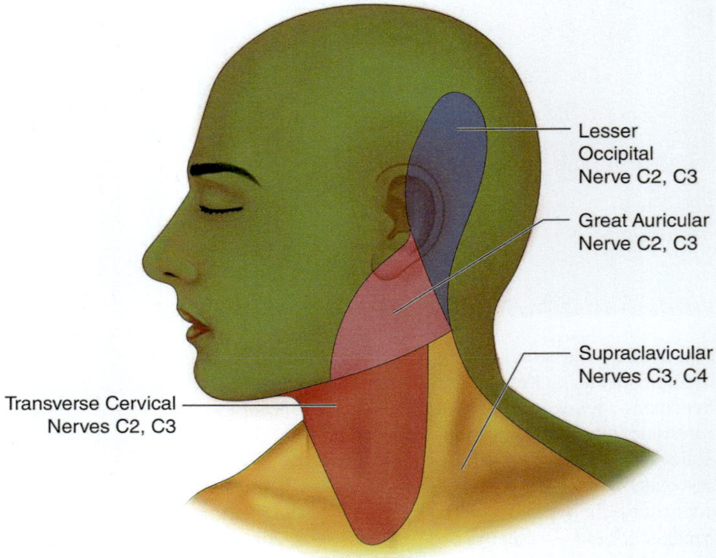

Fig. 2.186 The transverse cervical dermatomes C2, C3 are the basic dermatomes for the Keystone reconstructive technique

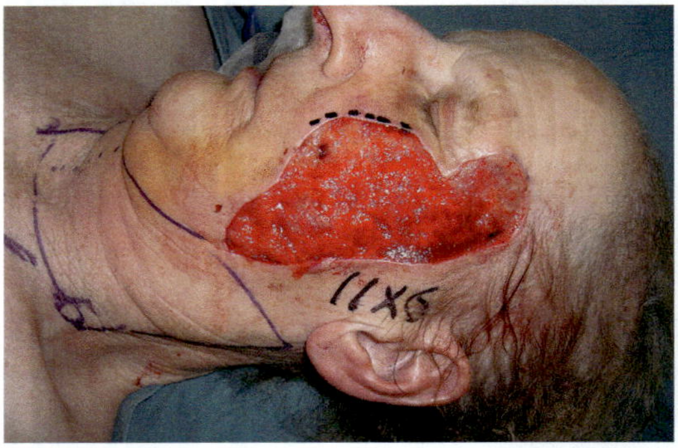

Fig. 2.187 The cervical Keystone is defined. This 11 × 6 cm defect of L cheek, the highlight of the nasolabial alignment, was the site of incomplete excision – hence the value of the DRAPE procedure

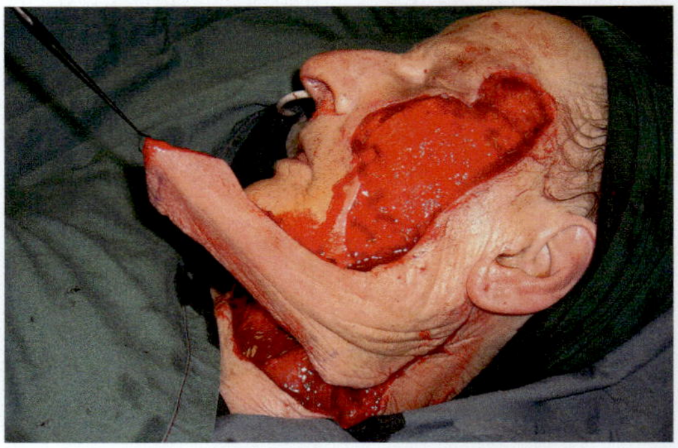

Fig. 2.188 The raising of the cervico-submental flap as an island of tissue to reach up to the level of the L temple. Even the hyperaemia of the apex of the flap is noted and based on sterno-mastoid perforators which is the site of one third deep attachment

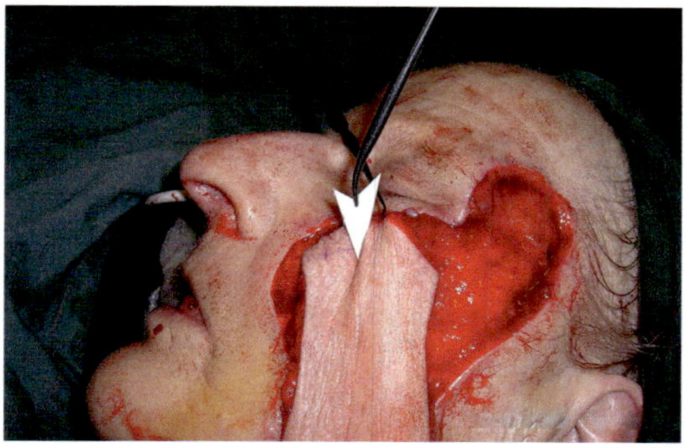

Fig. 2.189 A further stage in the reconstruction and the arrow confirms the reflex hyperaemia stage

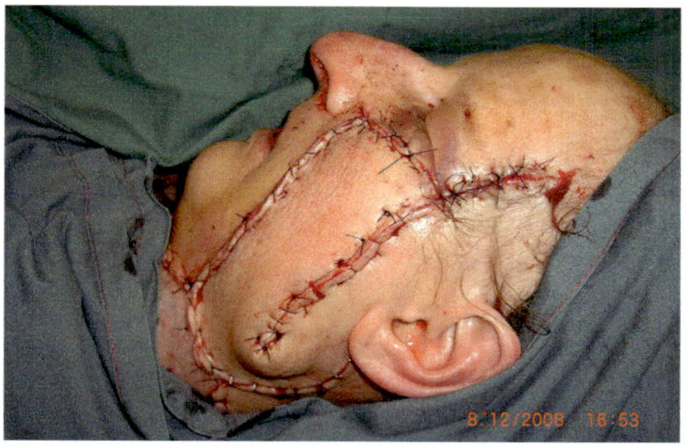

Fig. 2.190 The wound closure is completed using the standard single layer 3-phase nylon suture technique. One should note the suture line in the L infraorbital region is angled upwards to minimise any ectropion pull and the 'dog ear' superiorly has been excised leaving the later part for further adjustment

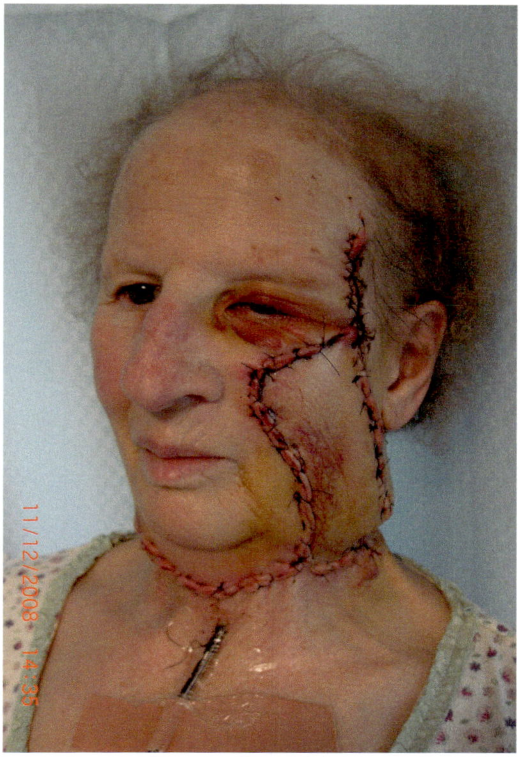

Fig. 2.191 Appearance at 3 days. Note the cervical suture crosses the midline. The P.A.C.E.S. characteristics of the Keystone were all exemplified in this island flap repair. The aesthetic outcome is seen in Fig. 24.8

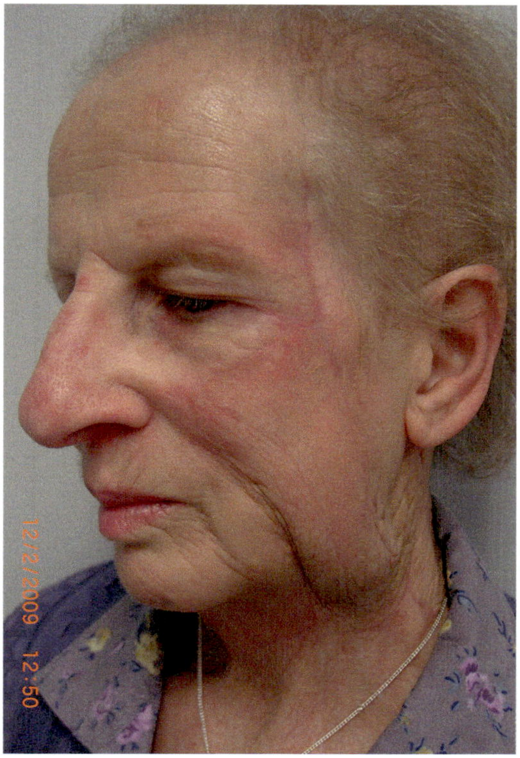

Fig. 2.192 The aesthetic appearance at 2 months. Note the absence of ectropion of the L lower eyelid, the suture line is barely visible using this 3-phase suture technique. The redundancy next to the angle of the jaw could have been revised but the patient refused given her age

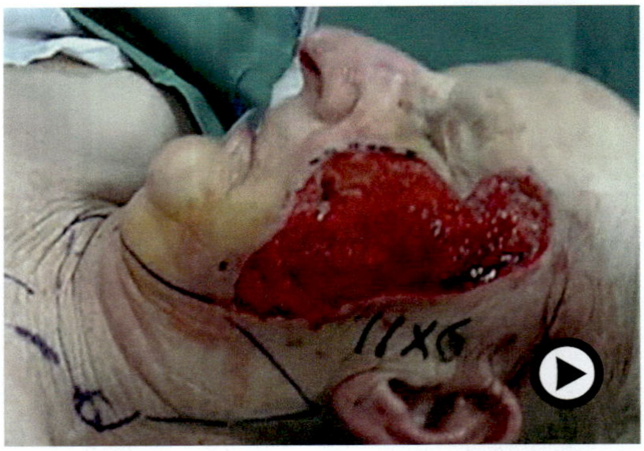

Fig. 2.193 Operative sequence (▶ https://doi.org/10.1007/000-b55)

2.1.7.5 Case 25: L Lower Cheek Keystone in the Elderly – Age Is Not a Contraindication

Melanoma of the L cheek over the L angle of the mandible in this 97-year-old male confirming age is not a contraindication in major surgery using this simple reconstructive tool of the Keystone repair (see Figs. 2.195, 2.196, 2.197, 2.198, and 2.199).

In summary, age is not a contraindication in this 97 year old and the speed of execution without complications exemplifies the P.A.C.E.S. characteristics.

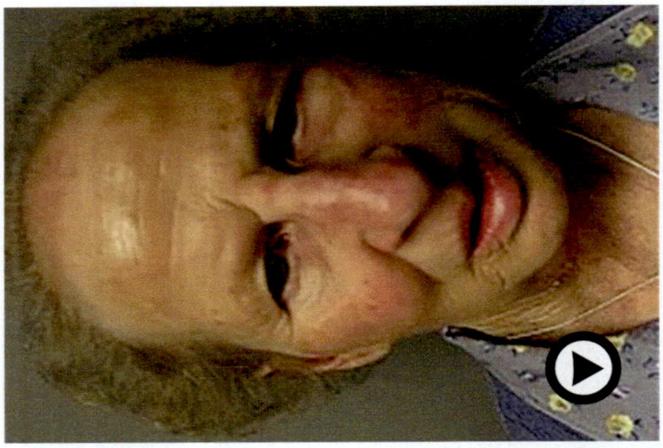

Fig. 2.194 Postoperative – patient perspective (▶ https://doi.org/10.1007/000-b56)

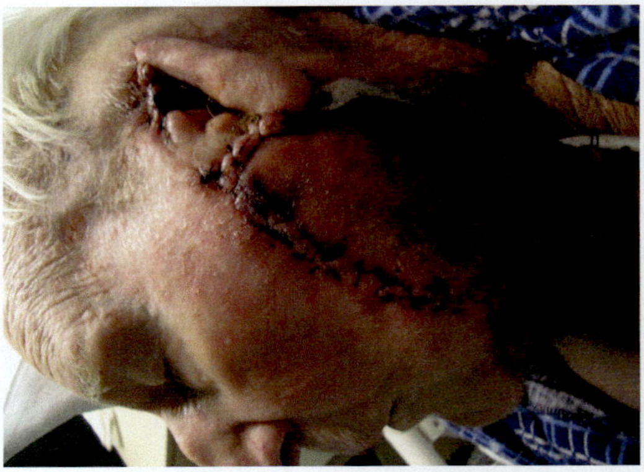

Fig. 2.195 Postoperative appearance during the wound dressing phase

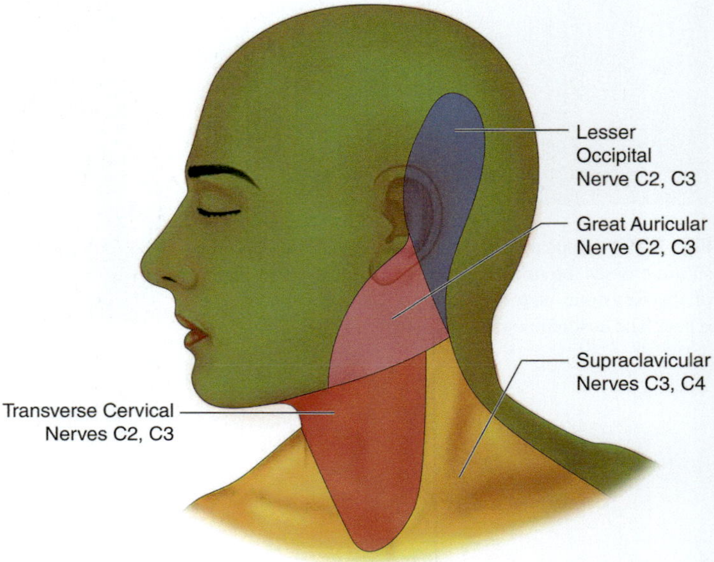

Fig. 2.196 The dermatomal mark out is the guide for the location of the random perforators coming through the fascia

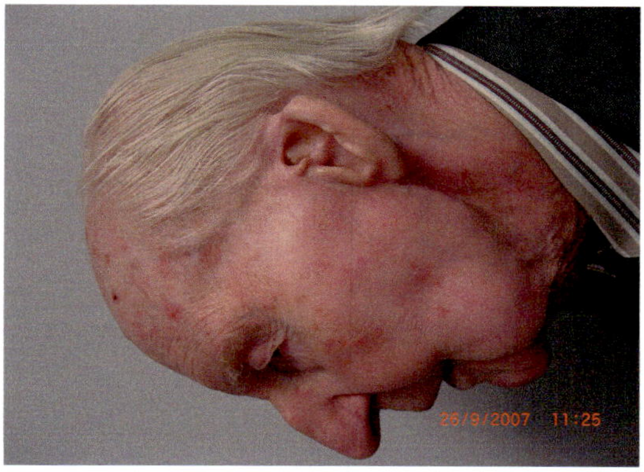

Fig. 2.197 Appearance at 9 months. Totally asymptomatic, clear of disease, no initial or postoperative pain, aesthetically acceptable, complications nil and the timeframe of 60 min for the procedure is economical in a 97-year-old confirming all the P.A.C.E.S. characteristics of the Keystone Island Flap

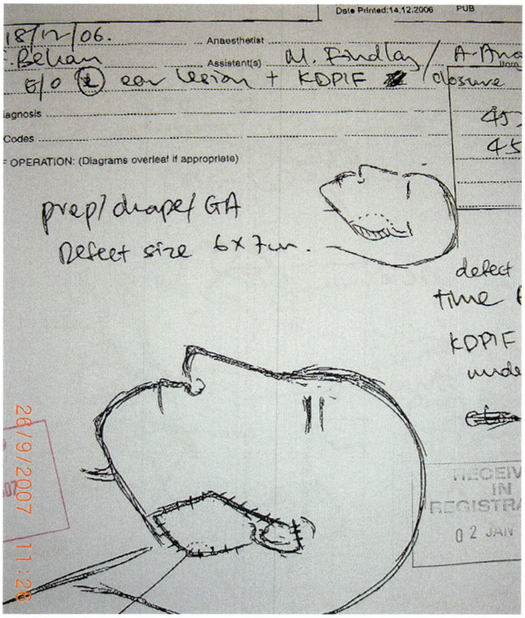
Date Printed:14.12.2006 PUB

18/12/06. Anaesthetist

Assistant(s) M. Findlay / A-Ana

E/O ear lesion + KDPIF closure

iagnosis

Codes

OPERATION: (Diagrams overleaf if appropriate)

prep/drape/ GA

Defect size 6 x 7cm.

defect

time

KDPIF

RECEIV

IN

REGISTRA

0 2 JAN

26/9/2007 11:26

Fig. 2.198 Operation page details – age is not a contraindication

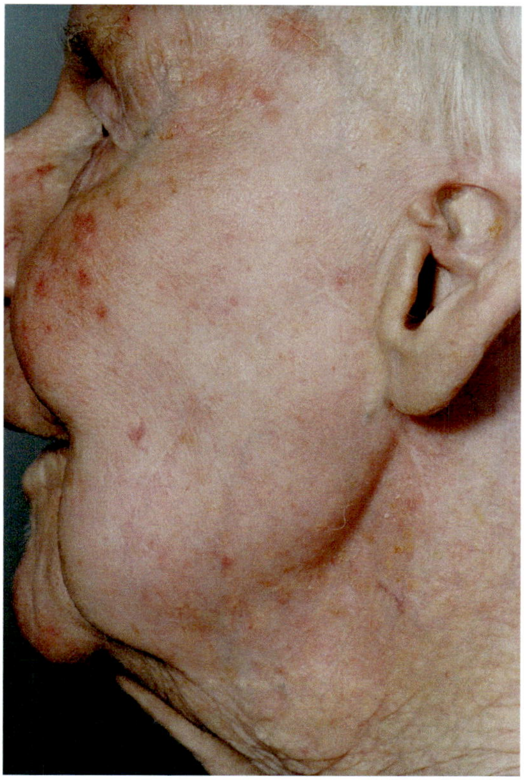

Fig. 2.199 The barely discernible scar

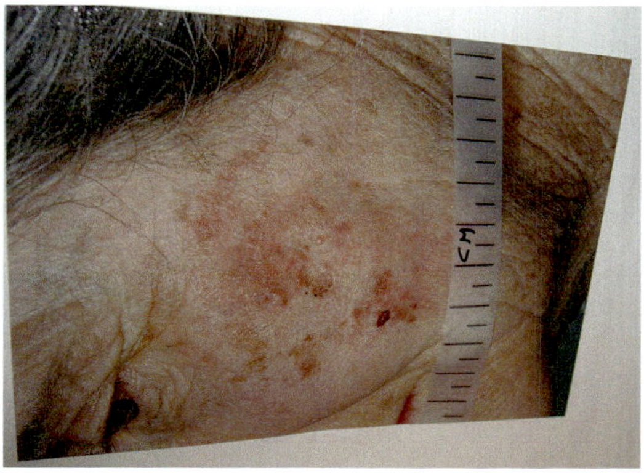

Fig. 2.200 The hyperpigmented spot in the HMF on the L cheek anterior margin lower third with a level I melanoma

2.1.7.6 Case 26: L Cheek Hutchinson's Melanotic Freckle

An HMF L cheek Clark Level I thin Melanoma with a 6 × 6 cm cheek defect in a 76-year-old female (see Figs. 2.200, 2.201, 2.202, 2.203).

In summary, the P.A.C.E.S. charactristics of the Keystone were all exemplified in this island flap repair and noting that large size defects

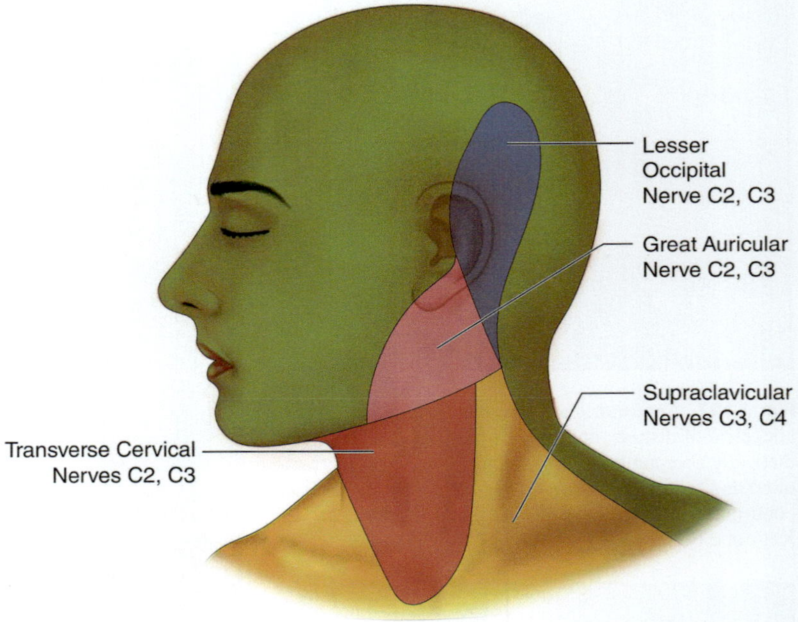

Fig. 2.201 The L cheek and angle of jaw flap was based on the greater auricular dermatome C2, C3 and the neck flap using the transverse cervical dermatome C2, C3 as an outline for the flap design

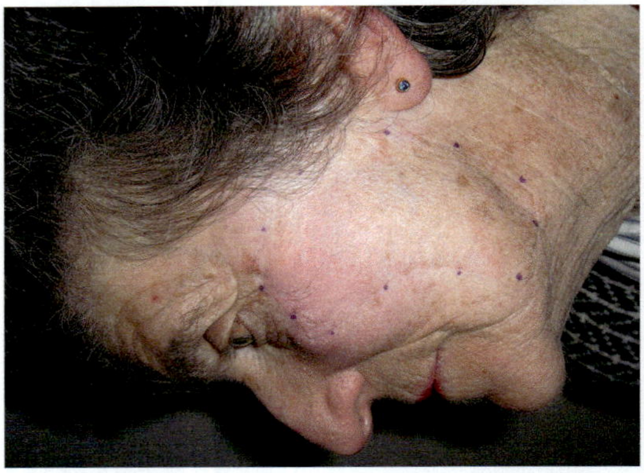

Fig. 2.202 Postoperative appearance following tumour removal measuring 6 × 6 cm of the L cheek. The scar line is outlined with blue dots as it is indiscernible using the standard 3-phase single layer nylon suture technique

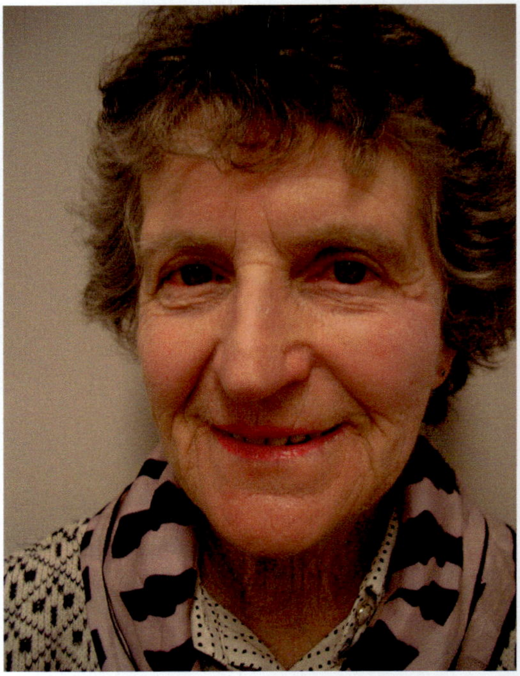

Fig. 2.203 The patient is extremely pleased with the aesthetic outcome

(6 × 6 cm) are difficult to reconstruct and the Keystone provides a solution.

2.1.8 Lip

The topical landmarks of a normal lip involve the external or dry vermilion, the wet mucosal approaching the oral lining, the total commissure with the philtral columns and governed by the orbicularis oris muscle. The input of the superior and inferior labial arteries is noted and the trigeminal and neural input V2 for upper (infraorbital innervation) and V3 for the lower (mental innervation).

Traditionally, direct closure is possible with the loss of 30% of the lip but most prefer 25% with a layered approximation of the various components, muscle, mucosa internally, vermilion superiorly and cutaneous externally.

The triangulate defect – A-shaped – creates a T image on direct closure. Bilateral advancements of the upper or lower create triangular remnants and the trimming of Burow's triangle are an essential in the lateral extremes, simplistically (taking out dog ears).

In the case of a total vermilionectomy, to close the mucosal defect is wrong in principle as this brings hear bearing tissue into the vermilion alignment in an internal direction. In this case here, it was wiser to create a Keystone design of the mucosa of the internal lining of the lower lip which allows external wet vermilion alignment to sit as it formerly did along the dry margin and the secondary defect in the buccal sulcus is allowed to mucosalise, taking up to 10 days. Grafting is avoided because of the dissimilarity between mucosal structures and the external integument and the clinical inconvenience of intraoral skin grafts needs no elaboration.

There are multiple flaps used to fix full thickness lip loss, up to 50%, (the Webster flap, the Gillies fan flap and the Karapandzic which retains the neurovascular axis) and local tissues are generally inadequate for repair of lower lip defects exceeding 75% of lip length [20]. The Abbe flap is a gesture of sharing where the upper or lower, based on the labial neurovascular structures, is turned on itself to fill the defect when the vascular division between the upper and lower lips is divided at a secondary stage at 2–3 weeks (S Lander a similar concept to the Abbe takes tissue from the lateral aspect of the upper lip into a mirror image site of the lower lip). When tissues beyond these limits are needed, microvascular free flaps may be required.

2.1.8.1 Case 27: Hutchinson's Melanoma of the Lower Lip

HMF of the lower lip in a farmer (see Figs. 2.204, 2.205, 2.206, 2.207, 2.208, 2.209, and 2.210).

In summary, the P.A.C.E.S. charactristics of the Keystone were all exemplified in this island flap repair. Mucosalisation of the secondary defect precludes the problem of tight closure and bringing in hair bearing tissue of the integument to achieve lip seal. The new vermilion has a normal alignment with the hair bearing tissue of the lower lip.

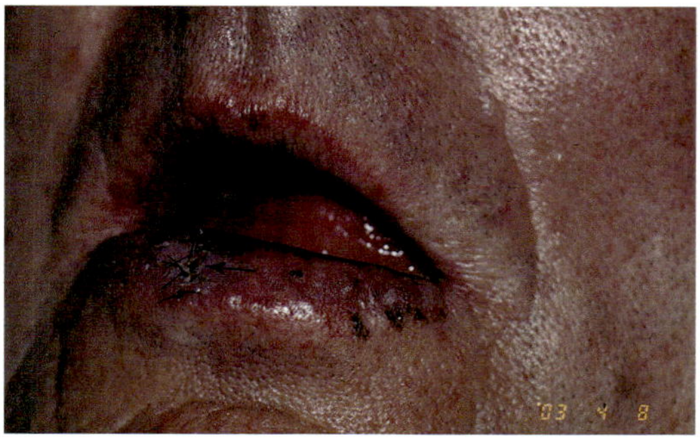

Fig. 2.204 The pathology confirmation of the HMF is noted with the suture line (arrowed)

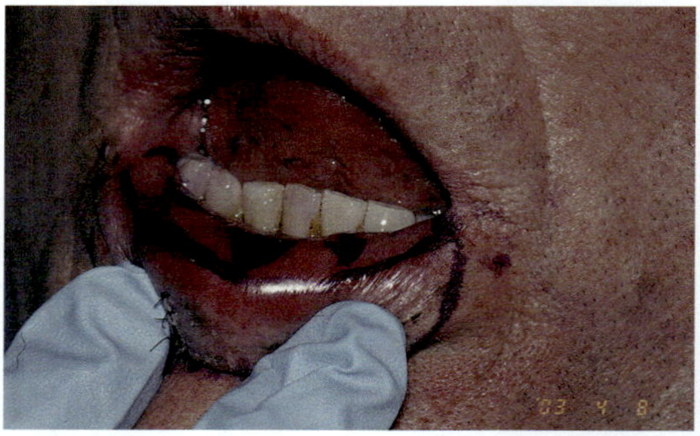

Fig. 2.205 The surgical excision of the total vermilionectomy from angle to angle of the lower lip. Direct closure brings the hair bearing tissue of the lower lip almost into an intraoral location which has an adverse effect on shaving comfort

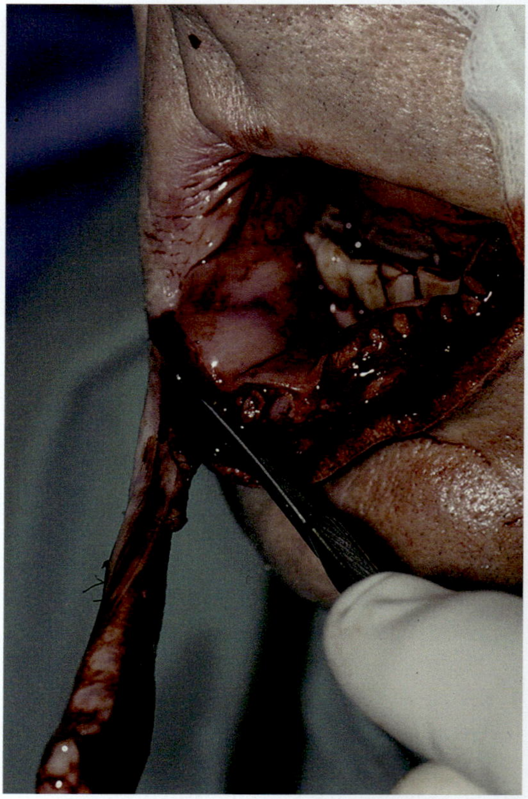

Fig. 2.206 In transit procedure removal of the lower lip vermilion margin

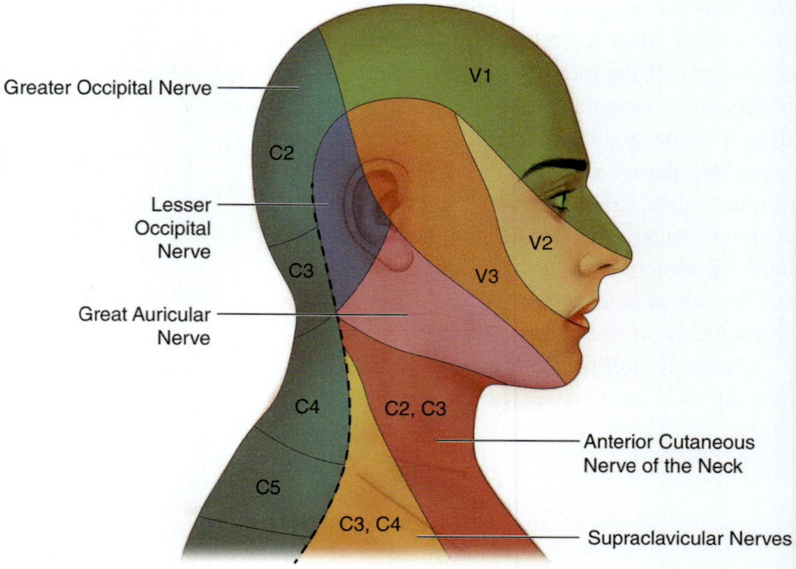

Fig. 2.207 The V3 dermatome joins across the lower lip from R and L sides and this is the basis of the Keystone mucosal Island from the intraoral lining of the lower lip to close the defect. The secondary defect below is not closed but left to mucosalise

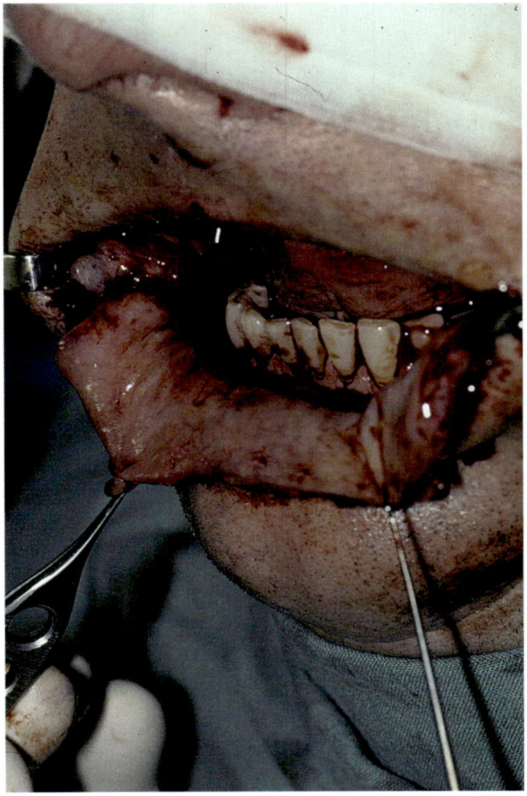

Fig. 2.208 The advancement as a Keystone of the internal lining of the lower lip to create the new vermilion. The secondary defect in the internal lining of the lower lip just above the buccal alveolar sulcus is left to mucosalise by secondary intention to avoid complications of hair bearing tissue dragged into the intraoral arrangement

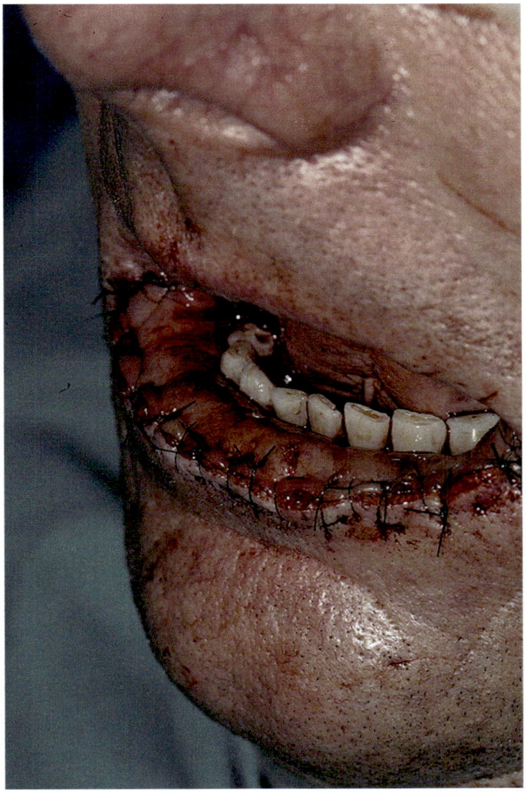

Fig. 2.209 The completed wound with the secondary defect left unsutured in the buccal alveolar succus

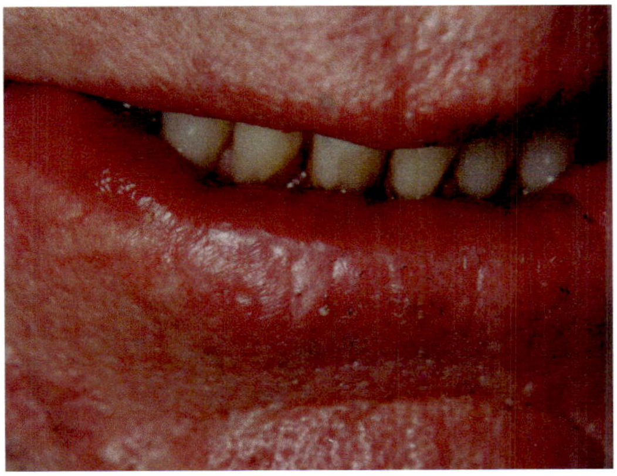

Fig. 2.210 The final appearance with lip seal achieved and the patient totally satisfied

2.1.8.2 Case 28: Mitotic Lesion Removing Two Thirds Lower Lip with Neck Gland Clearances

See Figs. 2.211, 2.212, 2.213, 2.214, 2.215, 2.216, 2.217, 2.218, 2.219, 2.220, 2.221, 2.222, 2.223, 2.224, and 2.225

The video of the patient talking in the supplement, with full articulation and movement and functional mastication producing a satisfactory outcome.

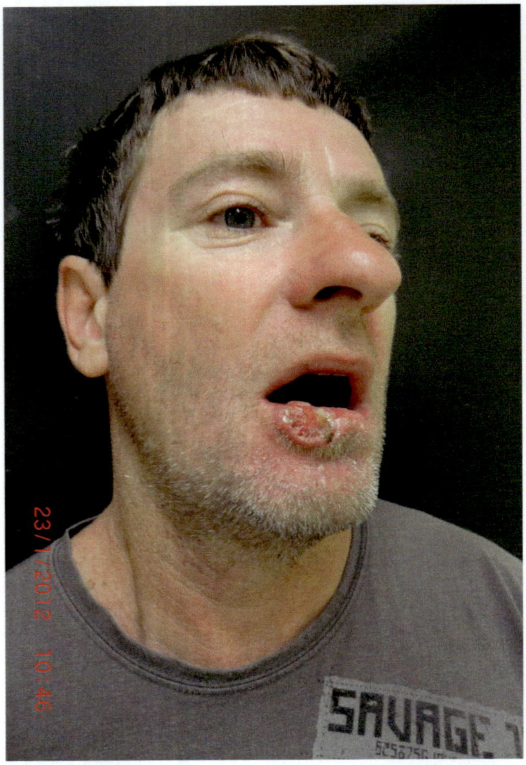

Fig. 2.211 The 2.5 cm lesion in the lateral side of the lower lip

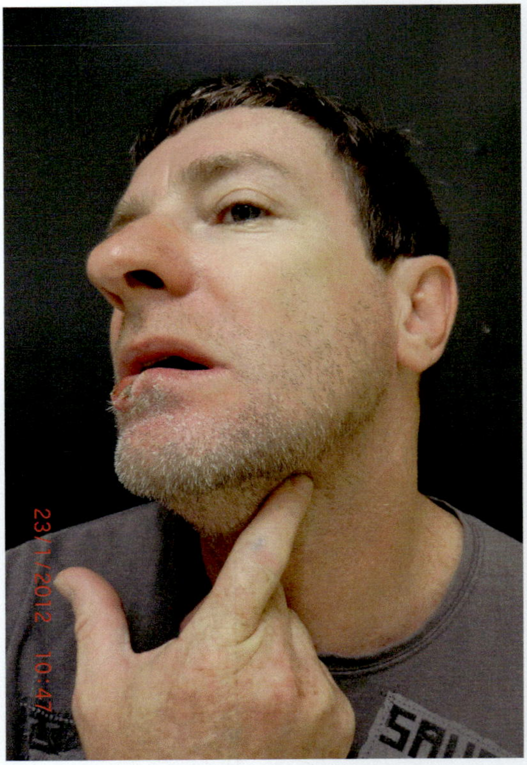

Fig. 2.212 The patient gesturing to the L submandibular nodal dissemination

In summary, functional normality has been achieved in lip seal and articulation reverting back to the embryological mark outs of the V3 dermatome and any microstoma is overcome by bringing a fresh island of mucosa from the lax tissue of the oral cavity and the inner lining of the L cheek. The P.A.C.E.S. characteristics of the Keystone were all exemplified in this island flap repair.

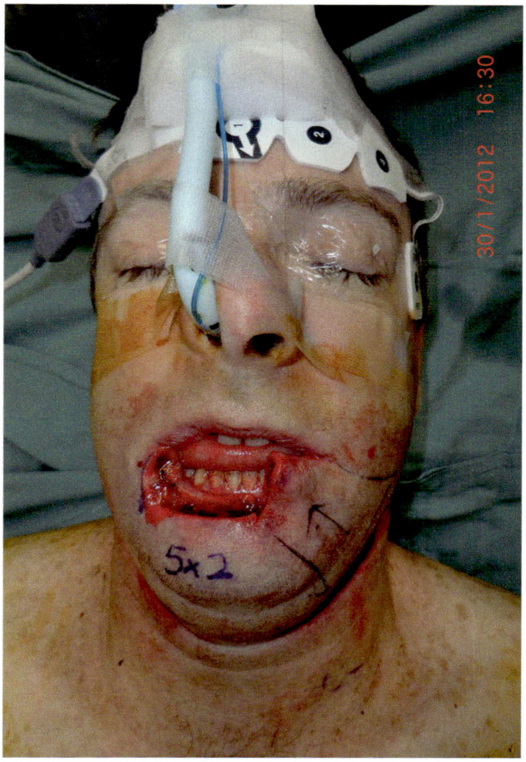

Fig. 2.213 The 5 × 2 cm full thickness loss and on the L the vermilion on the L side, based on the Keystone design, along the L mental eminence to advance to the right angle of the mouth

2.1.9 Neck

The Keystone application in neck reconstruction becomes a bonus for its simplicity, avoiding free flap reconstruction on most occasions. The line of the clavicular perforators above and the intercostal perforators below and posteriorly are the random sources of neurovascular axes without reverting to angiographic investigations which is a cost-saving exercise. Most cutaneous eruptions are associated with metastatic deposits and often there is severe undermining of the flaps for oncological access. The range of cases used show the application of the Keystone when its characteris-

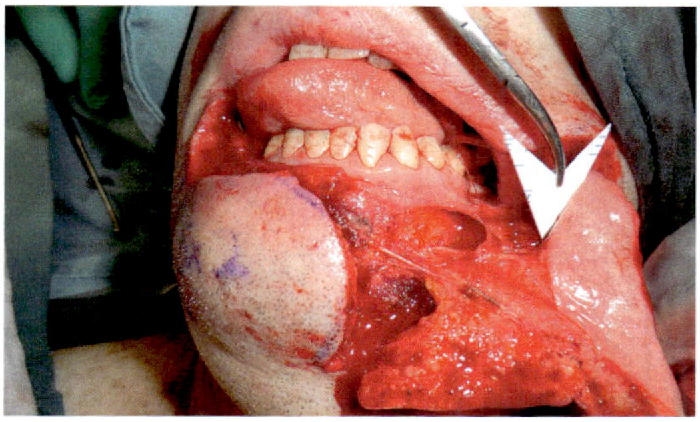

Fig. 2.214 The neurovascular structures emerging from the mental eminence in this mucosal lined lower lip reconstructive flap based on a quadrangular Keystone design

Fig. 2.215 The dermatomal mark out is the guide for the location of the random perforators coming through the fascia

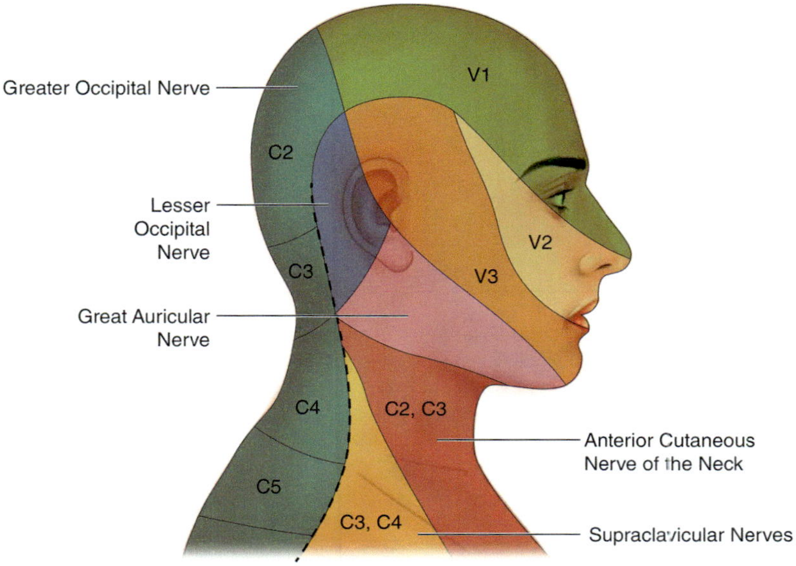

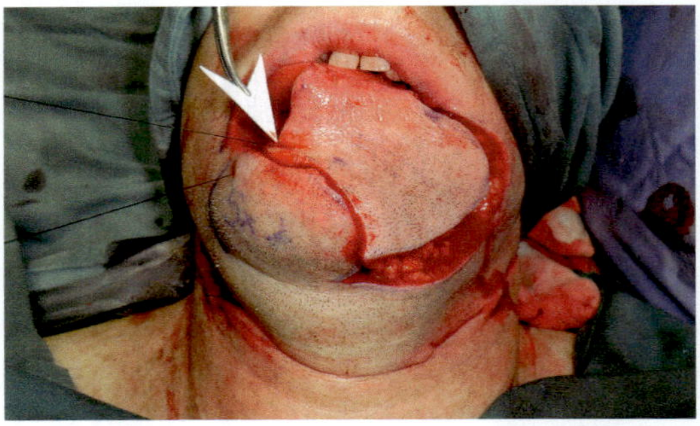

Fig. 2.216 Vermilion alignment at the right angle of the mouth as a layered closure. Mucosal, muscle and external epidermal alignment

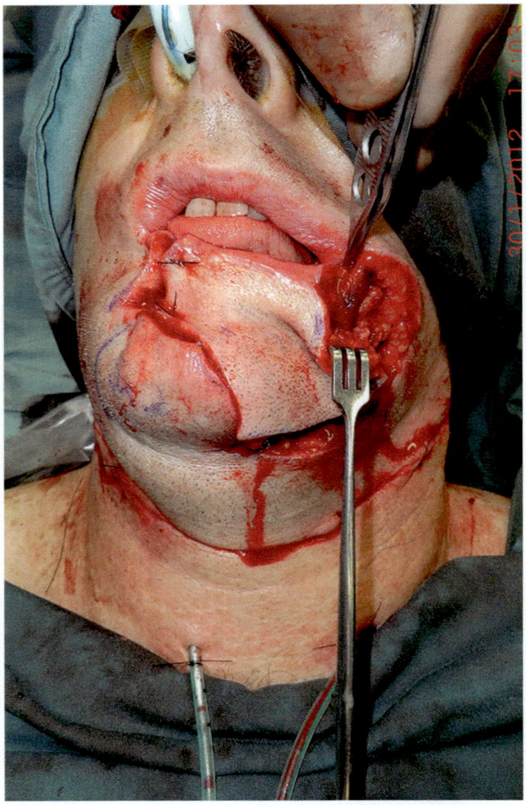

Fig. 2.217 Direct closure would have caused a micro-stoma and the vermilion replacement of approximately 2 cm is achieved by bringing an intraoral mucosal island flap, adjacent to the parotid duct, to fill this space and avoid a micro-stoma which would occur if direct closure had been employed

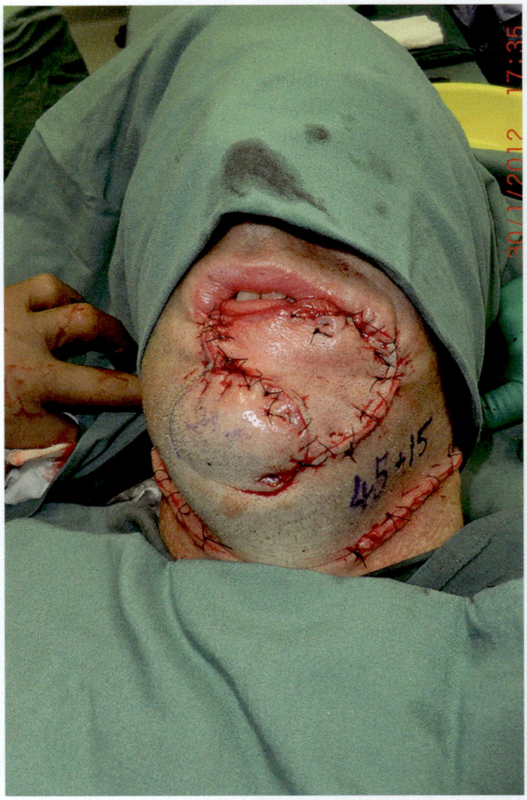

Fig. 2.218 Total timeframe for repair 60 min as indicated on the submandibular

tic facilities are evident from a clinical perspective. The undermining of the first case is part of the secondary dissemination means the Keystone, using the advantage of loose neck skin, is hypervascularised by creating an island and with deep attachment and perforators dotted along the clavicle, leaving one third deep attachment attached is the basis for its success. Yes, even closing under tension with Redi-Vac drainage installed.

The melanoma on the nape of the neck is closed using a similar random perforator design along the margin of the T1, T2 intercostal circulation, randomly placed but the island reflecting Keystone characteristics allows adequate closure under tension.

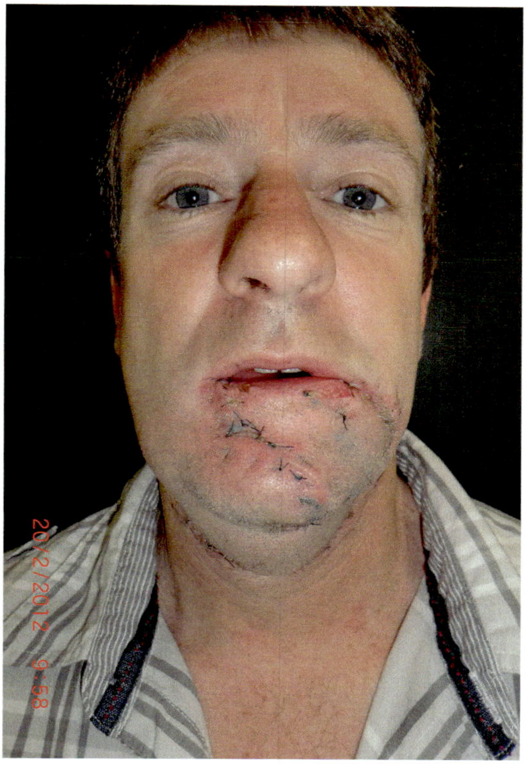

Fig. 2.219 Appearance at 2 weeks with two thirds of the sutures removed. Note the normal vermilion appearance and no micro stoma

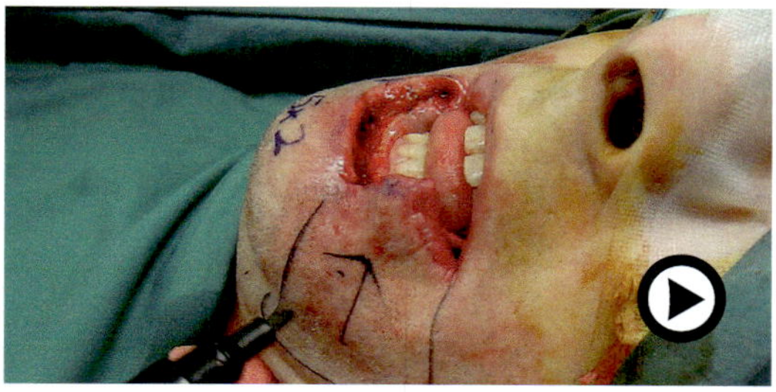

Fig. 2.220 Operative sequence (▶ https://doi.org/10.1007/000-b57)

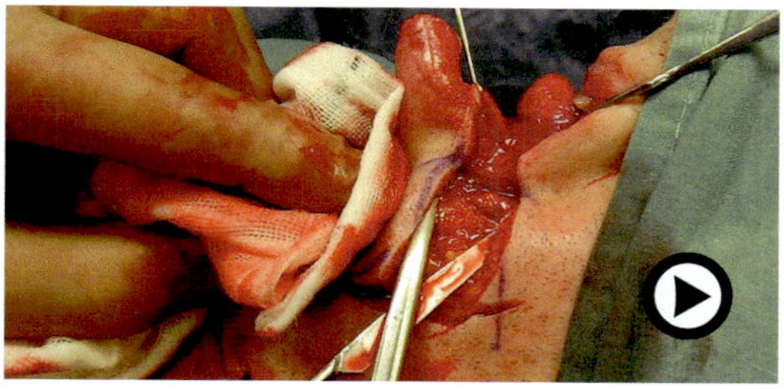

Fig. 2.221 Operative sequence (▶ https://doi.org/10.1007/000-b58)

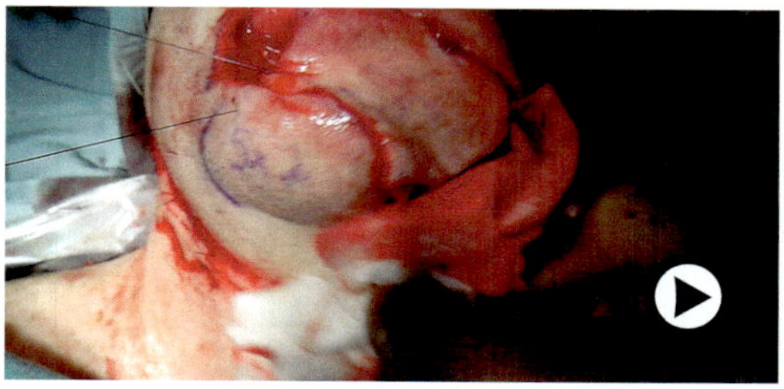

Fig. 2.222 Operative sequence (▶ https://doi.org/10.1007/000-b59)

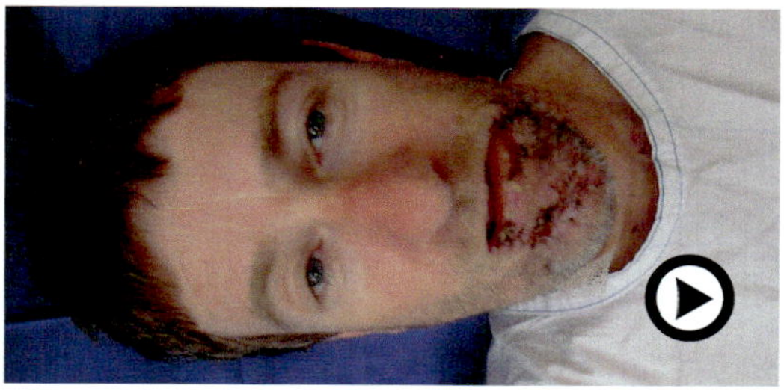

Fig. 2.223 Postoperative 7 days – patient perspective (▶ https://doi.org/10.1007/000-b5a)

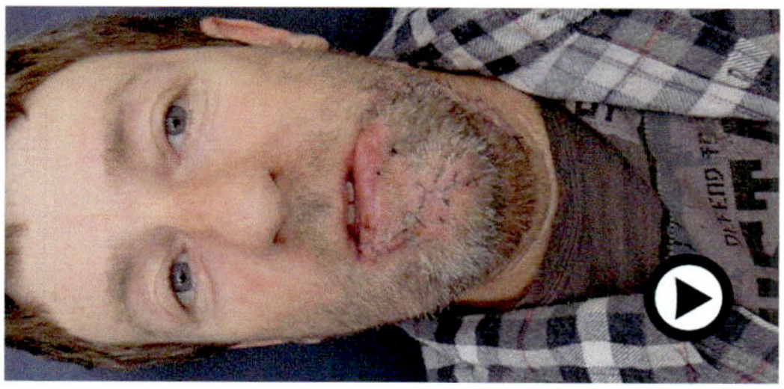

Fig. 2.224 Postoperative – patient perspective (▶ https://doi.org/10.1007/000-b5b)

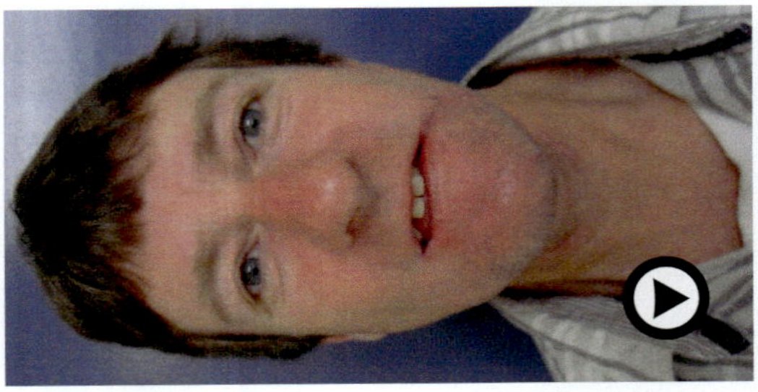

Fig. 2.225 Postoperative – patient perspective (▶ https://doi.org/10.1007/000-b5c)

The neck closure over the mastoid region following nodal excision is evident in the series but one outstanding commentary is warranted, the facial tissues are hypervascularised by islanding through the V2 dermatome to ensure a period of healing without necrosis and this ensured vascular perfusion helps this guarantee.

2.1.9.1 Case 29: Infraclavicular Keystone for Closing a Defect of the Anterior Neck Following a Neck Dissection

Recurrent melanoma of the L neck in the supraclavicular region part of the neck clearance levels I–IV in an 80-year-old male with a past history of CVA. His comorbidities indicate time on the theatre table is of the essence (see Figs. 2.226, 2.227, 2.228, 2.229, 2.230, 2.231, 2.232, 2.233, and 2.234).

In summary, the P.A.C.E.S. characteristics of the Keystone were all exemplified in this island flap repair. Random perforators along the infraclavicular alignment guarantees the vascular support to achieve wound closure and successful healing.

2.1.9.2 Case 30: Posterior

Level II neck melanoma over the prominence of C7 (see Figs. 2.235, 2.236, 2.237, 2.238, 2.239, 2.240, 2.241).

In summary, the P.A.C.E.S. characteristics of the Keystone were all exemplified in this island flap repair.

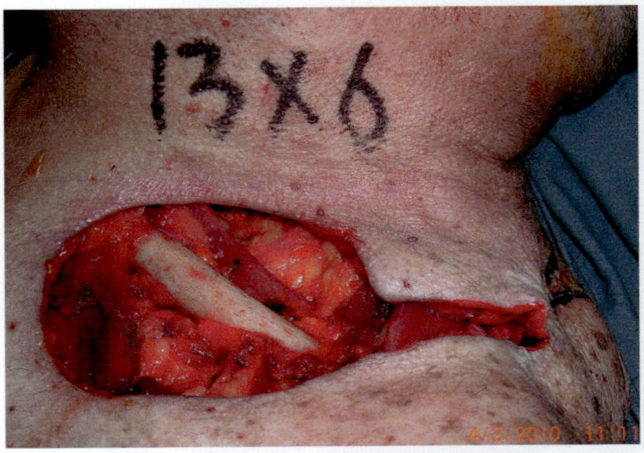

Fig. 2.226 The oncological defect of 13 × 6 cm following nodal clearances of levels I–IV. The exposed clavicle has caused undermining. The posterior extension of the wound is merely to facilitate clearence of level IV nodes

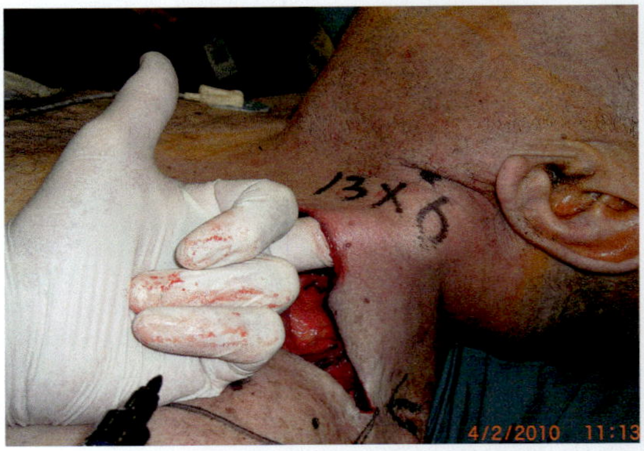

Fig. 2.227 The limits of undermining of the flaps to achieve oncological nodal clearence are indicated by the L middle finger which reaches to the L mastoid

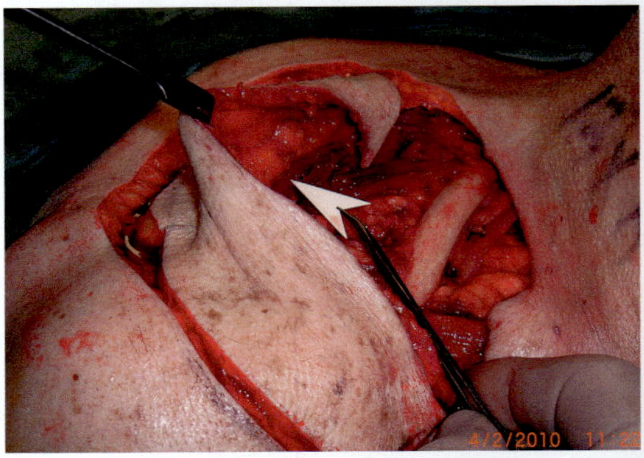

Fig. 2.228 The undermining of the inferior limits of the defect is indicated by the arrow in the vicinity of the intercostal sternal perforators which have not been dissected intentionally

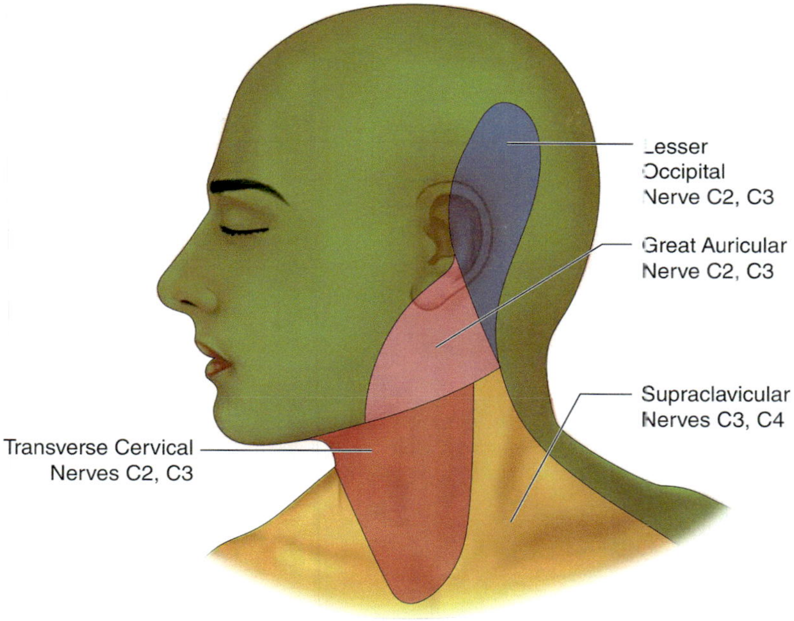

Fig. 2.229 The Keystone flap along the lines of the C4, C5 dermatome is the basis of the random perforator supply including intercostal sternal perforators to achieve reconstructive closure

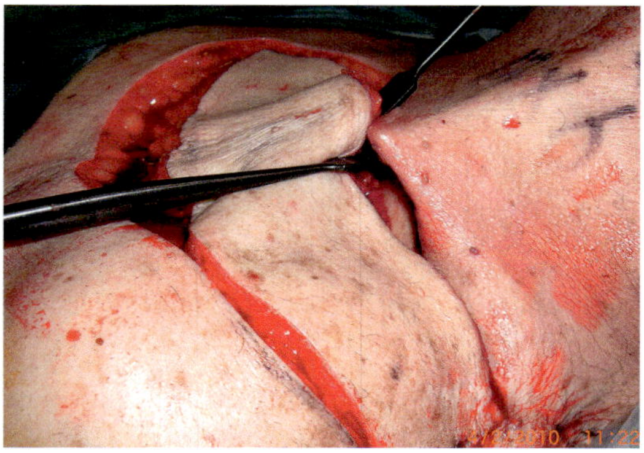

Fig. 2.230 The design mark out of the Keystone for neck closure

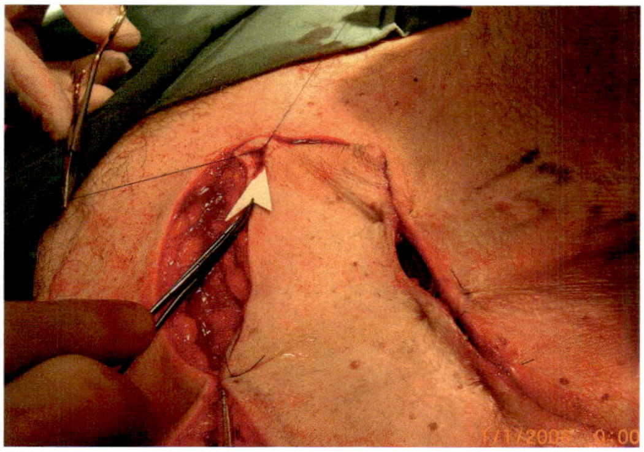

Fig. 2.231 Progress wound closure using the 3-phase single layer nylon suture technique. The arrow indicates the hyperaemia along the medial side of the flap indicating the major contribution from the intercostal perforators

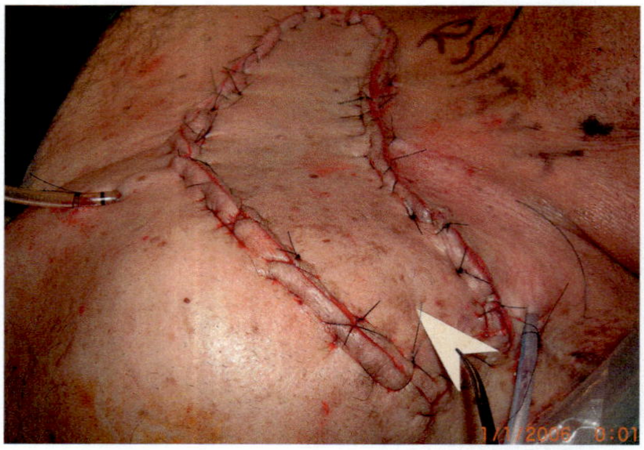

Fig. 2.232 Wound closure after 60 min. Redi-Vac installation and the hyperaemic flow without any lines of tension and potential necrosis have been overcome by the suprafascial and infrafascial support of this Keystone based on clavicular perforators

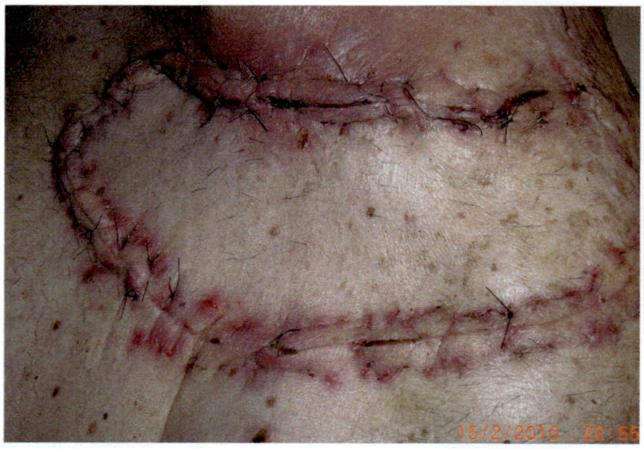

Fig. 2.233 Appearance at 10 days with the staged suture removal technique with the cutting of the continuous nylon and some of the interrupted units. The wound dressing is completed at 3.5 weeks for what is really tight wound closure.

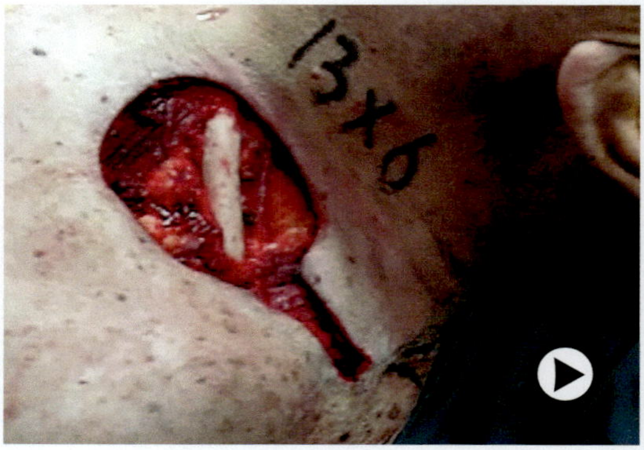

Fig. 2.234 Operative sequence (▶ https://doi.org/10.1007/000-b5d)

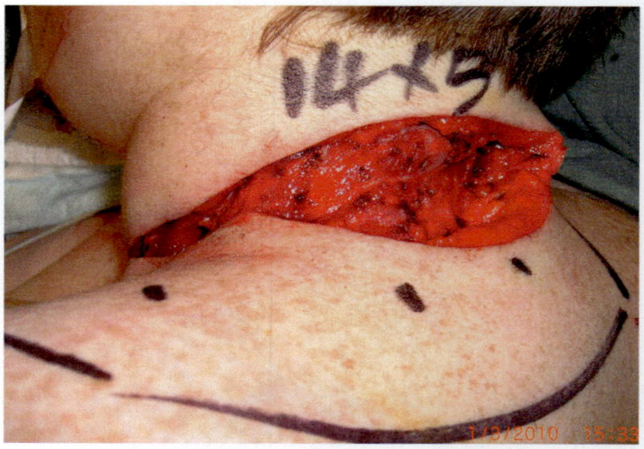

Fig. 2.235 A level II melanoma in the nape of the neck overlying the C7 spinal prominence. The short hair factor may have been an aeteological link in the development of the melanoma. The biopsy confirmed the wide 2 cm clearence margin. The Keystone mark out on the inferior limit of the defect is highlighted and the dots represent random perforator support in the C5, C6 dematome, the basis of its vascular support and these random intercostal perforators in the vicinity of the spine of the scapular on either side do not need identification

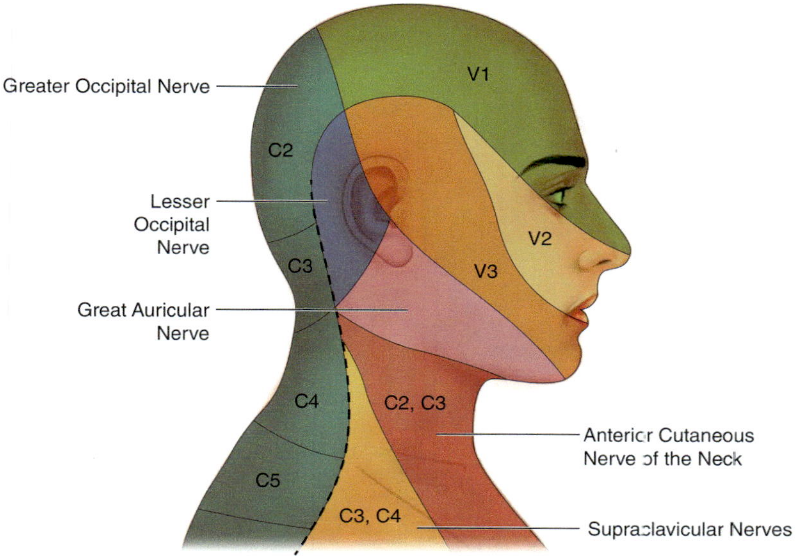

Fig. 2.236 The dermatomal mark out is the guide for the location of the random perforators coming through the fascia

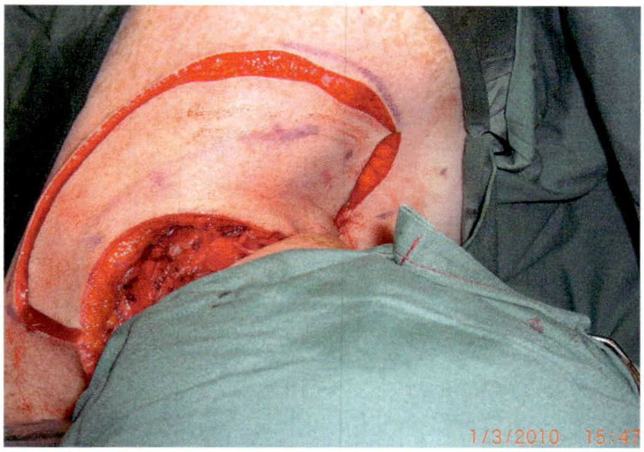

Fig. 2.237 The Keystone mark out of the flap where the medial and lateral parts of the island design are at the epidermal dermal level and the central part has retained deep attachment

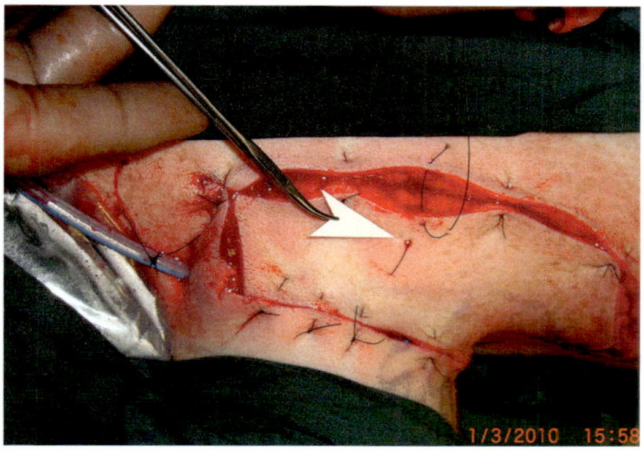

Fig. 2.238 In transit closure with some extension of the neck the V-Y points on either extreme close the flap medially and laterally and the arrow indicates the Red Dot Sign indicating its hyperaemic phase to ensure sound healing

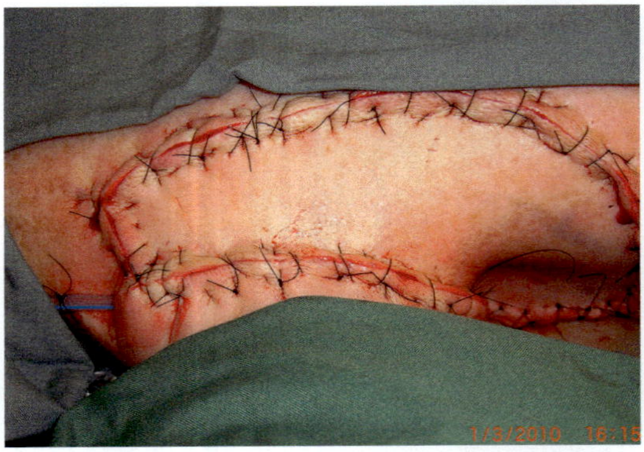

Fig. 2.239 The 3-phase single layer suture technique using locking mattress sutures at the maximum tension points. Ordinary matress sutures for wound closure and a continuous nylon for epidermal seal. Wound dressing technique follows the same 3 week cycle of cutting the loops at 7 days, some of the mattress sutures at 14 days and the tension sutures removed at 21 days or longer if they bleed. If this is the case leave these in another week

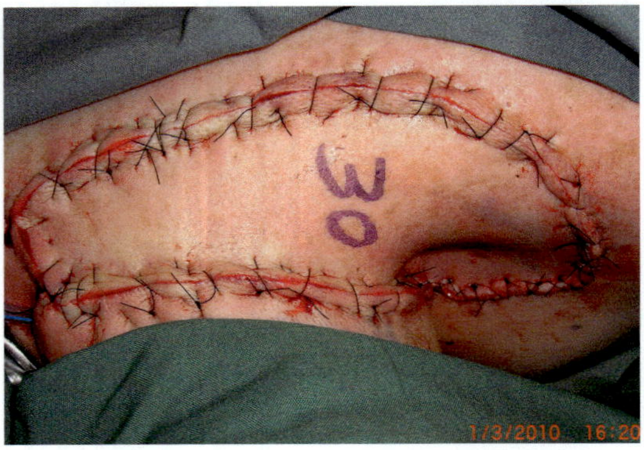

Fig. 2.240 The timeframe for repair of this defect is 30 min. Note the hyperaemia indicating the hypervascular phase evident in this Keystone island flap technique to ensure sound healing

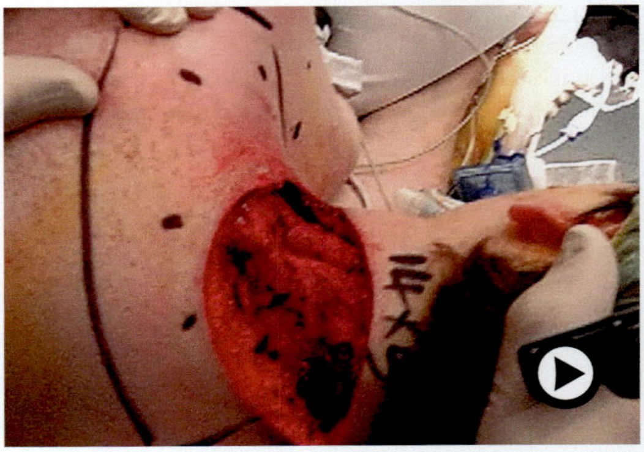

Fig. 2.241 Operative sequence (▶ https://doi.org/10.1007/000-b5e)

2.1.9.3 Case 31: L Mastoid Region

Level II melanoma over mastoid and parotid areas in this 78-year-old male with gross comorbidities. The defect size was 12 × 6 cm (see Figs. 2.242, 2.243, 2.244, 2.245, 2.246, 2.247, 2.248, and 2.249).

In summary, the hyperaemic phase of the Keystone principle has ensured vascular perfusion and therefore healing in this melanotic excisional defect in a 78 year old with extreme comorbidities.

2.1.9.4 Case 32: Supraclavicular Melanoma L Neck – Unknown Primary

Salvage procedure of undermined neck dissection flaps C2, C3 neck dissection. The Keystone principles are created by the island design as illustrated. This island flap obviates the development of any tissue necrosis in this neck dissection

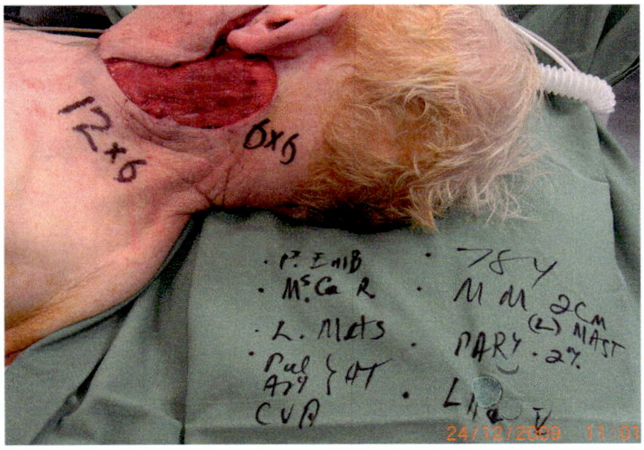

Fig. 2.242 A list of the comorbidities including vascular abnormalities (see video supplement)

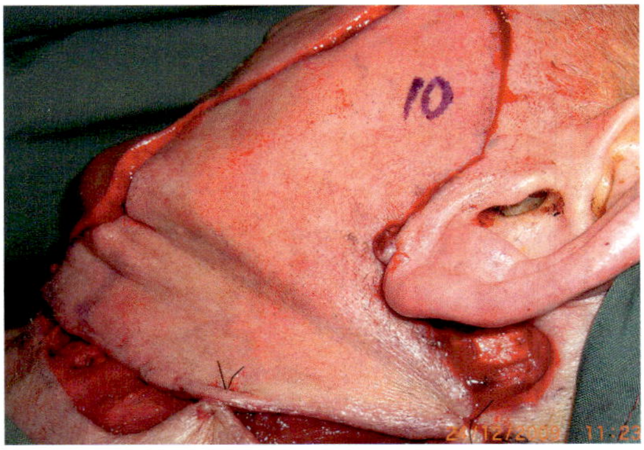

Fig. 2.244 The island Keystone is closed at various tension points as indicated

Fig. 2.243 The dermatome mark outs of transverse cervical C2, C3 and part of the great auricular dermatome C2, C3

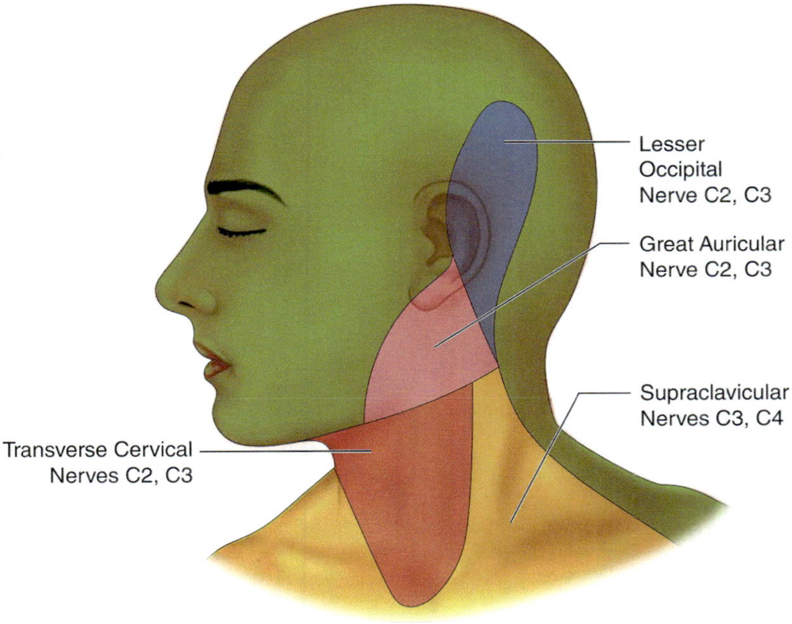

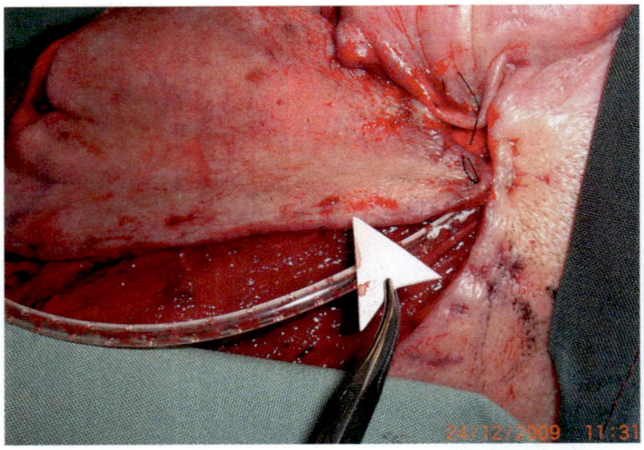

Fig. 2.245 The closure of the neck wound overlying the Redi-Vac drainage system and the arrow indicates the Red Dot Signs on the cervical tissue which is an indicator of the hyperaemia created by the island flap design and an endorsement of potential safe postoperative healing

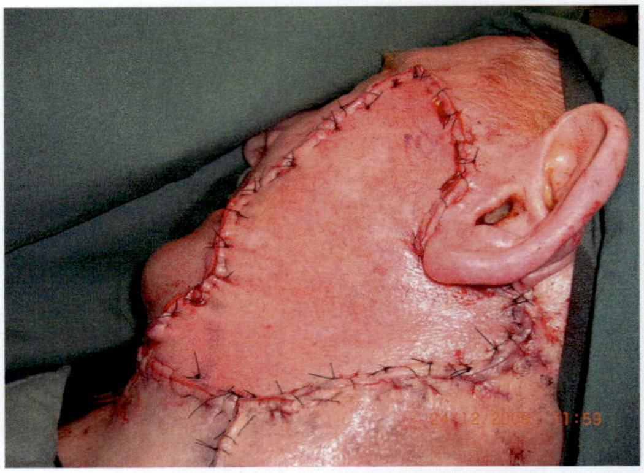

Fig. 2.247 The postoperative appearance at approximately 60 min later after employing the 3-phase single layer suture technique for closure. The outline of the flap including neck tissue and cervical extension becomes hyperaemic ensuring sound wound healing

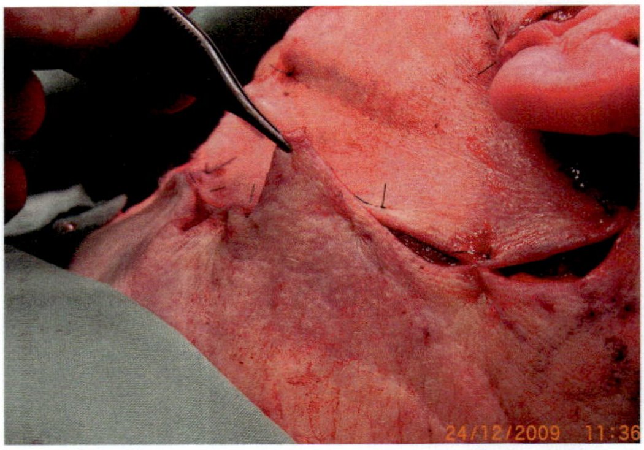

Fig. 2.246 Refining the closure by closing off excess tissue. Note the comparison of the hyperaemic phase of the Keystone used in the wound closure and the somewhat tardy circulatory flow with the neck tissue where the cyanosis of the attached neck tissue provides remarkable contrast of the undermined island flap

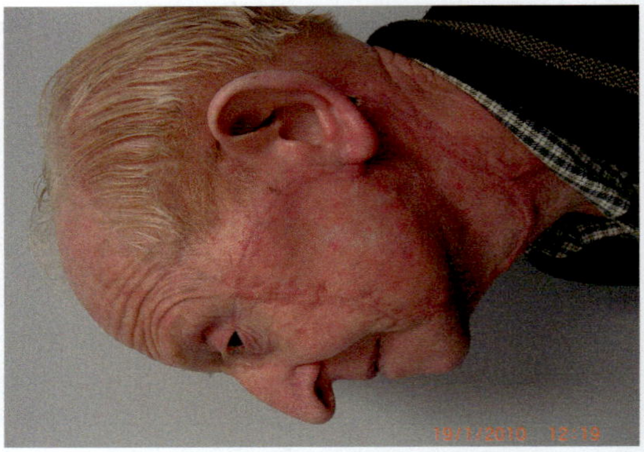

Fig. 2.248 The postoperative appearance at approximately 3 weeks. The P.A.C.E.S. characteristics of the Keystone were all exemplified in this elderly male with extensive comorbidities

in association with the tumour mass removal. This would otherwise happen with closure under tension at this oncological site in this 66-year-old male (see Figs. 2.250, 2.251, 2.252, 2.253, 2.254, 2.255, and 2.256).

In summary, epidermal islanding tissue leaving one third deep attachment of the undermined flap (Fig. 2.253) allows the loco-regional flap of the integument to achieve surgical healing in this melanoma of an unknown primary by reason of hyperaemic hypervascularity. All the P.A.C.E.S. charactristics are again exemplified.

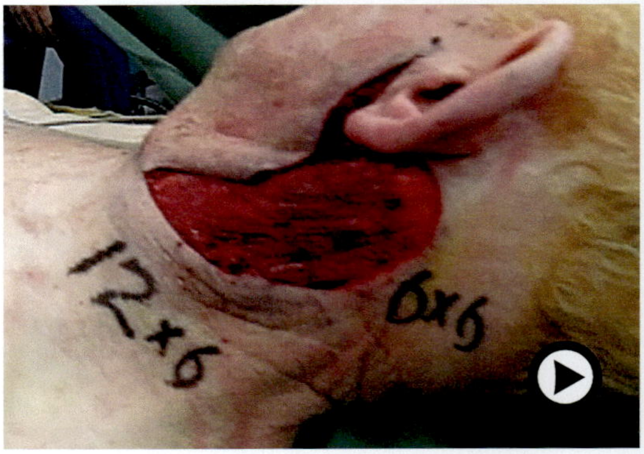

Fig. 2.249 Operative sequence (▶ https://doi.org/10.1007/000-b5f)

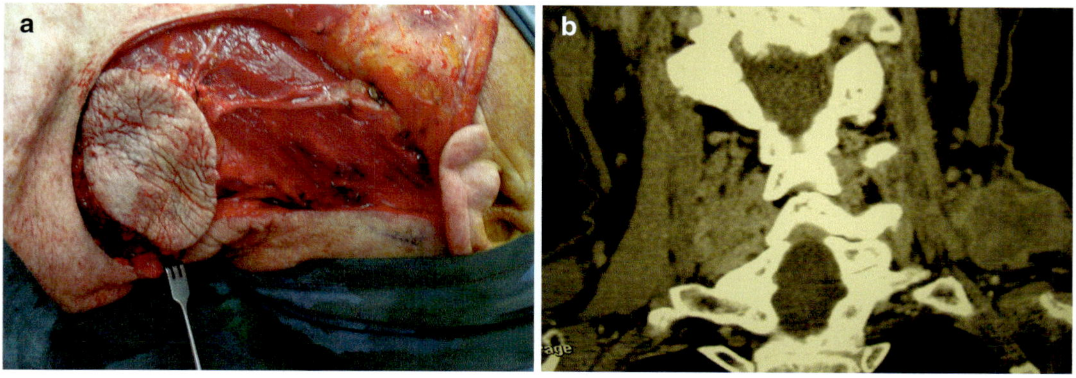

Fig. 2.250 (**a**) The surgical defect 9 × 8 cm. (**b**) CT confirmation

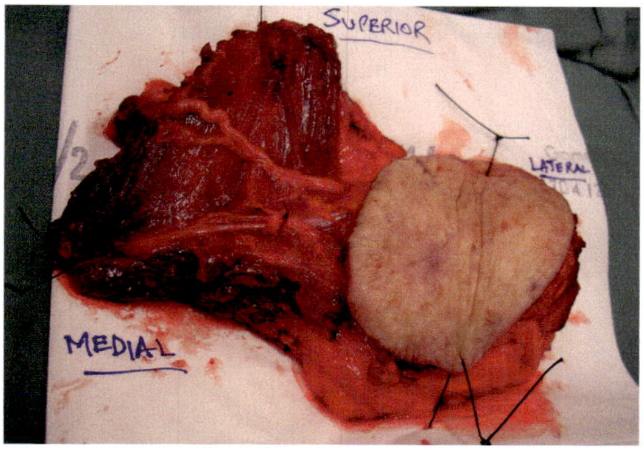

Fig. 2.251 Pathology specimen including nodal clearance from levels II, III and IV

Fig. 2.252 The dermatomal mark out is the guide for the location of the random perforators coming through the fascia

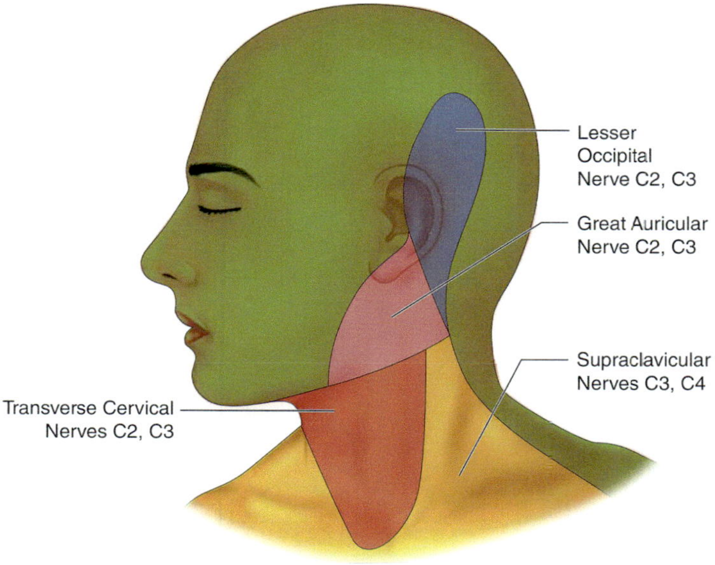

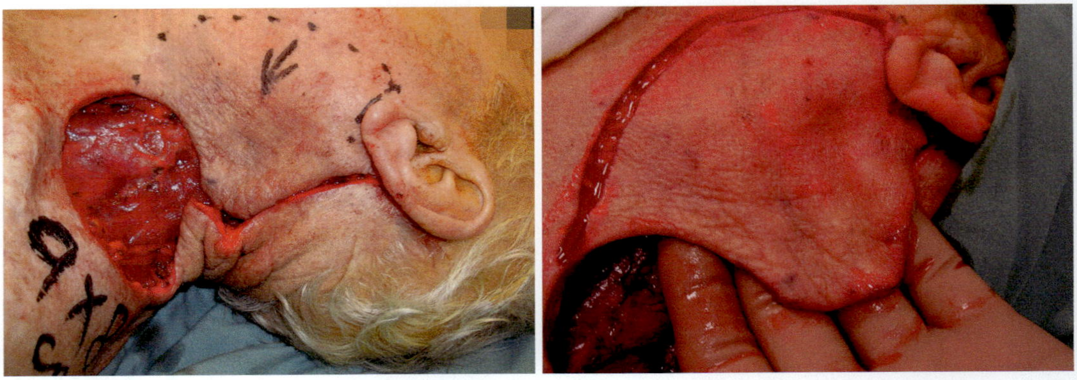

Fig. 2.253 This is the important slide as the undermined area of the flap is cyanotic and arrowed. To overcome this problem, the cervical neck flap is islanded at the epidermal level only leaving one third of deep attachment. It becomes hypervascularised with increased flow, eliminating the cyanotic appearance. The operator's digits are placed under the undermined flap leaving one third deep attachment. The reflex hyperaemia takes 10–15 min to develop this vascular change. This allows closure under tension for the 9 × 8 cm defect

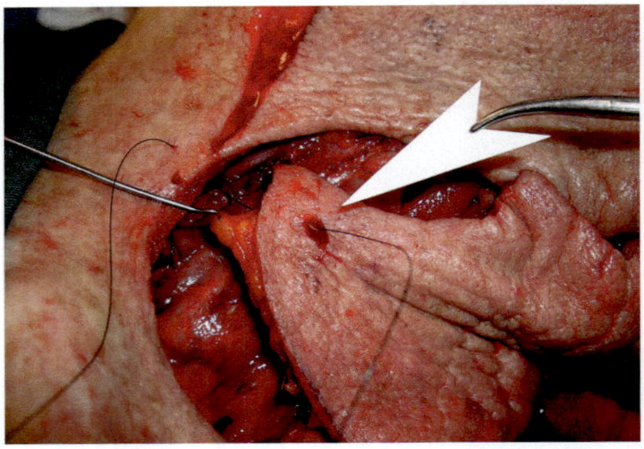

Fig. 2.254 The Keystone characteristic Red Dot Sign indicates the hyperaemia bleeding more on the flap side than the receiving site. This is an integral part of the excellent healing evidenced in Keystone reconstruction

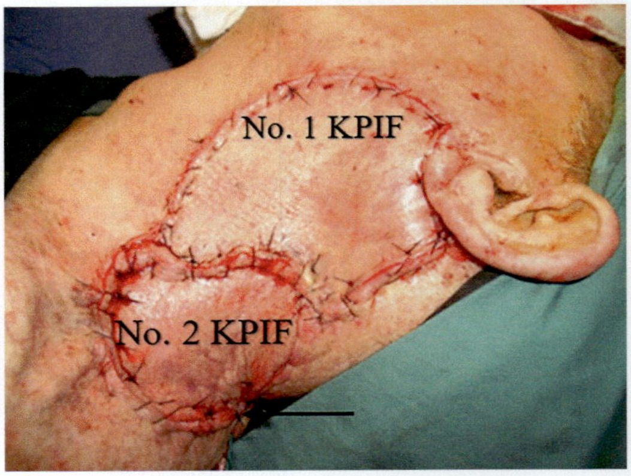

Fig. 2.255 A second Keystone with Redi-vac drainage from the cervical region (C2, C3) helps to close the defect to eliminate any element of tension. Note the vascular suffusion through both flaps reflecting the hyperaemic phase in contrast to the appearance of the surrounding tissues

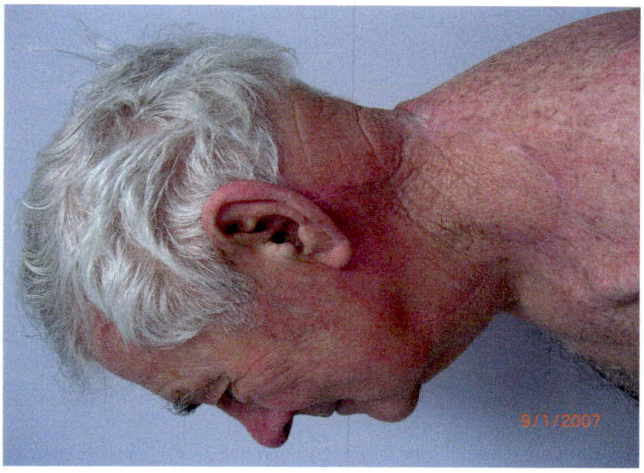

Fig. 2.256 Postoperative appearance. There is no indication of flap necrosis and the appearance of the facial expression mirrors his satisfaction

2.2 Adverse Outcomes Are Rare Complications of Keystone Flap Surgery

2.2.1 Hypertrophic Scarring Followed by Scar Revisional Surgery

This is a rare occurrence in Keystone reconstruction and reflects the nature of the physiology of the patient and ethnic background (Maltese origin). In this unusual case of hypertrophic scarring in a Keystone of the L neck along the line of the sternomastoid was the only case in this series of a large focus of head and neck reconstruction that experienced any hypertrophic element. The patient with this hypertrophic potential only develops this complication if there is that physiological tendency (see Fig. 2.257).

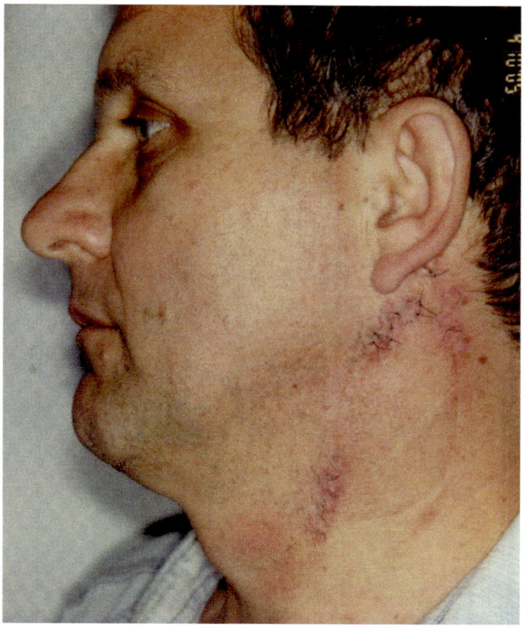

Fig. 2.257 Keystone L neck level II melanoma. Hypertrophic scar in a person with this potential

2.2.2 Dermal Necrosis in an Island Flap

Often when there is mitotic development in the integument, which is not evident clinically but present at the microscopic level, sometimes broaches the periosteum of the underlying tissue, this may have an anti angiogenesis factor operating and lead to superficial necrosis in any reconstructive flap and in this case in this 88-year-old male with a superficial temporal artery island flap covering a desmoplastic melanoma in the midline of the forehead (see Figs. 2.258, 2.259, 2.260, 2.261, and 2.262).

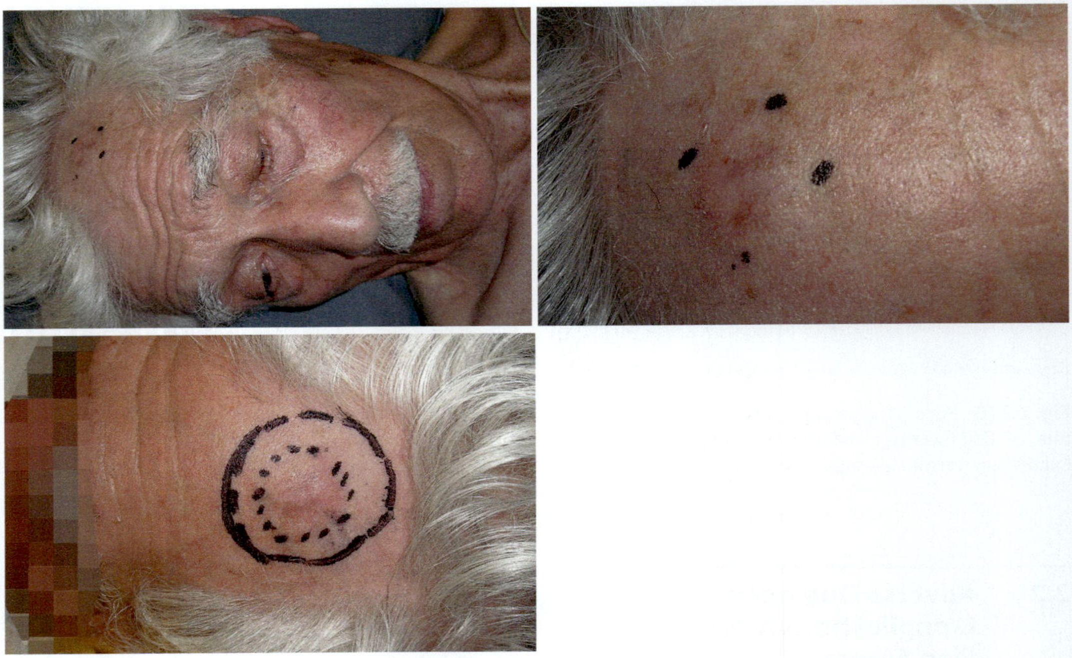

Fig. 2.258 Biopsy excision

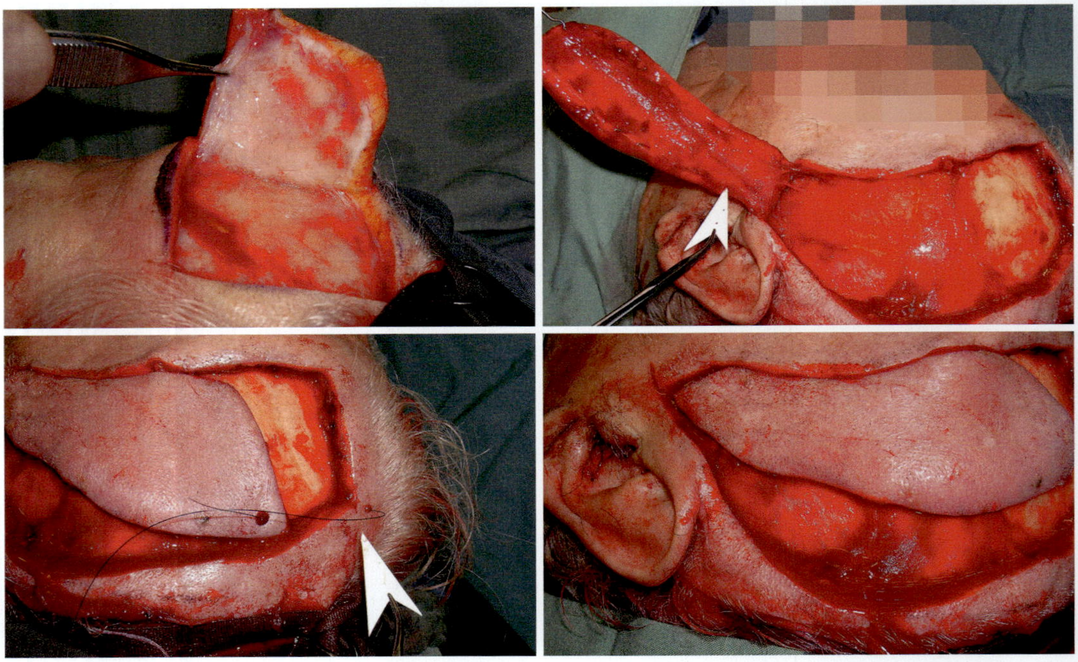

Fig. 2.259 Island flap on the superficial temporal artery (not skeletonised). Note the hyperaemia in the flap and the Red Dot Sign – Keystone characteristics

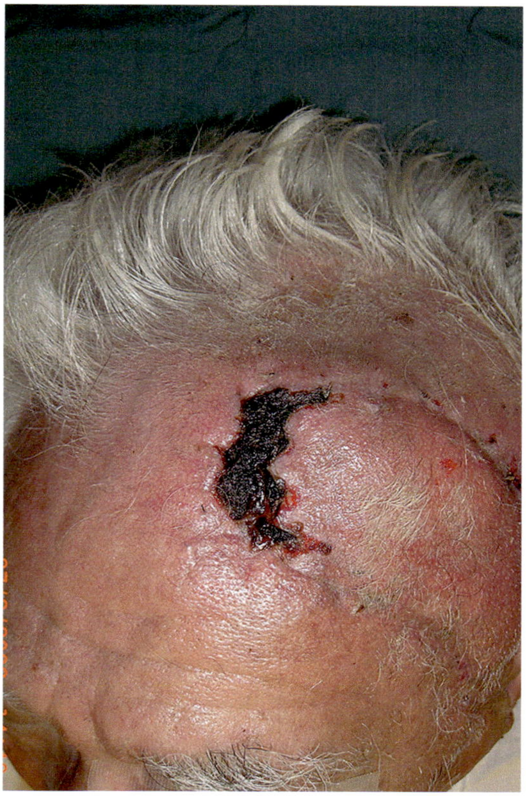

Fig. 2.260 Superficial distal necrosis in a viable flap is a rare finding and it most likely confirms a manifestation of underlying mitotic elements in the pericranium and impeding angiogenesis and tissue healing as part of the underlying pathology

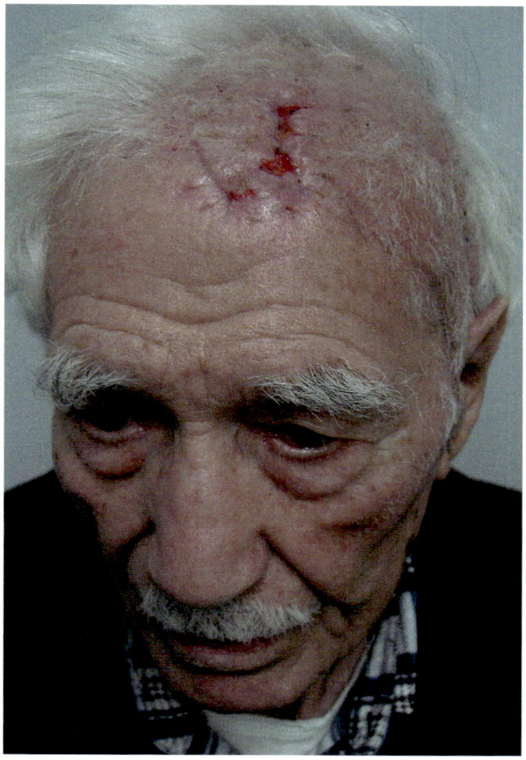

Fig. 2.261 Following debridement and wound closure

2.2.3 Complications of Wound Healing

Melanoma of the forehead in a patient with chronic lymphatic leukeamia which caused delay in the angiogenesis factor of wound healing which ultimately resolved (see Figs. 2.263 and 2.264).

2.2.4 A Microsurgical Reconstructive Alternative for Parotid Defects

The Keystone in the unit's experience provides an acceptable alternative to closure of defects in the vicinity of the parotid for melanoma and other mitotic lesions. The cases illustrated above reveal the surgical outcome where the P.A.C.E.S. characteristics are quite evident.

Free flaps with microsurgical technique become an option depending upon the experience of the operator and this case illustrates some of those limitations in relation to aesthetic outcome.

The widespread use of free flaps in head and neck reconstruction by plastic surgeons and non-plastic surgeons has its place but often at an economic and aesthetic reconstructive cost. This is emphasised where the burden of deformity for patients with poor facial reconstructions is considered (see Figs. 2.265 and 2.266).

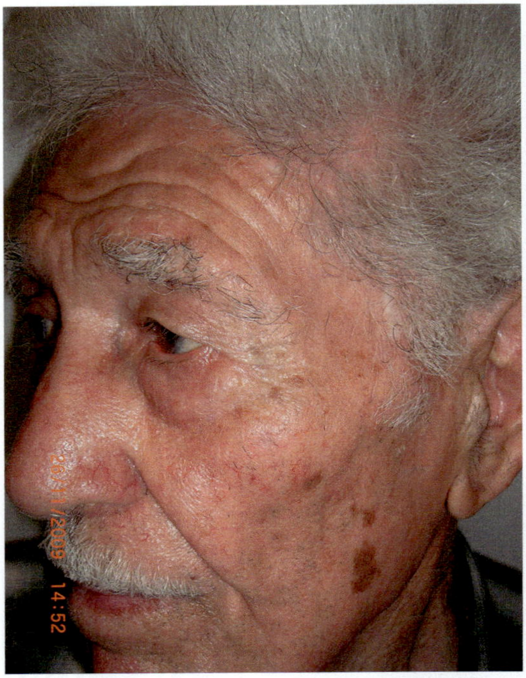

Fig. 2.262 The postoperative appearance – tumour-free interval at 18 months and no sign of integumentary recurrence

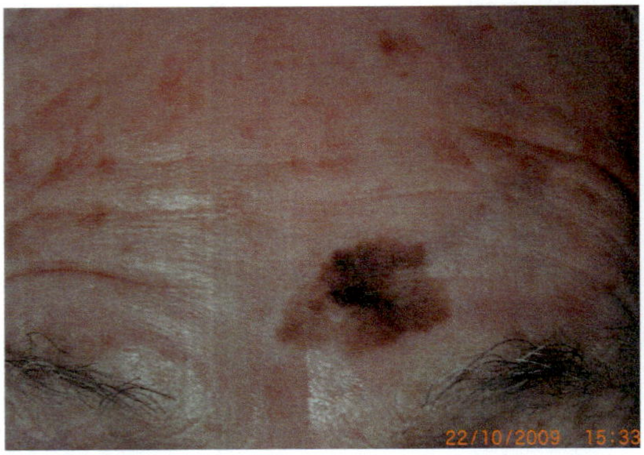

Fig. 2.263 The patient on presentation with a 3 × 3 cm lesion of the glabellar. Hutchinson's melanotic freckle level I melanoma

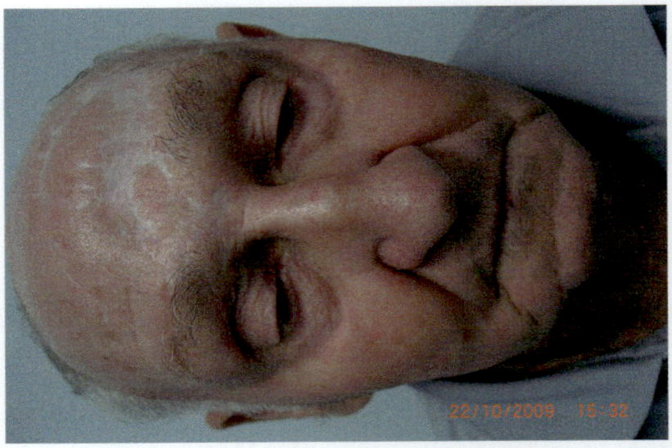

Fig. 2.264 Finally healed after secondary reconstruction

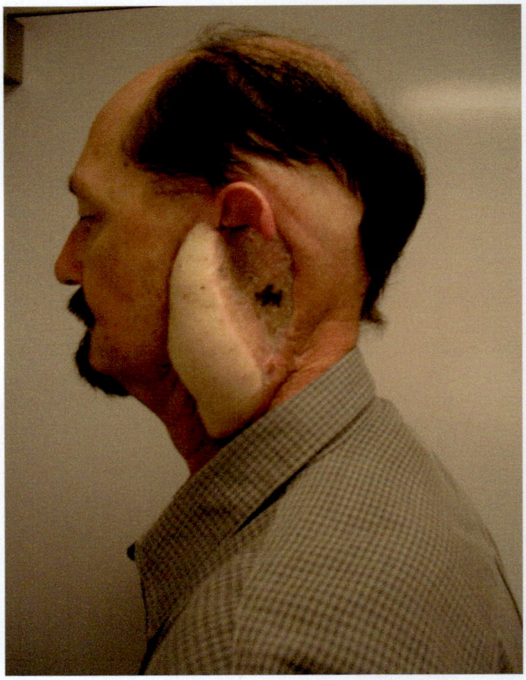

Fig. 2.265 This borrowed case from another unit with a free flap reconstruction helps to emphasise the poor aesthetic outcome for large parotid defects. In the parotid section, it makes valid comparisons with the Keystone closures for large melanoma defects over the parotid with or without subsequent radiation. This aesthetic deformity has created a psychological worry for the patient, so much so that he wears head gear to disguise the deformity when he goes out in public for social interchange, shopping, etc. becoming a social reject with its psychological implications.

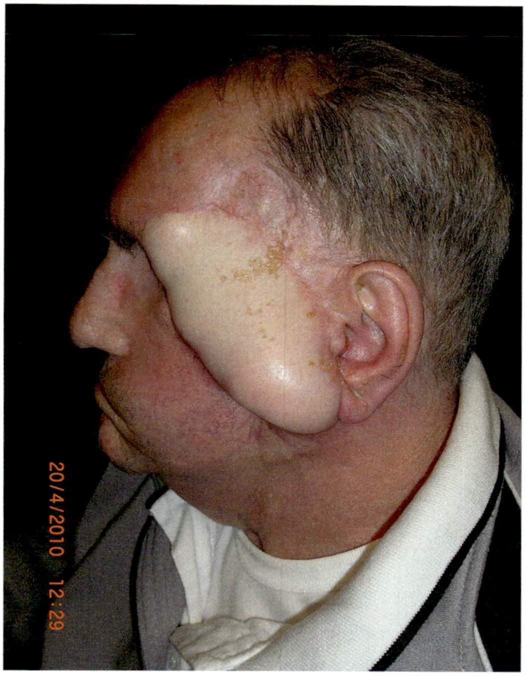

Fig. 2.266 A microsurgical alternative which needs no elaboration when one compares the P.A.C.E.S. outcomes of the Keystone perforator island flap concept

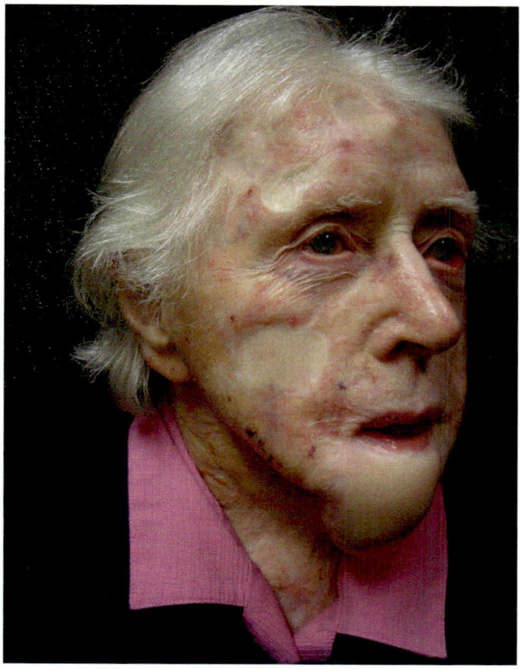

Fig. 2.267 An alternative method of lower lip reconstruction using a microvascular technique and this makes an interesting comparison for a similar defect in Case 28 using Keystone concepts. This could precipitate psychological changes when patients similarly treated become social outcasts

In summary, the psychological disturbance is something always to be considered by the oncological team involved with major head and neck reconstructions. This must be part of the preoperative consultation of informed consent (see Fig. 2.267, 2.268, and 2.269).

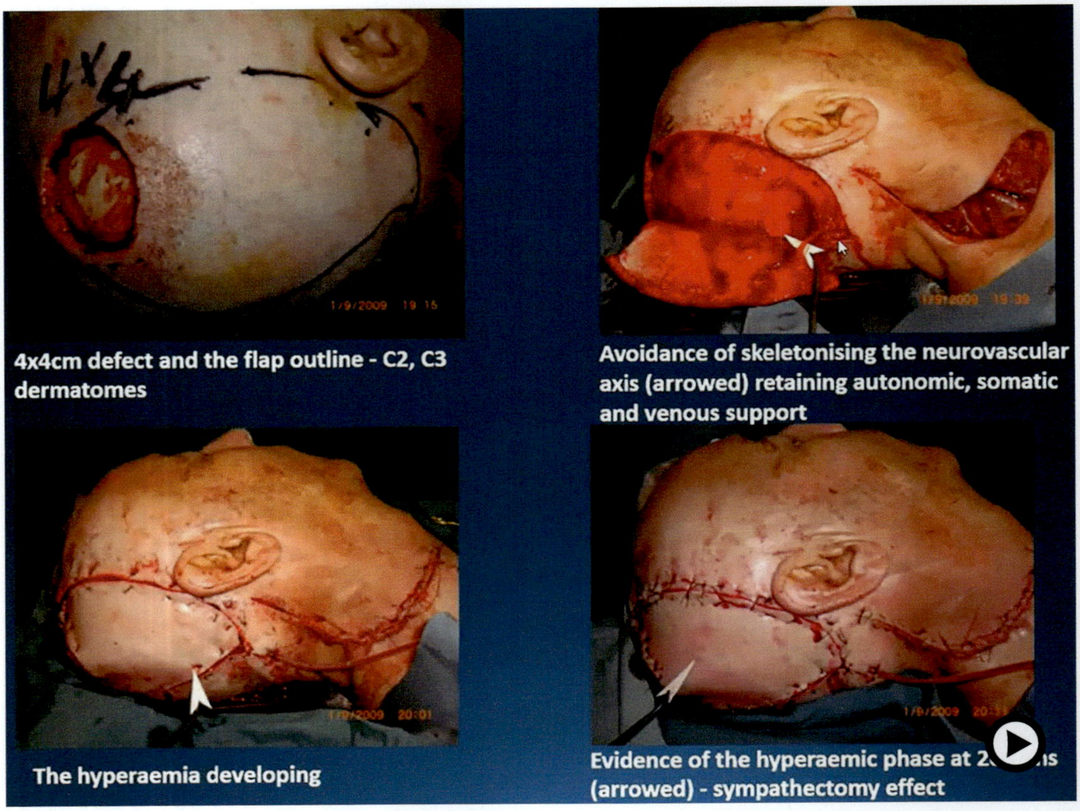

Fig. 2.268 Head and neck cases (▶ https://doi.org/10.1007/000-b4k)

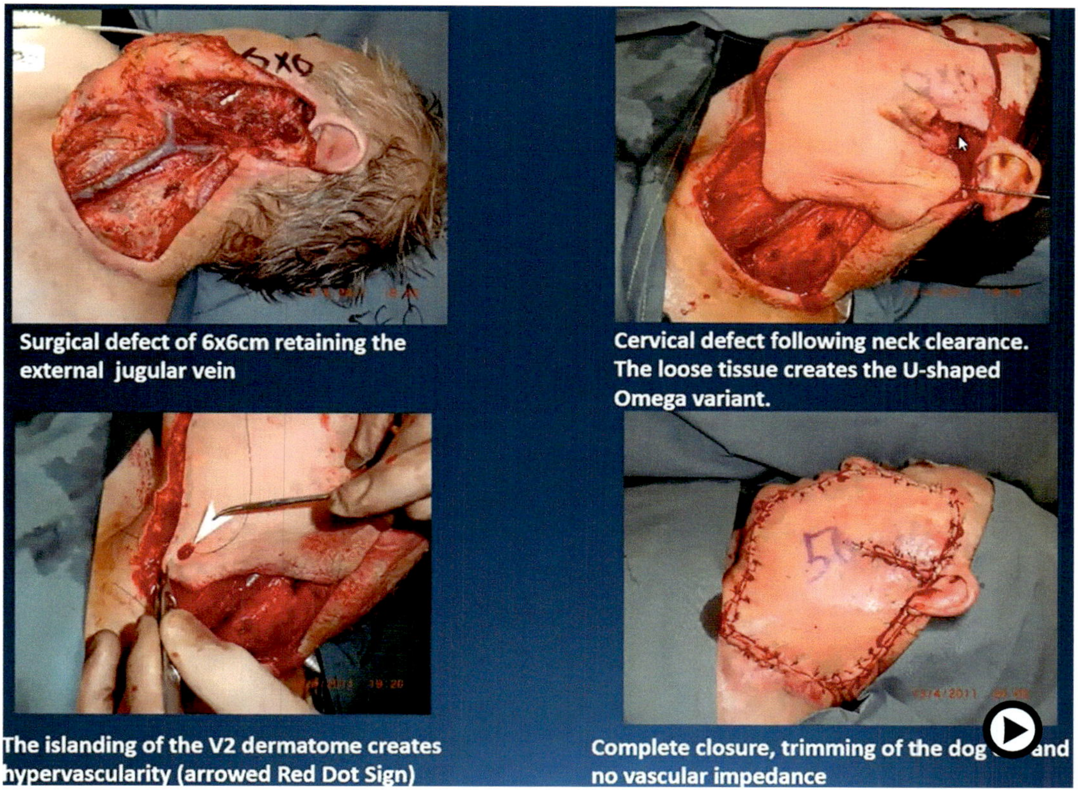

Fig. 2.269 Head and neck cases (▶ https://doi.org/10.1007/000-b5h)

References

1. Haddad-Tame, et al. Reconstruction of the aesthetics units of the face with microsurgery: experience in five years. Microsurgery. 2000;20:211.
2. Gonzalez-Ulloa M. Restoration of the face covering by means of selected skin in regional aesthetic units. J Plast Reconstr Aesthetic Surg. 1956;1226(56):80036–2.
3. Gonzalez-Ulloa M, Stevens E. Reconstruction of the nose and forehead by means of regional aesthetic units. Br J Plast Surg. 1960;13:305–9.
4. Gillies H, Millard D. The principles and art of plastic surgery. London: Butterworth; 1957.
5. Zimany A. The Bi-lobed flap. Plast Reconstruct Surg. 1953;11(6):424–34.
6. Dufourmentel C. Closure of limited loss of cutaneous substance. So-called "LLL" diamond-shaped L rotation-flap. Ann Chir Plast. 1962;7:60–6.
7. Belt PJ, Emmett A. Local transposition flap repair of the pectoralis major myocutaneous flap donor site. Plast Reconstr Surg. 2004;114(3):732–7.
8. Barron J, Emmett A. Subcutaneous pedicle flaps. Br J Plast Surg. 1965;18:51–78.
9. Nordstrom RE, Devine JW. Scalp stretching with a tissue expander for closure of scalp defects. Plast Reconstr Surg. 1985;75:578.
10. Lee B, Bickel K, Levin S. Microsurgical reconstruction of extensive scalp defects. J Reconstr Microsurg. 1999;15:255.
11. Beasley N, et al. Scalp and forehead reconstruction using free revascularized tissue transfer. Arch Facial Plast Surg. 2004;6(1):16–20.
12. Lipa J, Butler C. Enhancing the outcome of free latissimus dorsi muscle flap reconstruction of scalp defects. Head Neck. 2003;26(1):46–53. https://doi.org/10.1002/hed.10338.
13. TerKonda S. Concepts in scalp and forehead reconstruction. Otolaryngol Clin North Am. 1997;30(4):519–39.
14. Behan F, et al. Island flaps including the Bezier type in the treatment of malignant melanoma. Aust N Z J Surg. 1995;65(12):870–80.
15. Dufourmentel. Stag-beetle flap. Sliding island flap with plasty in VY. Ann Chir Plast. 1970;15(4):344–7.

16. Behan F, et al. Oncologic clearance with preservation of reconstructive options: literature review and the 'delayed reconstruction after pathology evaluation (DRAPE)' technique. ANZ J Surg. 2012;82(11):780–5.
17. McGregor JC. A critical assessment of the biolbed flap. Br J Plast Surg. 1981;34:197.
18. Driscol BP, Baker SR. Reconstruction of nsasal alar defects. Arch Facial Plast Surg. 2001;3:91.
19. Burget GC, Menick FJ. Aesthetic reconstruction of the nose. St Louis: Mosby-Year Book; 1994.
20. Balch C. Modification of cross-lip flap. Plast Reconstr Surg. 1978;61(3):457–8.

Major Trunk Defects Using the Keystone Perforator Island Flap Technique

3

Contents

Supplementary Information The online version contains supplementary material available at https://doi.org/10.1007/978-3-031-39868-1_3. The videos can be accessed individually by clicking the DOI link in the accompanying figure caption or by scanning this link with the SN More Media App.

3.1 Case Presentations

3.1.1 Case 33: 13 × 10 cm Defect in the Supraclavicular Region with Exposed Carotid Following a Neck Dissection

A supraclavicular mass in an 80 year old – a typical story of a secondary melanoma with an unknown primary (see Figs. 3.1, 3.2, 3.3, 3.4, 3.5, 3.6, 3.7, 3.8, 3.9, 3.10, 3.11, 3.12, and 3.13).

F. Behan, *Atlas of Keystone Reconstructive Technique in Melanoma Management*,
https://doi.org/10.1007/978-3-031-39868-1_3

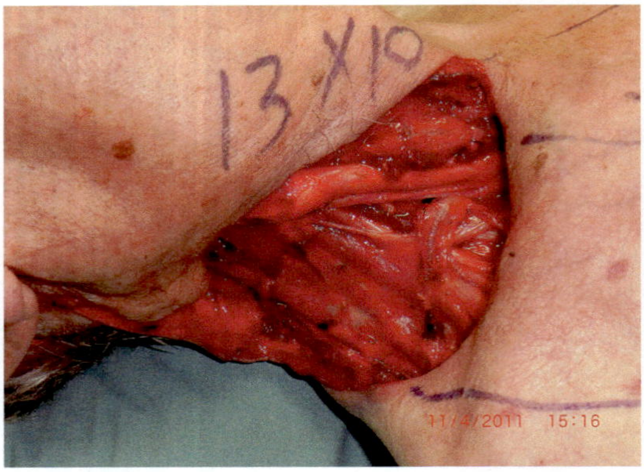

Fig. 3.1 Closure using a Keystone principle island flap based on an original pectoralis major design, i.e. islanding, and the hypervascularity that is produced ensures good healing

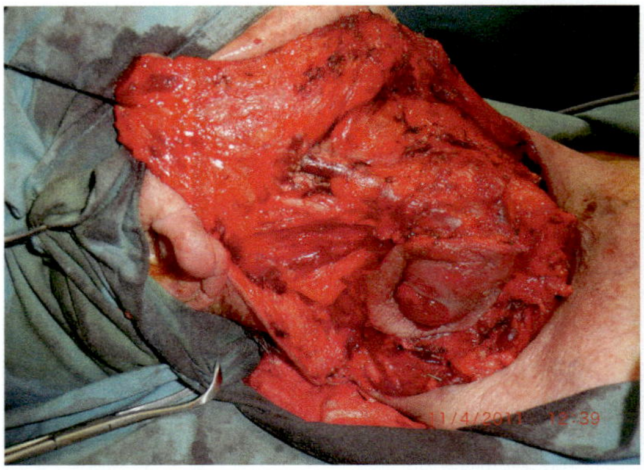

Fig. 3.2 Closure of a secondary defect employing Keystone principles on random intercostal perforators. 90 minutes for the oncological excision and 50 minutes for the Keystone variant of the pectoralis major. A fascial lined island flap within the dermatomal mark outs of the chest wall

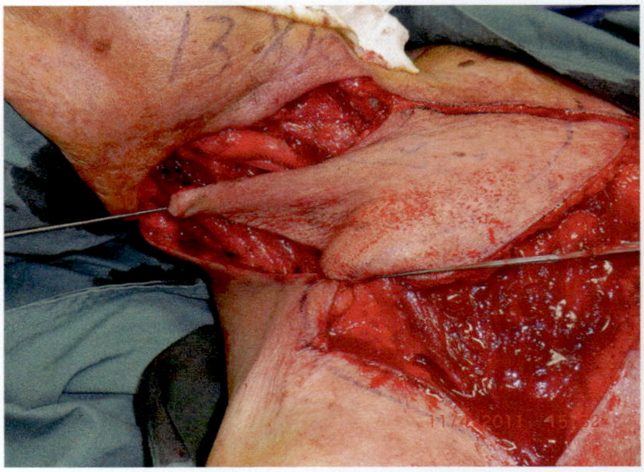

Fig. 3.3 The hypervascular stage of the pectoralis major island flap illustrating Keystone island principles of hyperaemia and hypervascularity

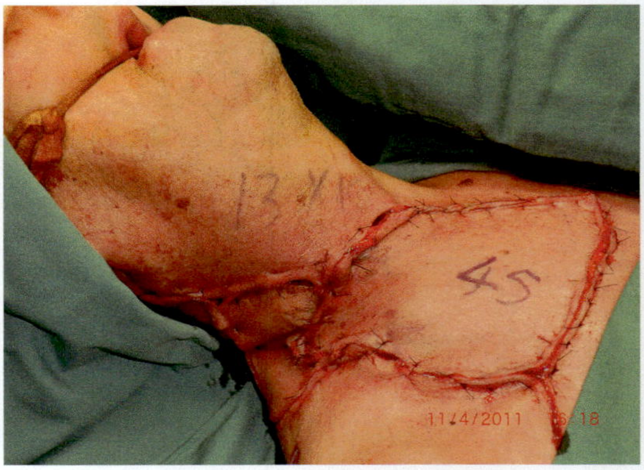

Fig. 3.4 The timeframe for closure under tension in an 80 year old meets with the approval of the anesthetic department – 45 minutes

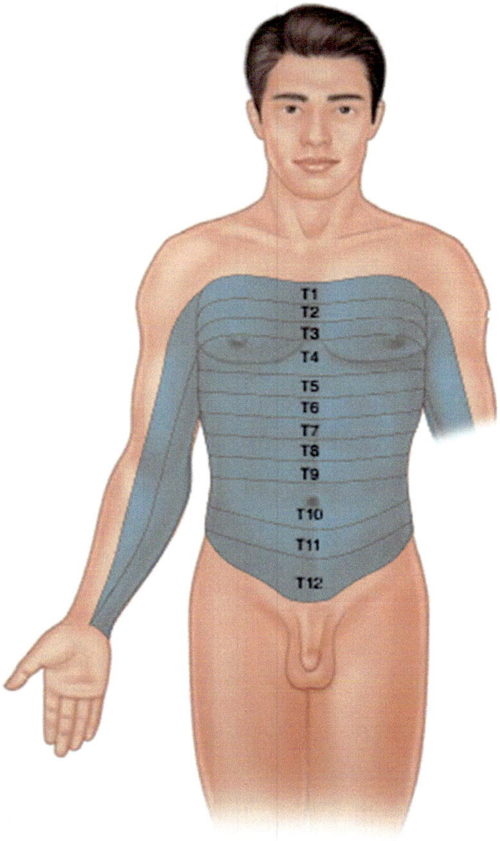

Fig. 3.5 The dermatomal mark out is the guide for the location of the random perforators coming through the fascia

In summary, the pectoralis major flap has been a standard reconstructive tool since Bakamjian's [1, 2] publications in the 1970s. The simple technique of creating an islanded tissue based on intercostal perforators in the Keystone principle guarantees almost universally perfusional dynamics. The 10% necrosis rate of delto pectoral flaps is part of surgical history, in other words islanding creates reliability with increased vascular perfusion when employed with the delto pectoral flap technique.

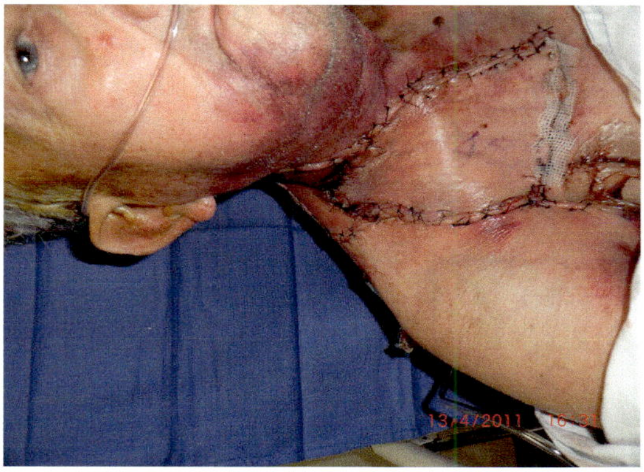

Fig. 3.6 Two days postoperative appearance showing full vascularity in the flap, no evidence of necrosis under drain tube support and the P.A.C.E.S. characteristics all applied when this wound is closed under tension employing the 3-phase single layer suture technique. The patient had continued his smoking habit throughout the healing phase reflected in the vascular changes in the flap.

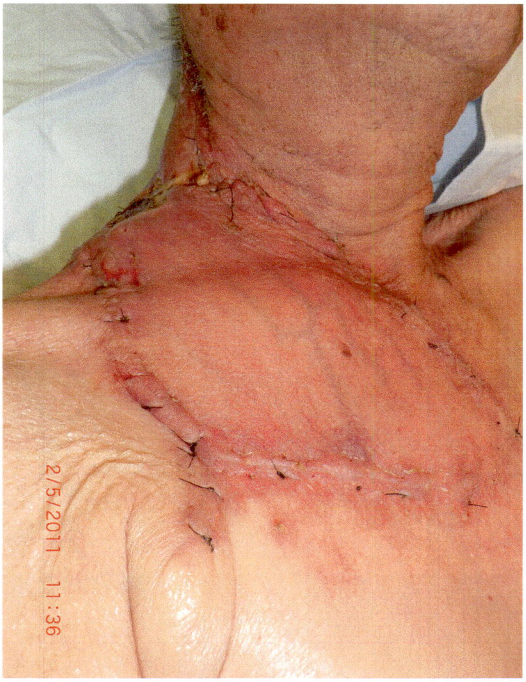

Fig. 3.7 Two weeks postoperative with staged removal of tension sutures

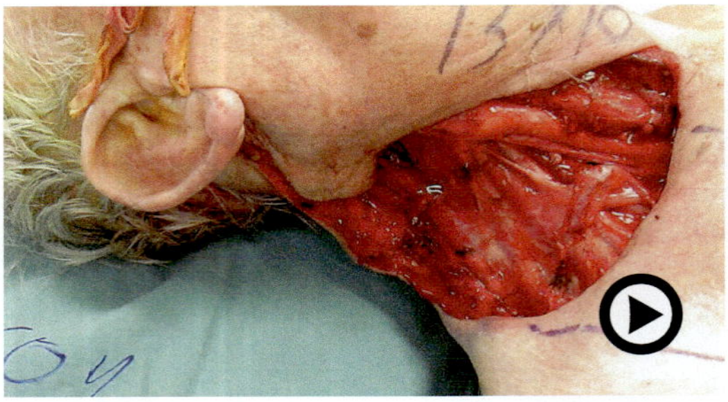

Fig. 3.8 Operative sequence (▶ https://doi.org/10.1007/000-b5q)

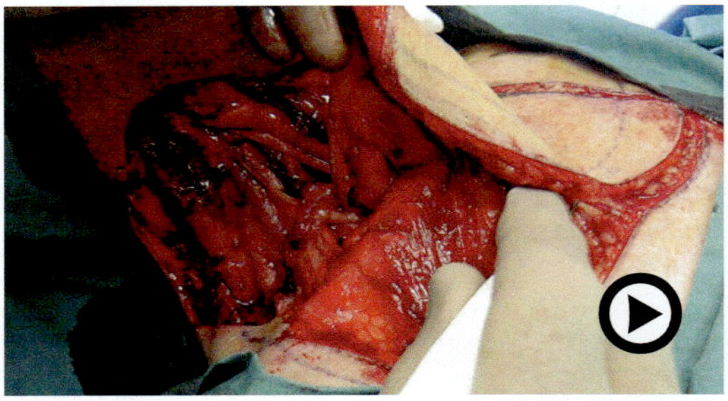

Fig. 3.9 Operative sequence (▶ https://doi.org/10.1007/000-b5k)

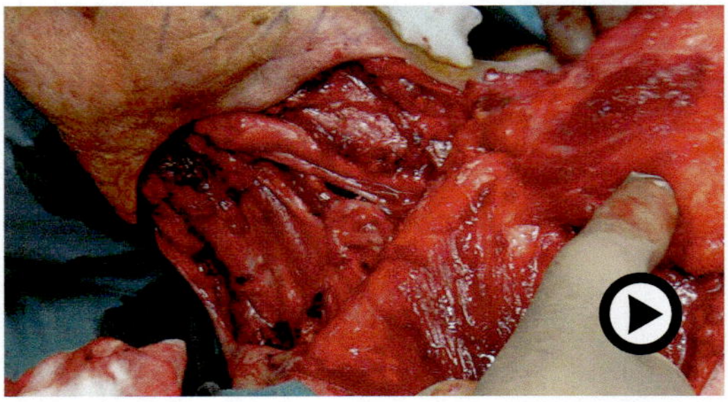

Fig. 3.10 Operative sequence (▶ https://doi.org/10.1007/000-b5m)

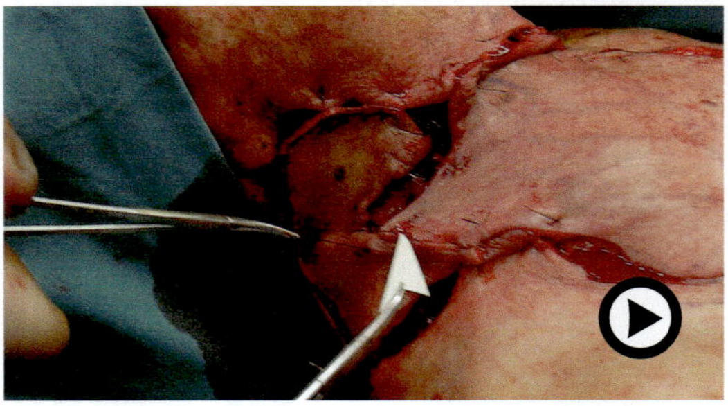

Fig. 3.11 Operative sequence – Red Dot Sign (▶ https://doi.org/10.1007/000-b5n)

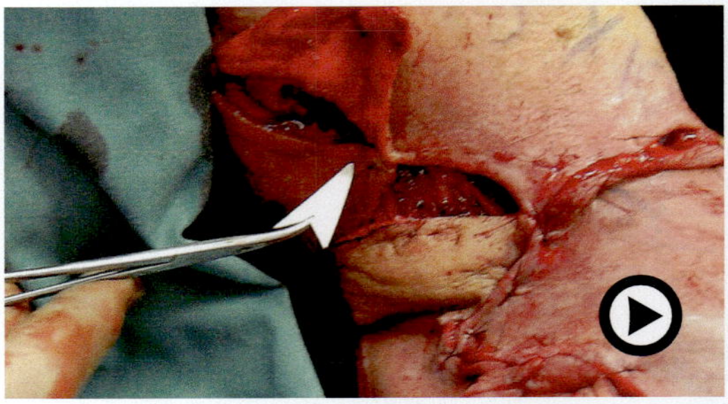

Fig. 3.12 Operative sequence (▶ https://doi.org/10.1007/000-b5p)

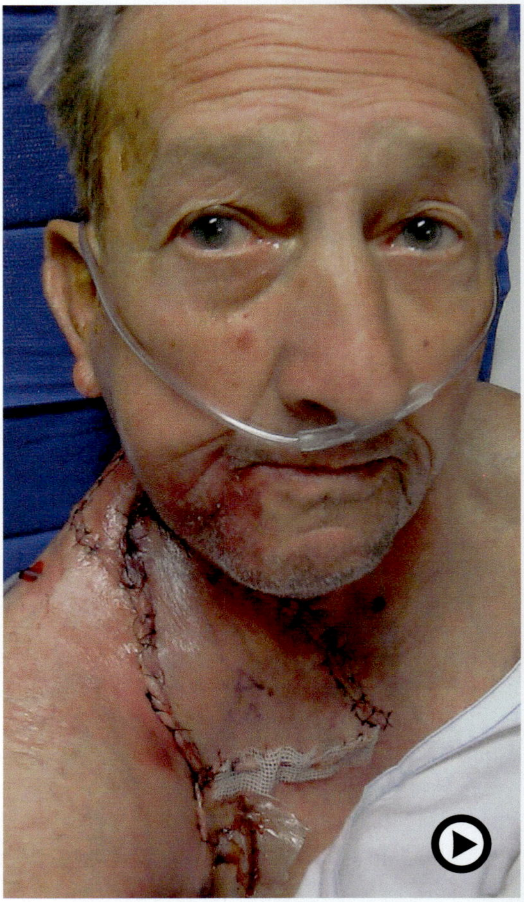

Fig. 3.13 Postoperative – patient perspective (▶ https://doi.org/10.1007/000-b5j)

3.1.2 Case 34: 11 × 5 cm Vertical Melanoma Defect Closed with a Standard Keystone Repair Bridging T4-T10 Dermatomes

Trunk posterior L infrascapular region. Melanoma of the trunk 3 mm Clark Level IV.

Keystone closure vertically aligned along the line spanning intercostal perforators T4-T10. Oncological defect 11 × 5 cm. Tumour-free interval seven years (see Figs. 3.14 and 3.15).

In summary, this Keystone covers three intercostal perforator sites and it is vertically orientated because it matches the excisional defect which also was vertically orientated.

3.1.3 Case 35: 7 mm Melanoma Excision DRAPE Procedure for Pathology Clearance then a Vertically Orientated Keystone Bridging T3 and T6

Refer again to case 41 in upper limb.

Melanoma of the R scapular in a 65-year-old male. Clark Level III, 7 mm. Delayed Reconstruction After Pathology Evaluation (DRAPE).

A guarantee for oncological/histological clearance before definitive closure (see Figs. 3.16, 3.17, and 3.18).

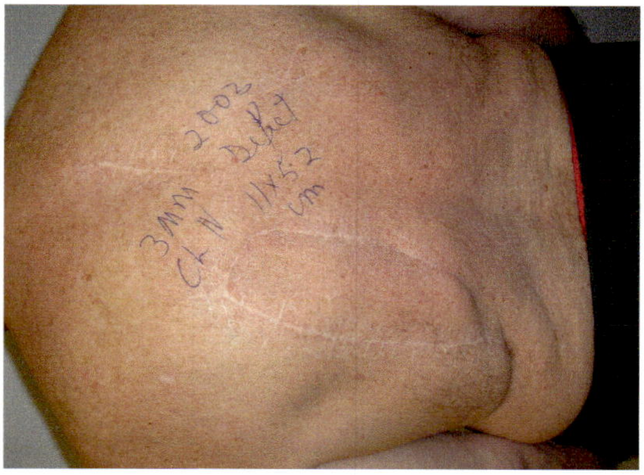

Fig. 3.14 Postoperative appearance and the P.A.C.E.S. characteristics all applied

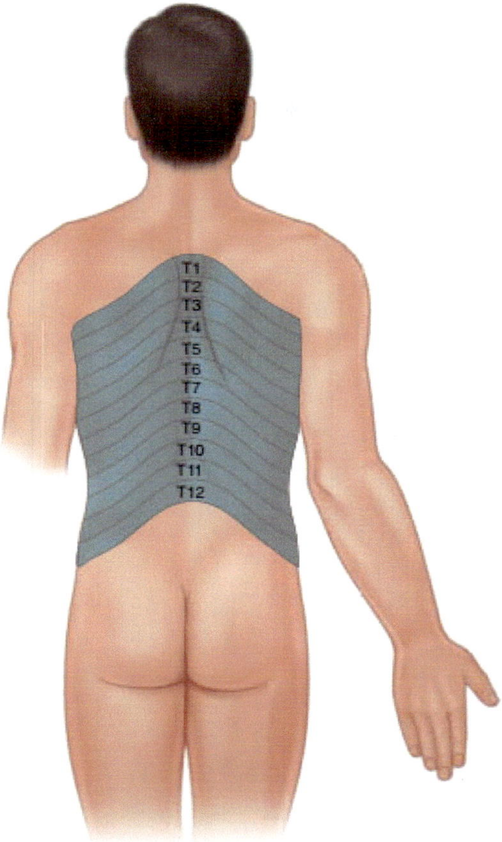

Fig. 3.15 The dermatomal mark out is the guide for the location of the random perforators coming through the fascia

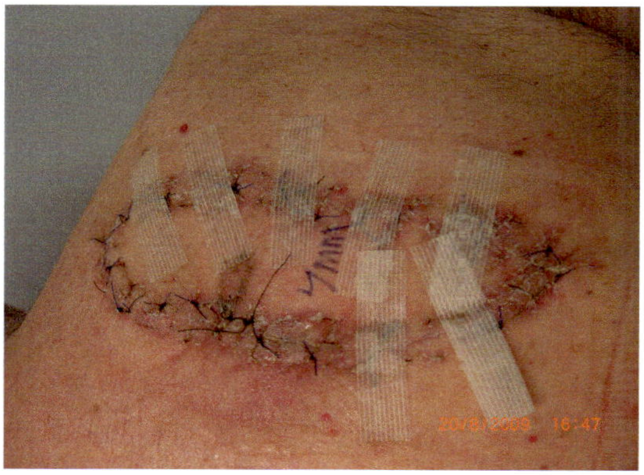

Fig. 3.16 Wound appearance at 7 days cutting the continuous nylon sutures and the 3-phase wound dressing technique also applies to save rupture. No appearance of necrosis and the hyperaemic flare is evident but fading after 7 days

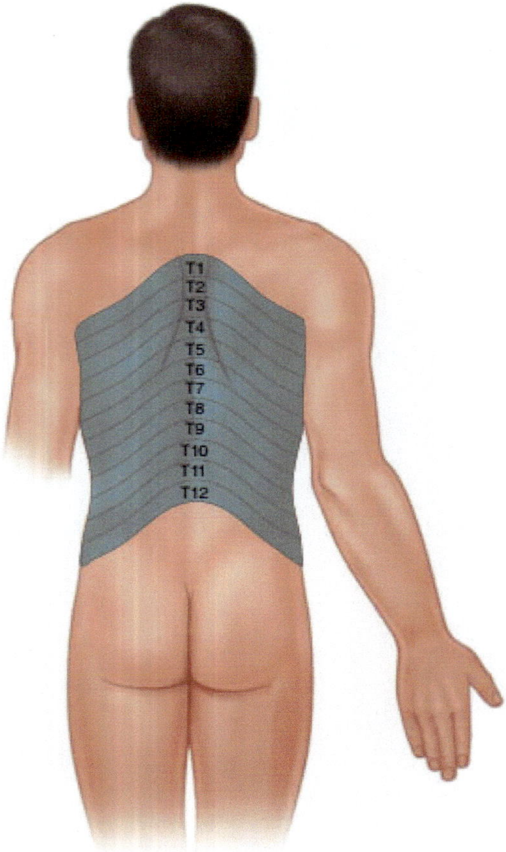

Fig. 3.17 The dermatomal mark out is the guide for the location of the random perforators coming through the fascia

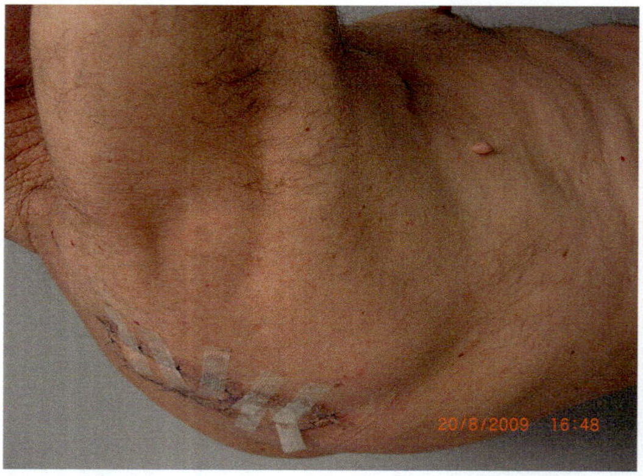

Fig. 3.18 Lateral view from the axillary region. Note the eversion of the surgical margins which is a guarantee of excellent wound healing, creating dermal apposition. Cutting the loops leaving the remnants in situ allows the wound to gradually settle

3.1.4 Case 36: L Infrascapular Melanoma After a Sentinel Node Investigation and the Circumferential Orientation of the Biopsy Creates the Ultimate Design for the Surgical Clearance in the Keystone Repair

Melanoma of the L infrascapular/lumbar region (see Figs. 3.19, 3.20, 3.21, 3.22, 3.23, and 3.24).

3.1.5 Case 37: 14 × 8 cm Defect over the L Scapular Region for a Melanoma/Sarcoma

Melanoma/sarcoma of the L scapular region in this 59-year-old male.

Confirmed histologically with associated axillary clearance performed by Professor Michael Henderson of the Peter McCallum Melanoma Clinic for nodal dissemination into the axillar

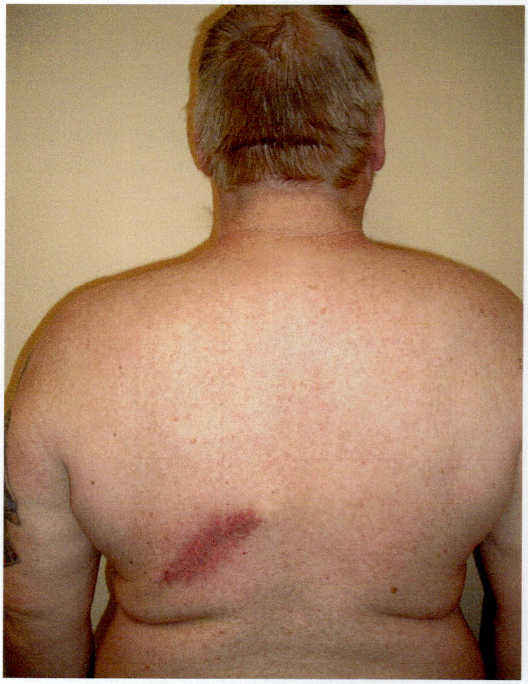

Fig. 3.19 Excisional biopsy prior to re-excision

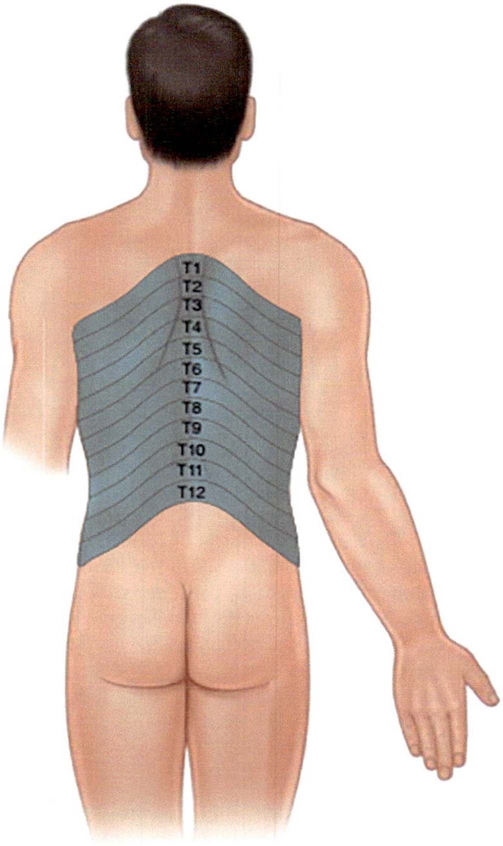

Fig. 3.20 T6-T8 intercostal perforator mark out alignment

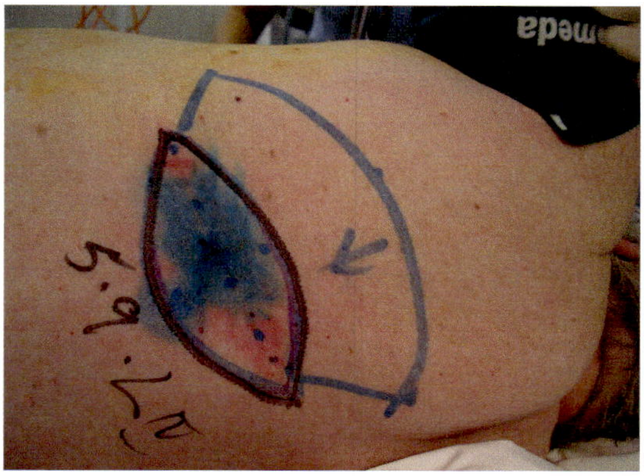

Fig. 3.21 Sentinel node investigation negative and the excision completed with the Keystone based on T6-T8 random intercostal and scapular perforators

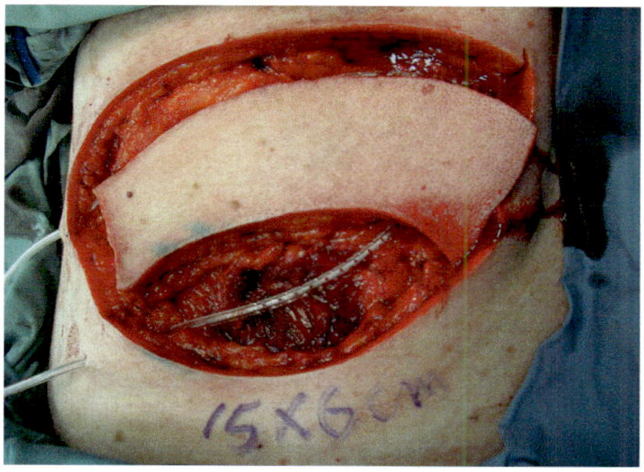

Fig. 3.22 The oncological defect size is 15 × 6 cm down to and including the deep fascia and needs drainage. The Keystone defect likewise needs drainage. Thus, from a technical point of view, the Redi-vac tubing is inserted in a u-shaped manner, draining two sites with a single tube which is just inserted beneath the Keystone with blunt dissection

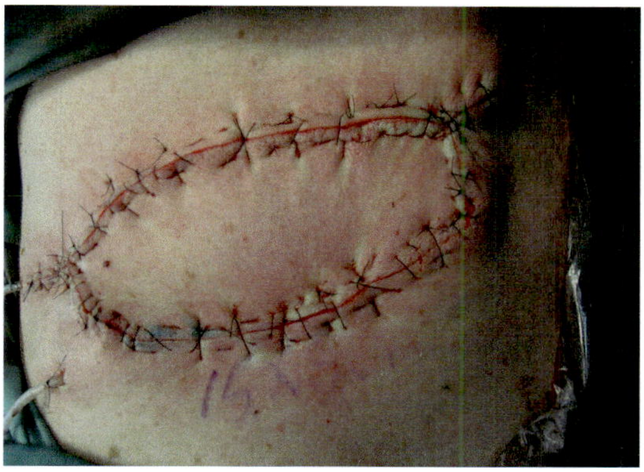

Fig. 3.23 The closure in theatre showing lines of tension with the 3-phase single layer suture technique. Tension locking sutures which stay in 3 weeks along the mid-section of each arc, ordinary mattress sutures to close the wound and stay in for 2 weeks and a single continuous nylon for epidermal seal cut at 7 days which gives an aesthetic suture line

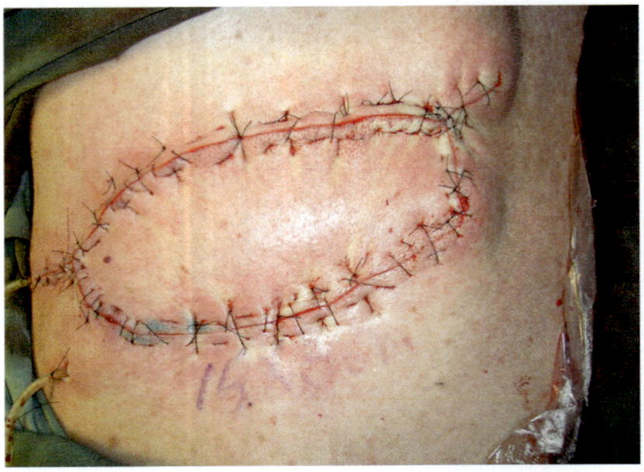

Fig. 3.24 At the completion of the procedure. Notice how these lines of white tension marks have disappeared reflecting the hyperaemia as the circulation is perforator based in the suprafascial and infrafascial compartments. Thus, they bypass any sluggish flow in the subdermal plexus – the cause of flap necrosis orientated towards the subdermal plexus

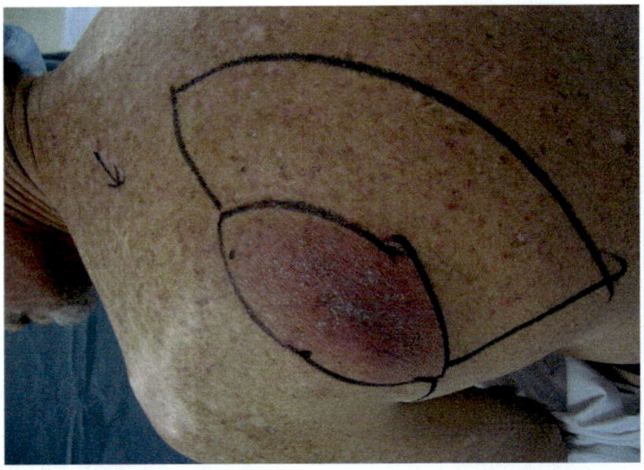

Fig. 3.25 Tumour mass approximately 14 × 8 cm. Note the Keystone mark out over the T2–T8 intercostal perforators the width matching the size of the tumour defect

(see Figs. 3.25, 3.26, 3.27, 3.28, 3.29, 3.30, 3.31, 3.32, 3.33, 3.34, and 3.35).

In summary, the Omega variant with the Keystone between T2 and T8 extending around the large surgical defect along the limits of the L

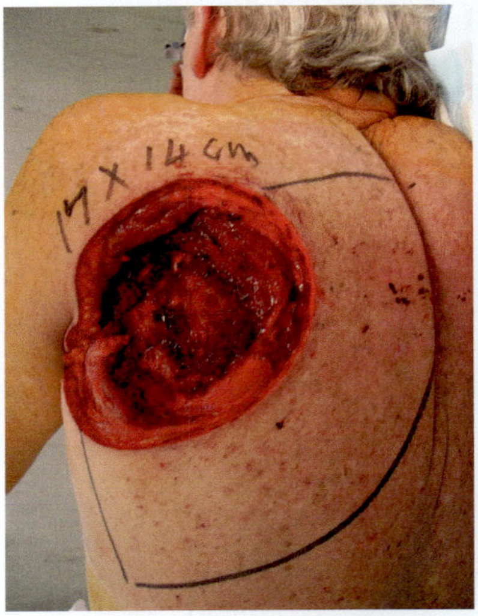

Fig. 3.26 The oncological defect of 14 × 17 cm down to the scapular fascia. The mark out of the Keystone along T2–T8 along the intercostal perforators. My working rule – an essential requirement for flap viability in all Keystones – is leaving one third deep attachment. The flap is attached in this middle area based on random intercostal perforators which are not defined. Whereas the upper and lower thirds both fascial lined and undermined ensure flap viability to the apices to complete the u-shape or omega variant closure

scapular associated with L axilliary clearance. The u-shaped variant facilitates closure and the patient healed well apart from draining a seroma from the L axilla at the tenth day which settled down perfectly.

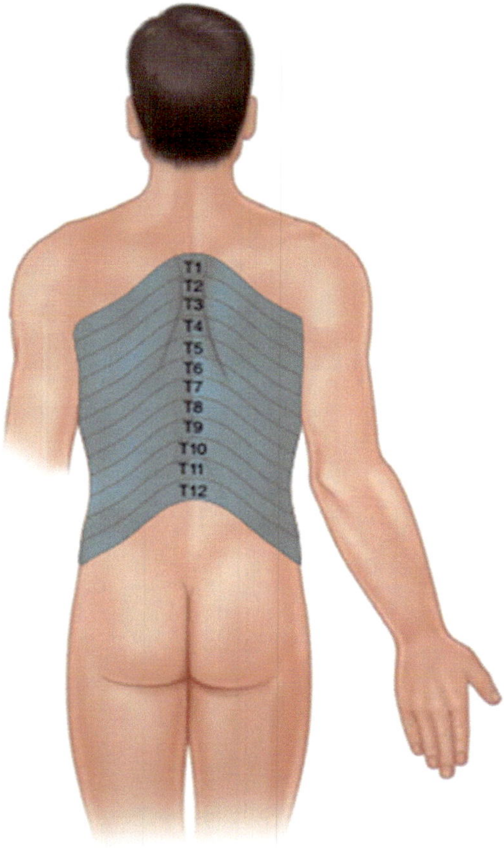

Fig. 3.27 The dermatomal mark out is the guide for the location of the random perforators coming through the fascia

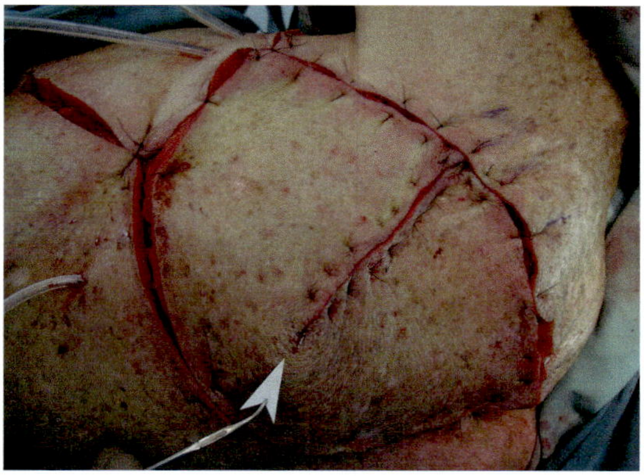

Fig. 3.28 Closure technique under Redi-vac drainage at the two sites and axillary is separately drained. Such is the reliability and the hyperaemia of these observed vascular changes the dog ears can be trimmed at the epidermal level in the acute phase down to the limits of the arrow because the flaps are fascial based and not dermally based. The postoperative appearance confirms this hypothesis, without any need for dog ear correction

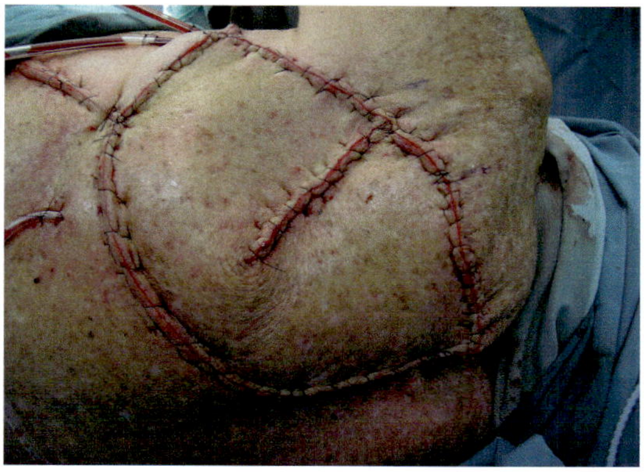

Fig. 3.29 The final specimen with double Redi-vacs in position one for the axilla and one for the Keystone repair. No evidence of cyanosis/necrosis occurred and the P.A.C.E.S. characteristics were all evident

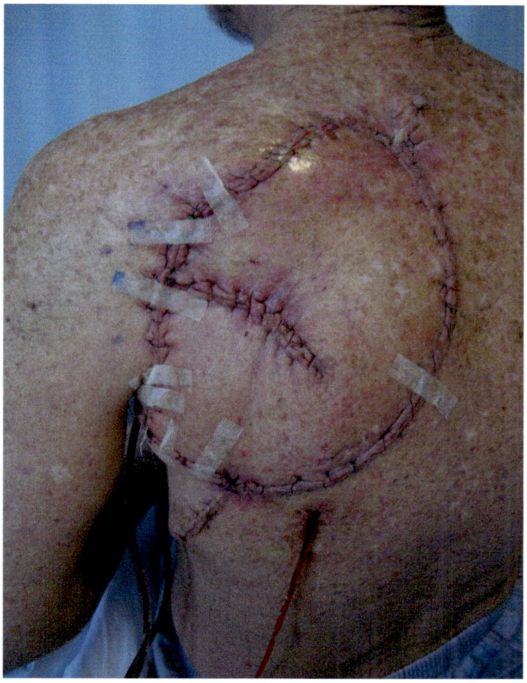

Fig. 3.30 Day 4 postoperative image. A drainage of the axillary collection became necessary following the removal of drain tube – perhaps movement was a factor and the patient had a personality to match it

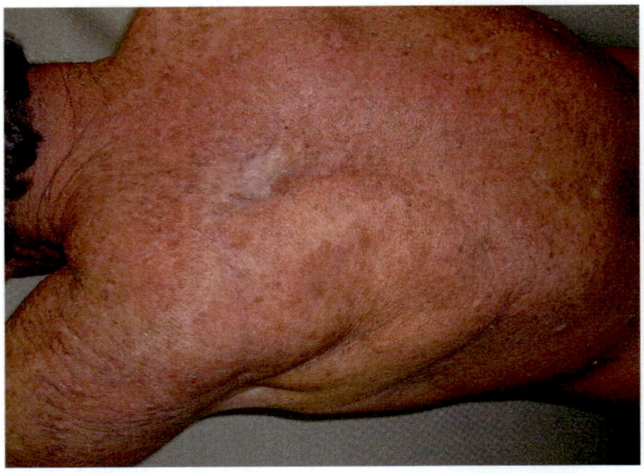

Fig. 3.31 Full functional rotation of the shoulder girdle without any pain or limitations of range of movement after 6 weeks – all pain free

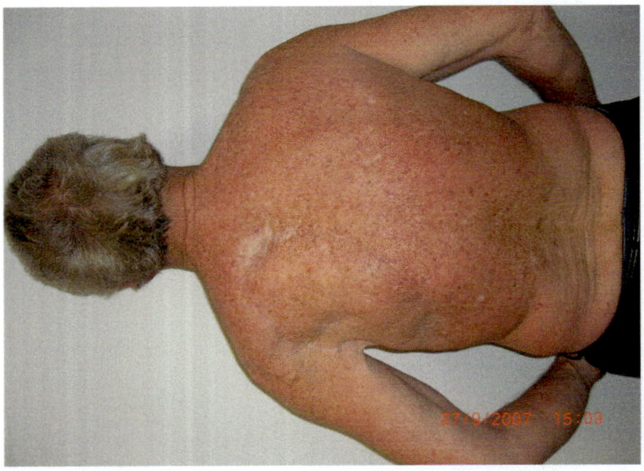

Fig. 3.32 Preparing to mountaineer in the Himalayas after 6 weeks

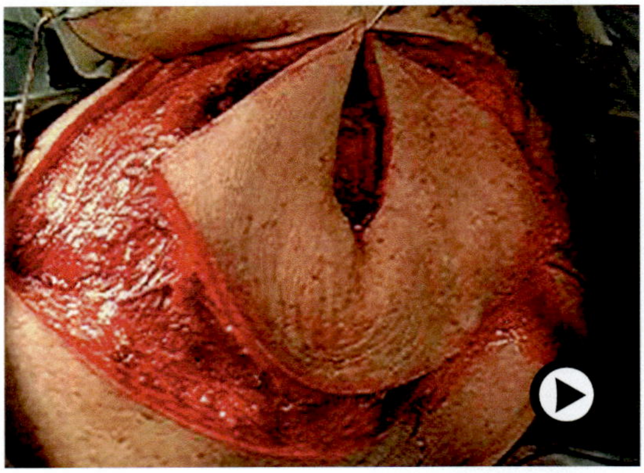

Fig. 3.33 Operative sequence (▶ https://doi.org/10.1007/000-b5r)

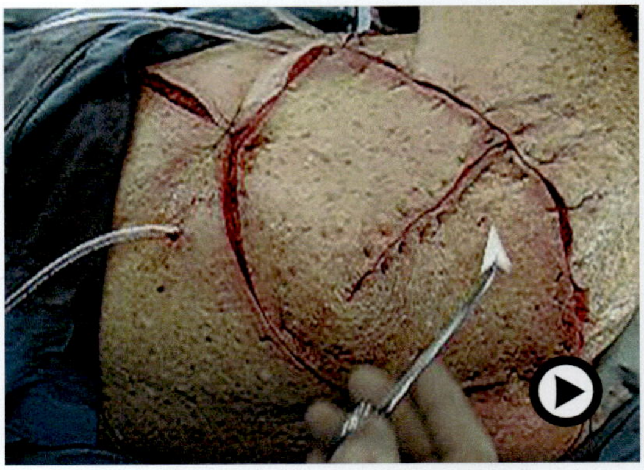

Fig. 3.34 Operative sequence (▶ https://doi.org/10.1007/000-b5s)

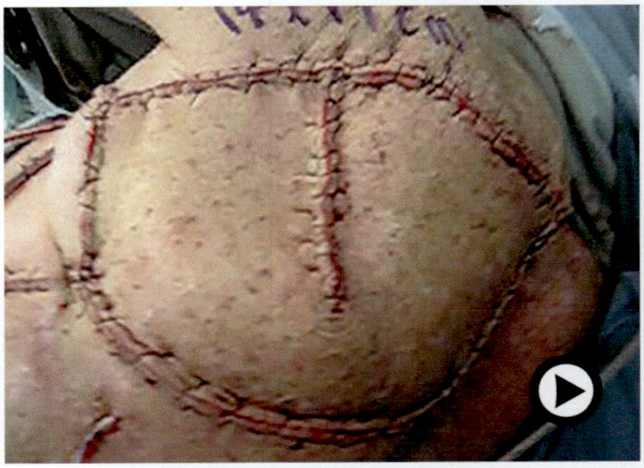

Fig. 3.35 Operative sequence (▶ https://doi.org/10.1007/000-b5t)

3.1.6 Case 38: 15 × 8 cm Defect Recurrent Malignant Melanoma Anterior Chest Wall in the L Supramammary Region

Recurrent malignant melanoma of the chest wall (see Figs. 3.36, 3.37, 3.38, 3.39, 3.40, and 3.41).

In summary, islanding lax tissue along perforator axes is a simple method for anterior trunk Keystone closures with all P.A.C.E.S. characteristics evident.

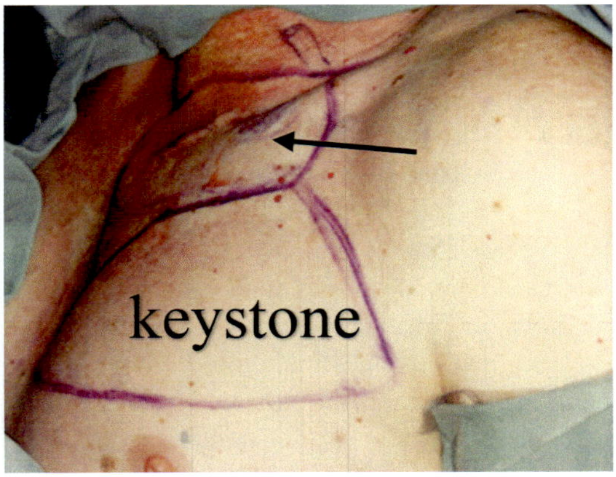

Fig. 3.36 The recurrent melanoma of the chest wall in the intra-clavicular region adjacent to the sternoclavicular joint. The Keystone mark out in the supramammary region overlies intercostal perforators 2, 3 and possibly 4th and rotated into the defect, clinically equivalent to an island deltopectoral flap based on the same 2, 3, 4 IC perforators

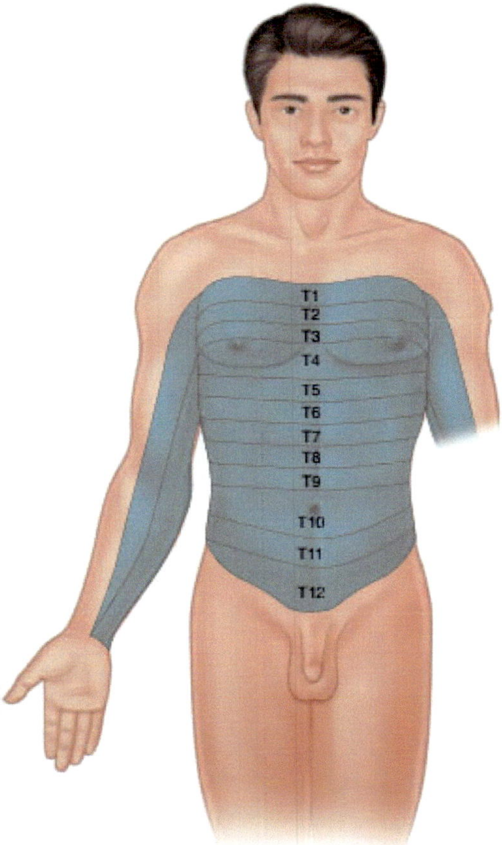

Fig. 3.37 The dermatomal mark out is the guide for the location of the random perforators coming through the fascia

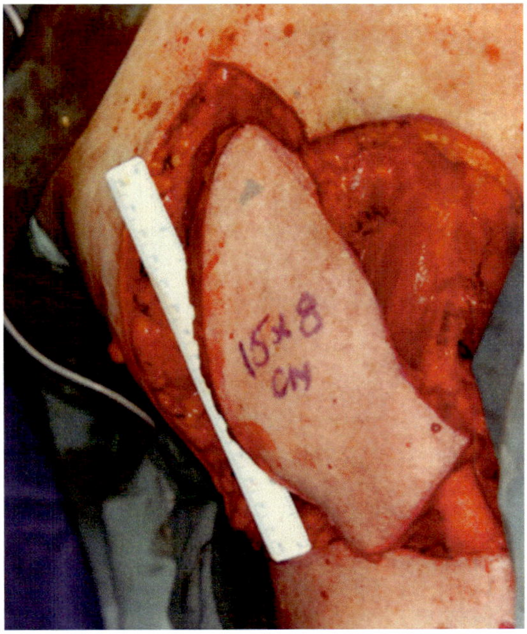

Fig. 3.38 The Keystone measuring 15 × 8 cm is swiveled on the random perforators (on the alignment of the nipple) at the T4 site. These perforators are randomly located and not individually skeletonised to preserve adventitial support containing somatic, autonomic and lymphatic supply. Thus, preserving a return to normality because of the retention here of the embryological components arising and accompanying the perforators

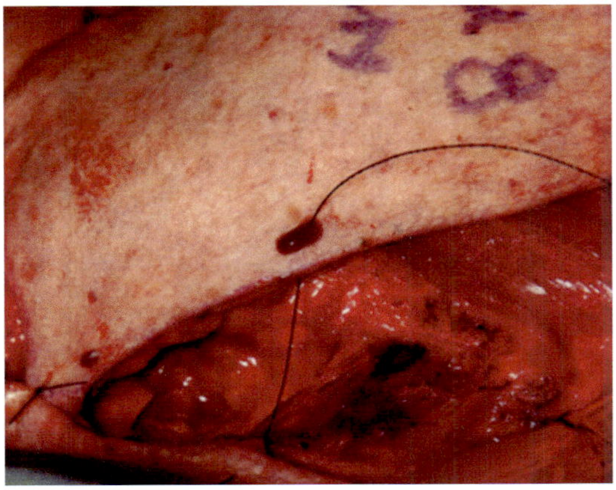

Fig. 3.39 The hyperaemic factor is indicated by the Red Dot Sign where the blood flow at the suture site over the Keystone bleeds more than the insertional attachment. Once more a confirmatory sign of the hyperaemic phase seen in Keystone reconstructions. This is a reflection of a sympathectomy effect by islanding the dermal epidermal mark out and with possible contributions from a hydrostatic component with venous drainage being directed down the perforator axes ensuring sound healing

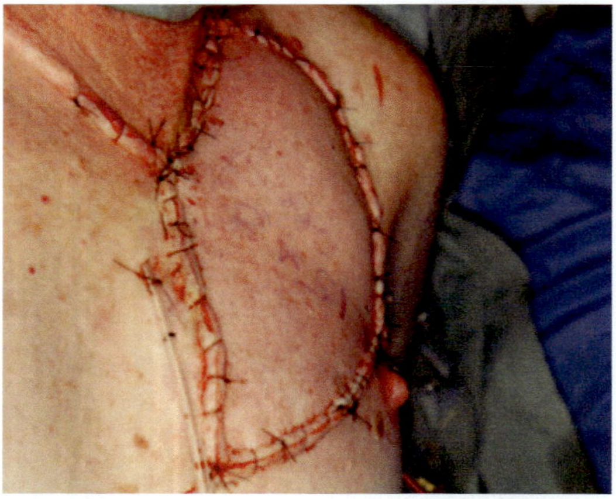

Fig. 3.40 The insertion of the Keystone flap reflecting the hyperaemia which usually surfaces in 10–15 min. The V-Y closure of the axillary defect and the rotation of the Keystone into the infraclavicular oncological defect region helps to close the surgical wound under Redi-vac drainage. The 3-phase single layer suture technique is used throughout all cases: Locking mattress sutures at the points of tension stay in 3 weeks; 2 weeks ordinary interrupted mattress sutures for wound closure; and continuous nylon for 1 week for epidermal seal

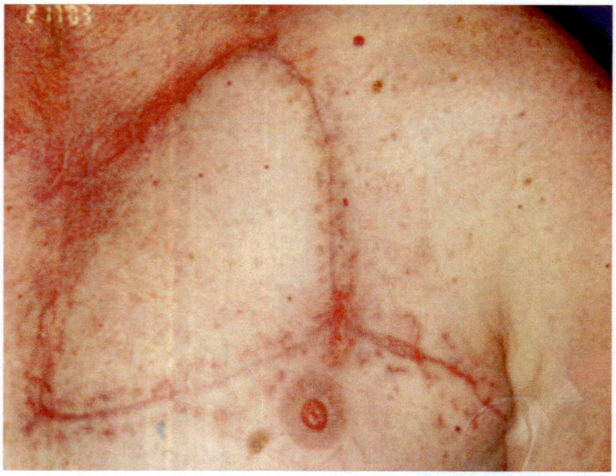

Fig. 3.41 The healed wound appearance at 4 weeks

3.2 Complications: Shoulder Girdle Activity

3.2.1 Premature Removal of Tension Sutures – Wound Breakdown

It is mandatory when wound dressings are referred to outside clinics and lacking experience in Keystone management that simple wound dressing instructions stipulating the 3-phase element of suture removal must be observed as the wound closures are all done under tension:

- Cut the continuous nylon at 1 week to 10 days and leave in situ.
- Take out half the mattress at week 2.
- Thirdly, the tension locking sutures stay in 3 weeks at least. Should bleeding occur on removal, even at this late stage, it does not matter to leave them in another week (see Figs. 3.42, 3.43, and 3.44).

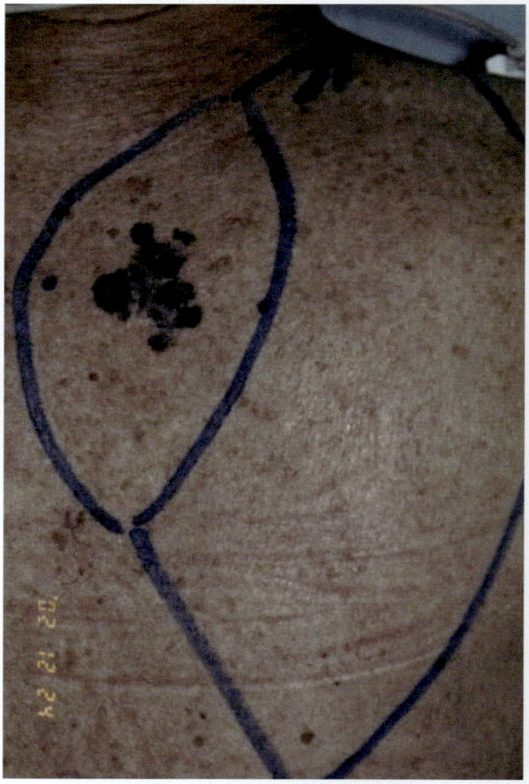

Fig. 3.42 Mark out of the Keystone for pathology in the midline of the back – Clark level IV 3.25 mm

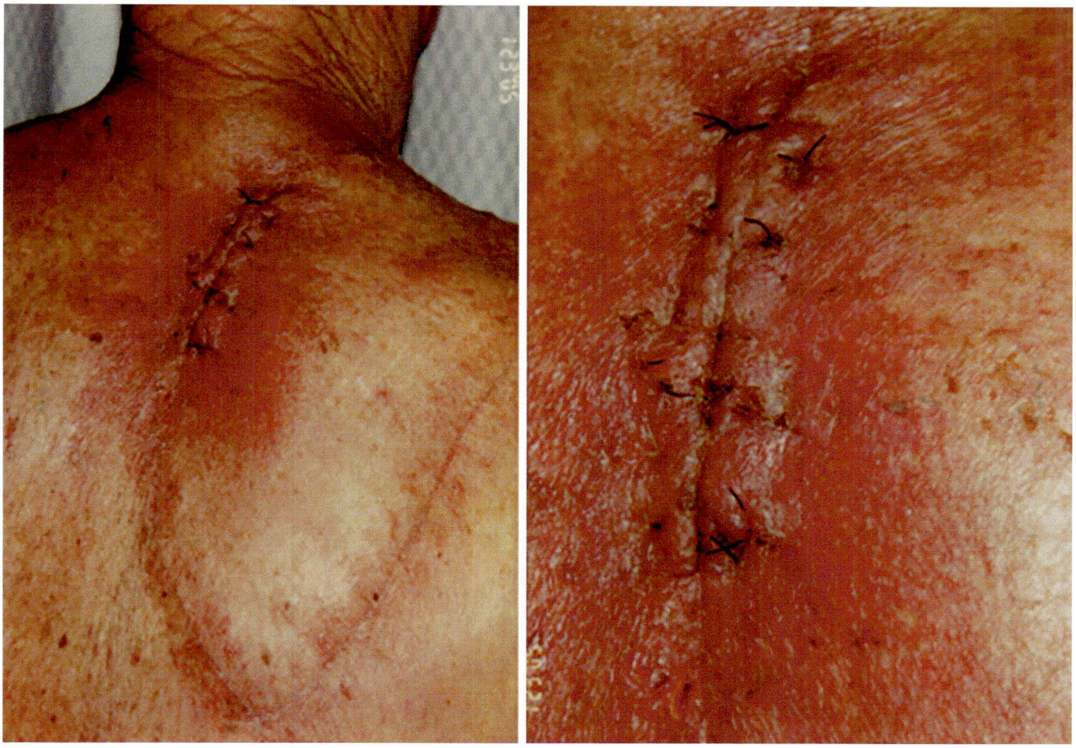

Fig. 3.43 The scapula Keystone on the medial side had the tension sutures prematurely removed at 2 weeks by an outside clinic where wound dressing techniques were not followed. This led to wound rupture and breakdown. The solution is a simple wound re-suturing using locking mattress sutures under local anaesthetic and left in situ for a further 3 weeks, a rare complication when supervision is lacking

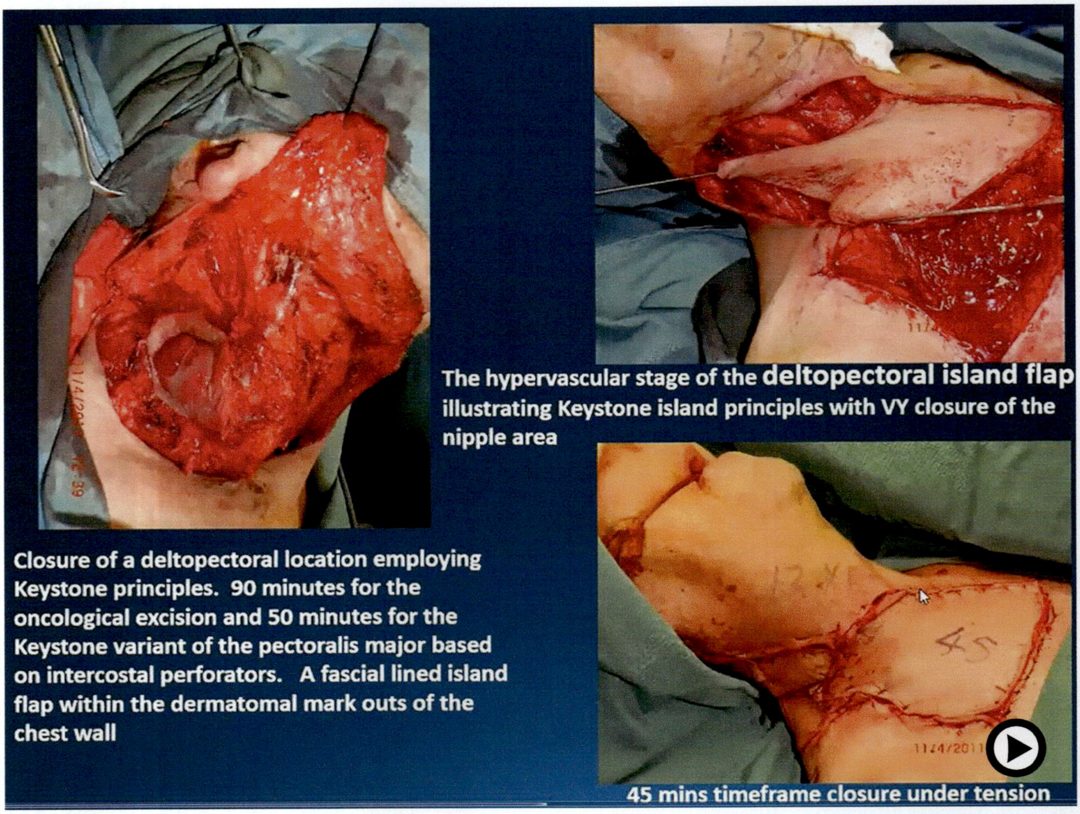

Fig. 3.44 Major truck (▶ https://doi.org/10.1007/000-b5v)

References

1. Bakamjian VY, Holbrook LA. Prefabrication techniques in cervical pharyngo-oesophageal reconstruction. Br J Plast Surg. 1973;26(3):214–22.
2. Bakamjian VY, Poole M. Maxillo-facial and palatal reconstructions with the deltopectoral flap. Br J Plast Surg. 1977;30(1):17–37.

Major Upper Limb Defects Using the Keystone Technique

4

Contents

4.1 Case Presentations

4.1.1 Case 39: Melanoma of the Arm – Over Biceps

Any melanoma with a longitudinal biopsy orientation is well managed with the Keystone concept reconstruction vertically orientated. The soft muscle bellies of the biceps and triceps areas facilitates closure under tension. In this case, the oncolological defect was 7 × 4 cm (see Figs. 4.1, 4.2, 4.3, 4.4, 4.5, 4.6 and 4.7).

In summary, an aesthetically acceptable outcome for a young lady wearing summer clothing and the P.A.C.E.S. characteristics are all exemplified.

Supplementary Information The online version contains supplementary material available at https://doi.org/10.1007/978-3-031-39868-1_4. The videos can be accessed individually by clicking the DOI link in the accompanying figure caption or by scanning this link with the SN More Media App.

F. Behan, *Atlas of Keystone Reconstructive Technique in Melanoma Management*, https://doi.org/10.1007/978-3-031-39868-1_4

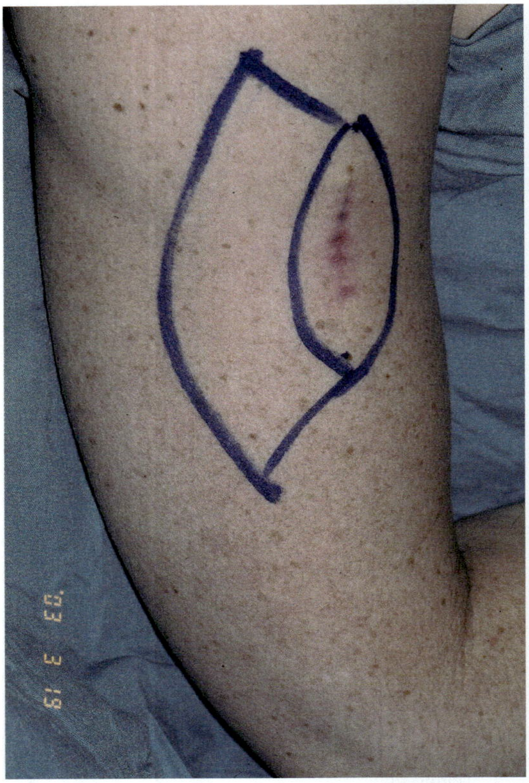

Fig. 4.1 In a well-presented young lady, fully aware of the problems of scarring deformity in her upper limb and the controversy such scarring produces mentally and physically is partially overcome with the Keystone concept. The alternative 'melon slice' scar deformity always raises questions over its lack of aesthetic appeal and resultant outcome – the shark bite comment surfaces regularly to describe their deformity, to the patient's embarrassment and dissatisfaction as well. The biopsy site and the Keystone flap mark out are illustrated between deltoid and the lower third of the arm is evident where a single flap closes two defects

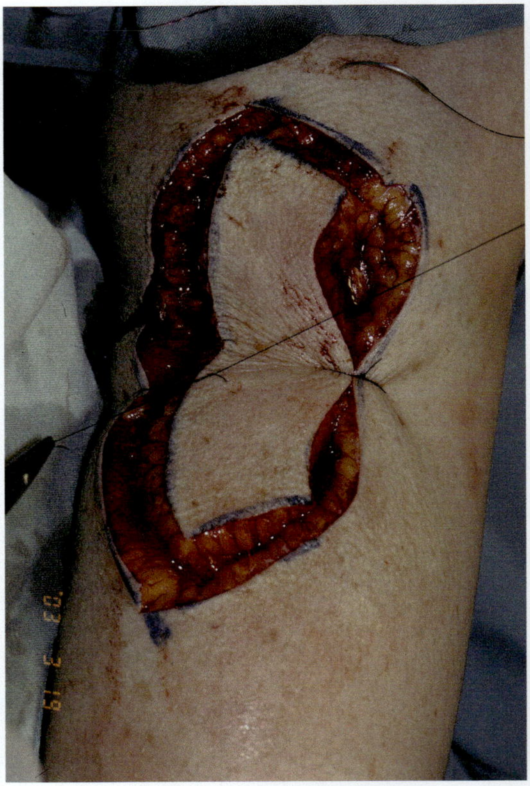

Fig. 4.2 The initial lines of maximum tension in this fascial lined island flap occur when the convex and concave sides are aligned. Note the pink flare reflecting hyperaemia and hypervascular perfusion in this island flap has been attributed to a sympathectomy effect at the epidermal level because of the island delineation. Random perforators in the suprafascial and infrafascial compartments are the source of its vascularity. There is no skeletonisation of any defined perforator axes and no undermining of the Keystone flap should this detract from the neural basis at the autonomic and somatic levels

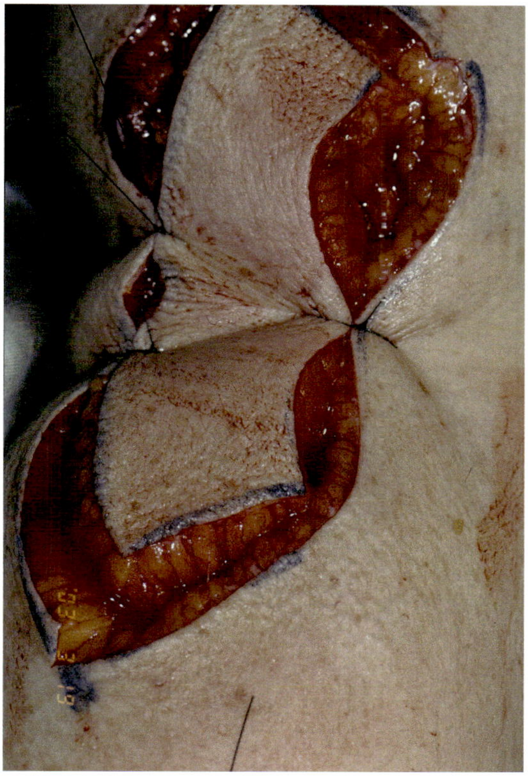

Fig. 4.3 Note the lines of tension – a contraindication in surgical wound closure as part of our teaching but these are not significant when adopting Keystone principles. Having broken this rule of surgery and used repetitively – it is because the circulation in the subdermal plexus is supported by the fascial perforators. The laxity of the muscle bellies facilitates the closure, achieved by compressing the biceps muscle volume

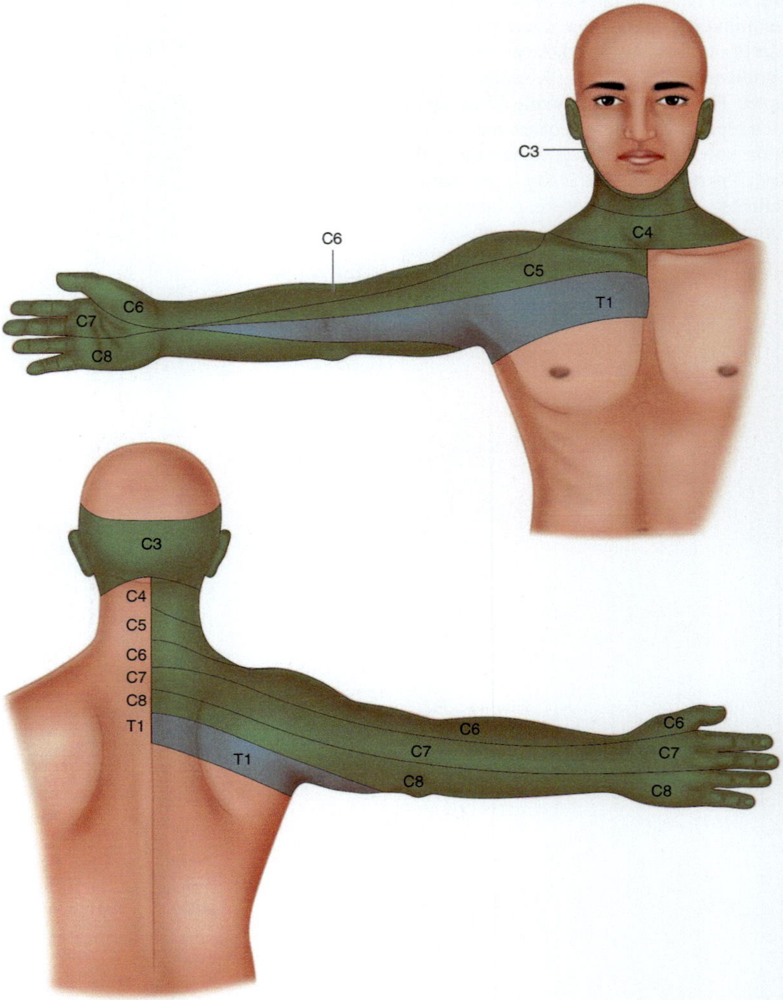

Fig. 4.4 The dermatomal mark out is the guide for the location of the random perforators coming through the fascia

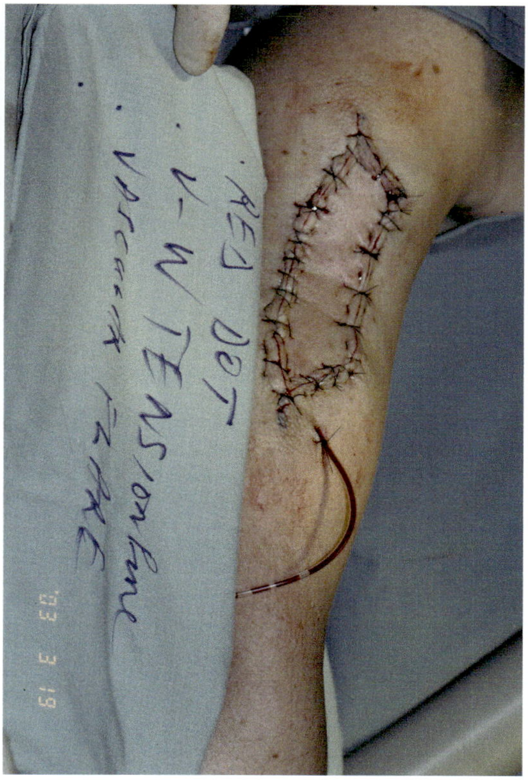

Fig. 4.5 Note the vascular flare, the lines of tension creases are disappearing usually in 10–15 min and the Redi-vac drainage is with the tubing bent in a u-shaped manner draining both surgical sites. The definitive closure – the simple 3-phase Keystone closure technique is applied where tension locking sutures in the epidermis in the centre of both arcs align the closure. There are no fascial deep layered sutures which may embarrass the circulation. Other mattress sutures complete wound margin closure accurately and the continuous nylon around the periphery achieves epidermal seal adding to its aesthetic outcome

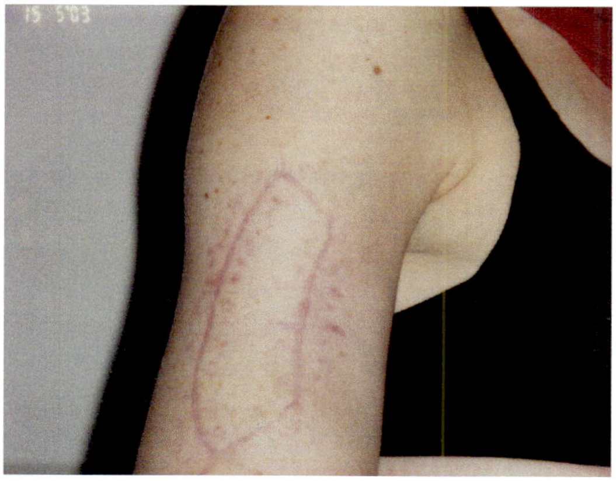

Fig. 4.6 The postoperative appearance after 3 years without any 'shark bite' appearance allowing her to wear full summer attire

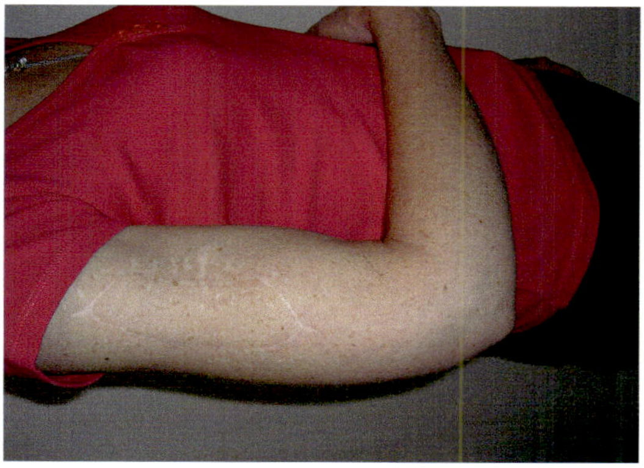

Fig. 4.7 An aesthetic outcome

4.2 Case 40: Melanomas Around the Elbow Region – Cubital Fossa

Keystone closure of the forearm adjacent to the cubital fossa without the need for skin grafting (see Figs. 4.8, 4.9, and 4.10).

The Keystone principles have been maintained and the aesthetic outcome using the C6 dermatome is repeated and is based on random perforators along the radial side below the elbow crease. The outline of the Keystone on the volar aspect of the forearm shows the acceptable aesthetic outcome without the cratiform deformity of a major split skin graft.

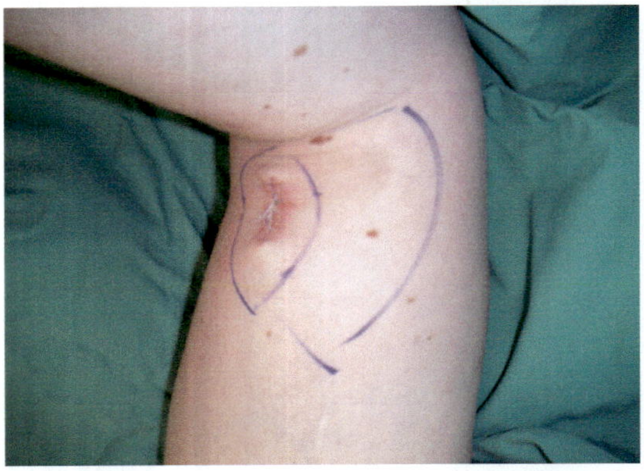

Fig. 4.8 Biopsy orientation. Lateral forearm Keystone mark out

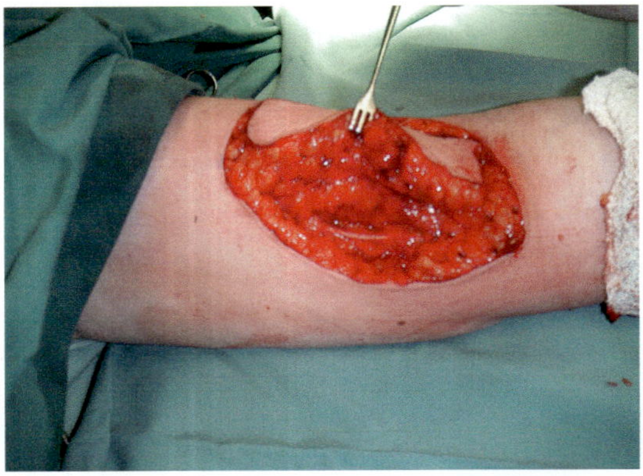

Fig. 4.9 Closure showing deep attachments underneath the Keystone which are not undermined

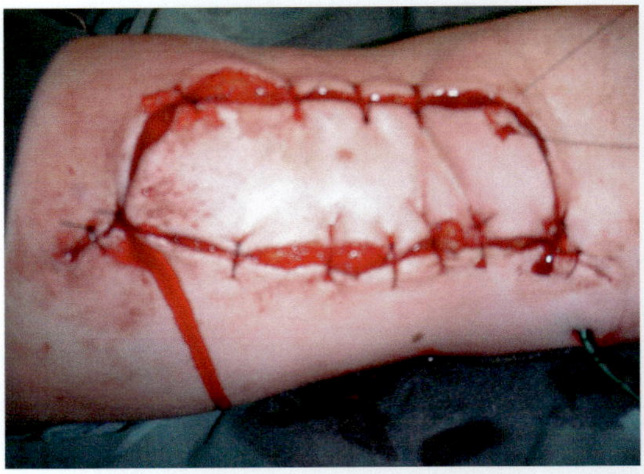

Fig. 4.10 Staged closure with the tension locking sutures in situ and the ordinary mattress around the periphery before the continuous locking suture is inserted. Note the Red Dot Sign in the flap margin which is hyperaemic and the Red Dot outside this margin is a little cyanotic

A postoperative L forearm melanoma repair showing the need for a split skin graft at the cubital fossa level because of the restrictions of closure and elbow movement (see Figs. 4.11 and 4.12).

4.2.1 Case 41: Complicated Areas of Reconstruction – Shoulder Girdle a Typical Site for a Male Industrial Worker

I have included this case over the posterior deltoid region because even though the Keystone application is ideal for reconstruction, the movement of the shoulder girdle is a definate contraindication if the patient is non-compliant. In other words, a firm shoulder splintage girdle using an orthoapaedic appliance holds the joint relatively immobile while healing continues over this 3 week period. This may help prevent any wound breakbown with premature removal of sutures

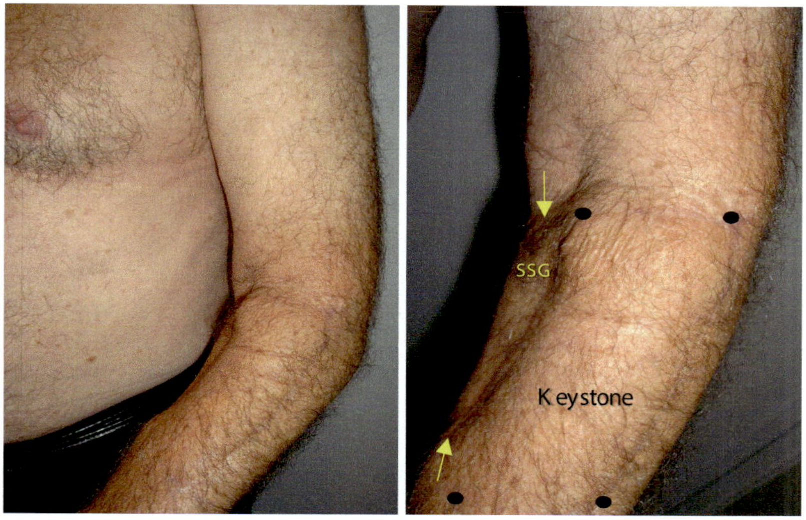

Fig. 4.11 The element of tension and the lack of elastic release in this elderly forearm warranted the use of a skin graft for the secondary defect (arrowed), the Keystone mark out is dotted in black

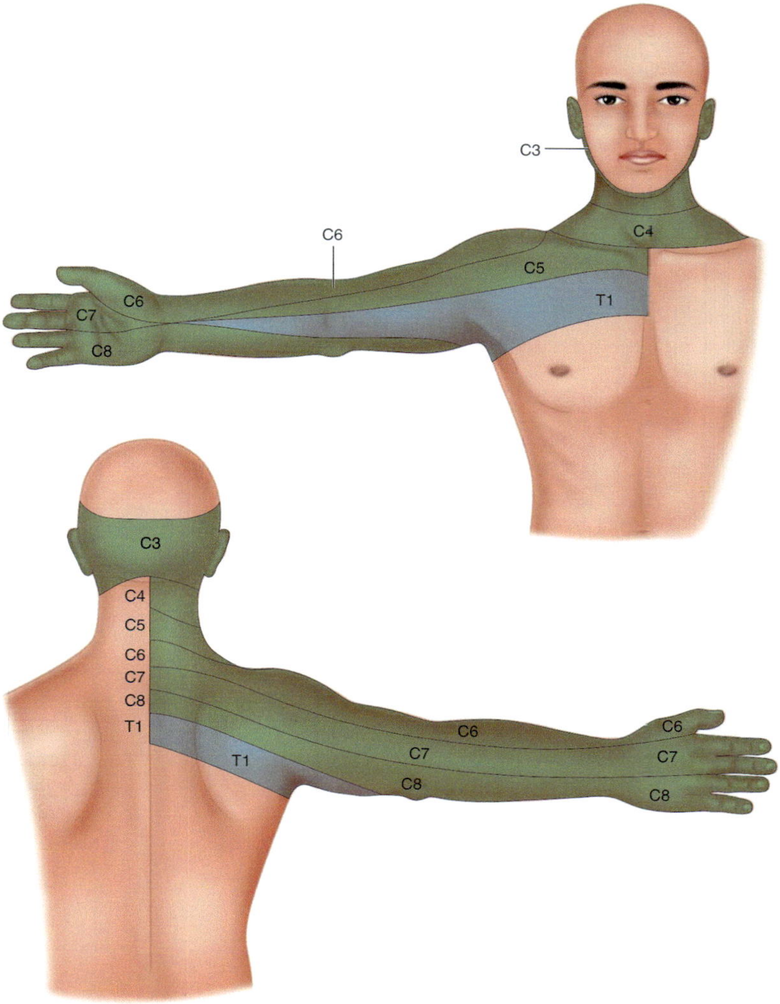

Fig. 4.12 The dermatomal mark out is the guide for the location of the random perforators coming through the fascia

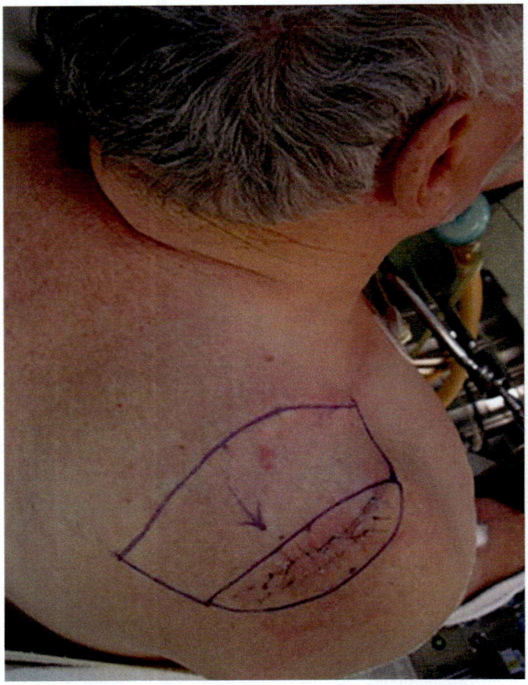

Fig. 4.13 Melanoma of the shoulder/deltoid region level III – > 1 mm. The Keystone flap mark out is indicated. The size is larger in transverse depth compared with the marked excisional defect

(see Figs. 4.13, 4.14, 4.15, 4.16, 4.17, 4.18, and 4.19).

In summary, stabilising shoulder movement goes some way to ensure wound healing but the pain-free recovery was the keynote of the repair and the P.A.C.E.S. characteristics were all exemplified.

4.2.2 Case 42: A Complicated Reconstruction in the Elbow Region – Inappropriate Biopsy Orientation

Melanoma R elbow complicated reconstruction as the Clark Level II 0.6 mm biopsy was done in a circumferential manner. Hence, the Keystone had to be circumferential in the supraepicondylar

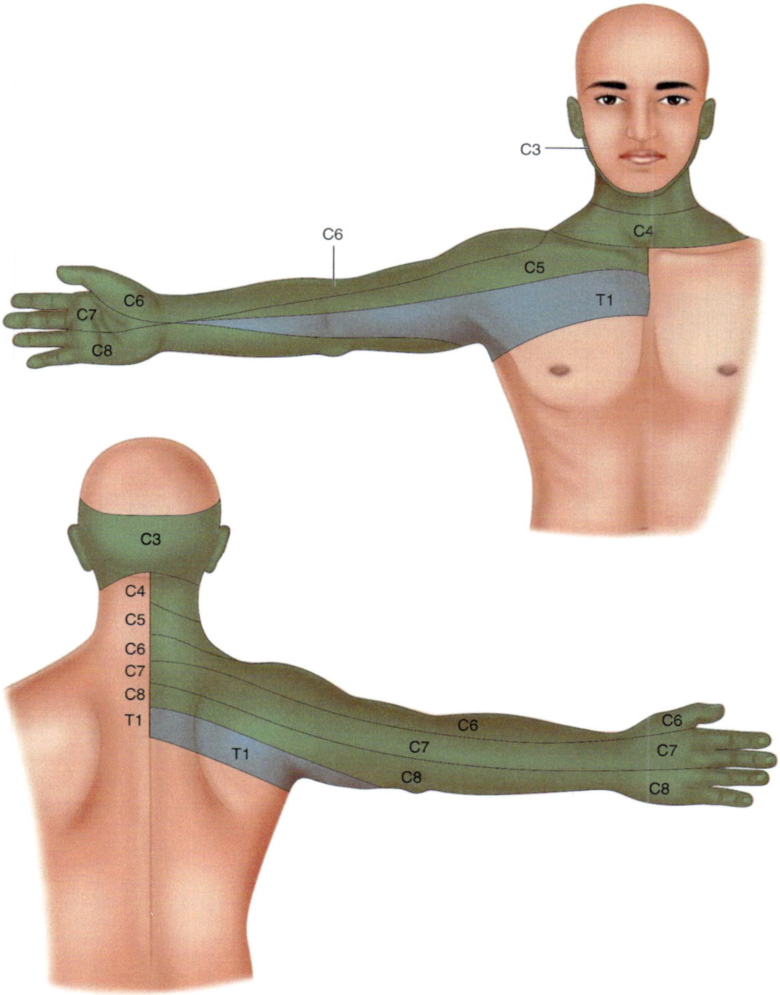

Fig. 4.14 The dermatomal mark out is the guide for the location of the random perforators coming through the fascia

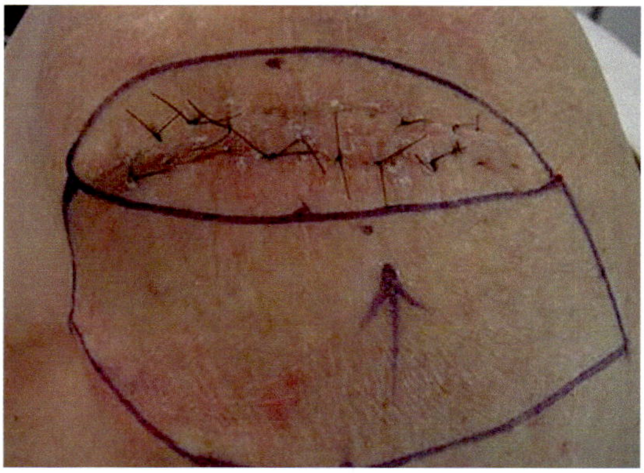

Fig. 4.15 A close-up of the planned Keystone design

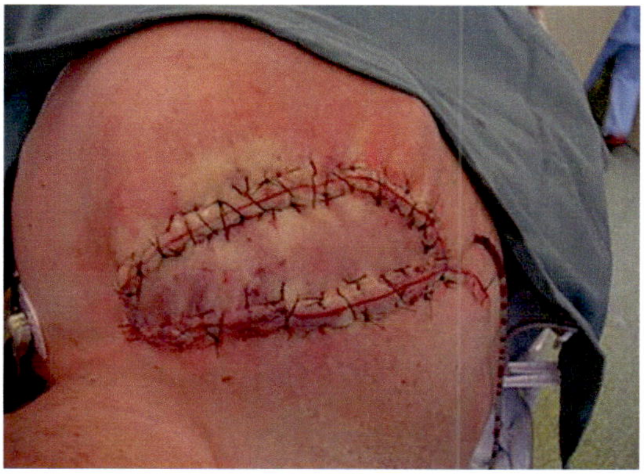

Fig. 4.16 The completed procedure. Note the area of hyperaemia throughout the flap slowly displacing the white lines of tension which reflect the changes in the subdermal plexus as the Keystone is fascially based on the deeper structures

region (see Figs. 4.20, 4.21, 4.22, 4.23, 4.24, 4.25, 4.26, and 4.27).

In summary, the reliability of the Keystone allows closure of tissue when the biopsy orientation is circumferential and not longitudenal. Its hyperaemia and slow suture removal ensures a complication free healing and reverted back to wearing summer attire.

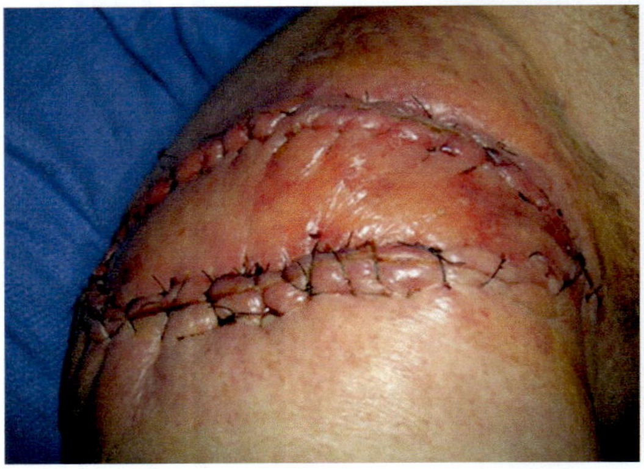

Fig. 4.17 Seven day appearance. A note of caution, note the wound oedema around the direct closure using the Keystone

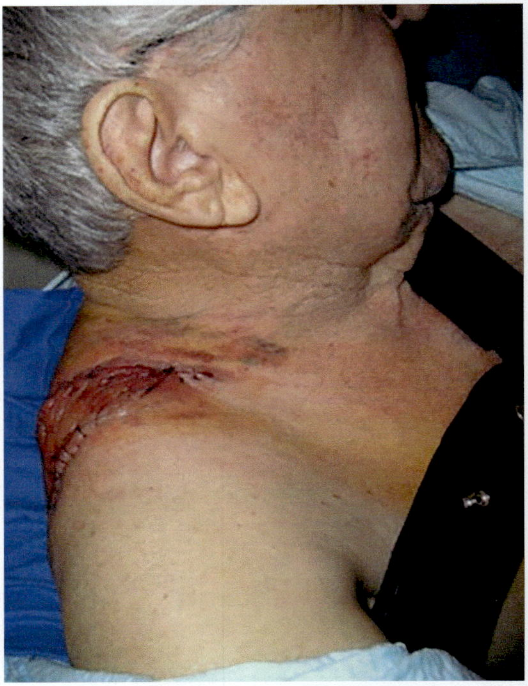

Fig. 4.18 Limb immobilisation splintage, a reflection of pain-free surgery

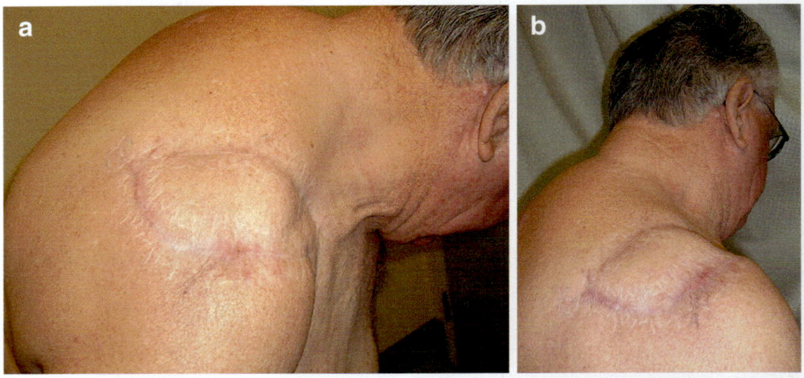

Fig. 4.19 (**a**) Postoperative outcome. (**b**) Postoperative outcome

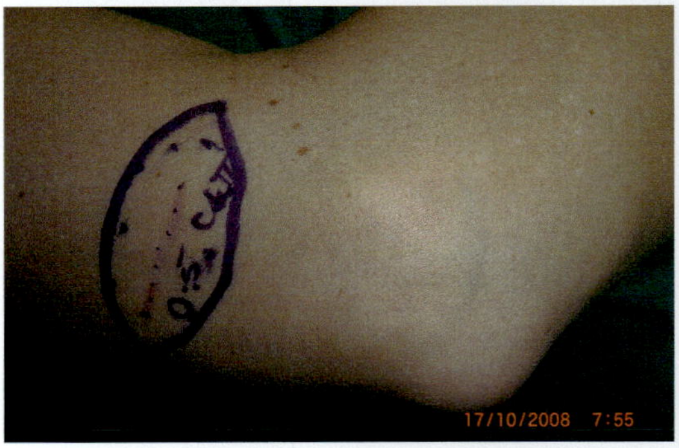

Fig. 4.20 Melanoma Clark level II 0.6 mm, bad circumferential biopsy, poor orientation

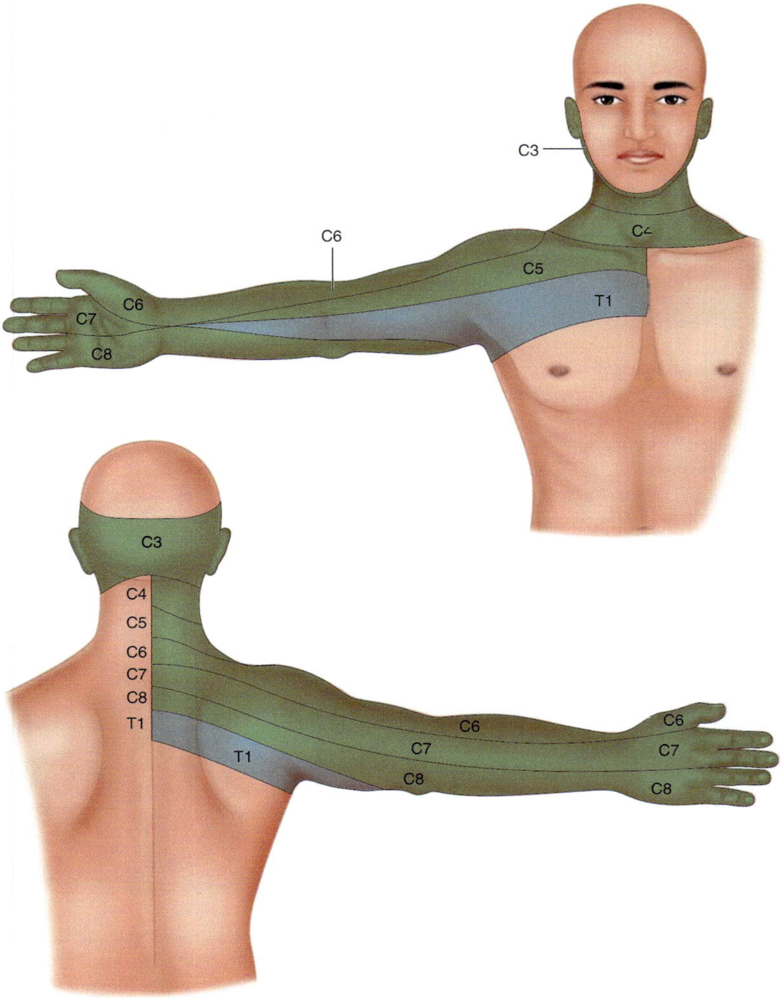

Fig. 4.21 The dermatomal mark out is the guide for the location of the random perforators coming through the fascia

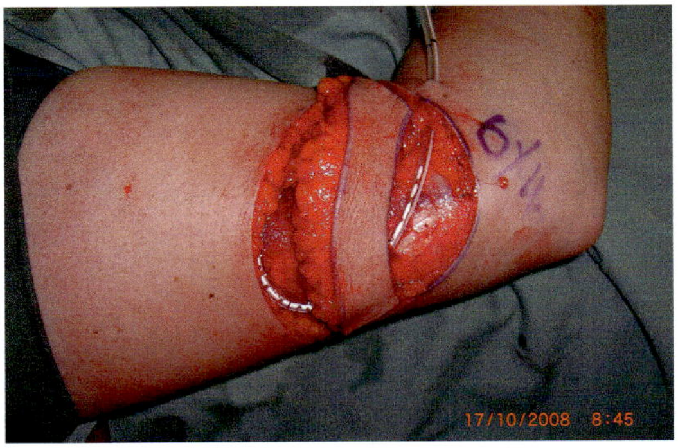

Fig. 4.22 6 × 4 cm excisional defect with a thinner 2 cm Keystone in the supraepicondylar region with a single Redi-vac tubing in a U-shaped design draining two surgical sites – oncological and Keystone sites

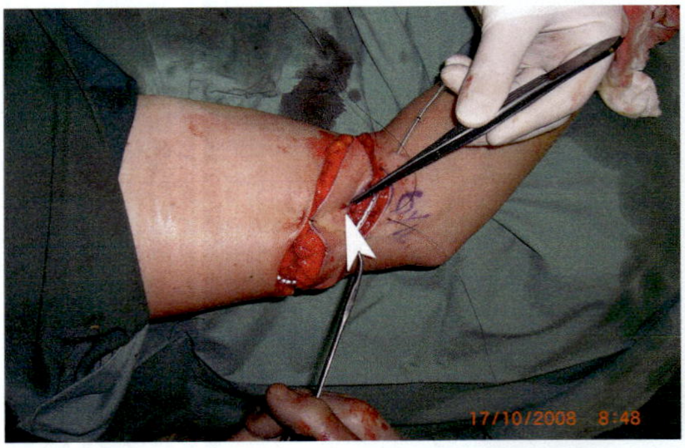

Fig. 4.23 Tensional closure is obvious with limited extension of R elbow. Note the Red Dot Sign (arrowed) confirms vascular integrity in spite of the restrictions of direct closure under tension. This technique breaks the obvious surgical rule of closure under tension but because there is random perforator circulatory support suprafascial and infrafascial avoiding dependence on the subdermal plexus. This maintains vascular integrity and minimises the possibility of necrosis

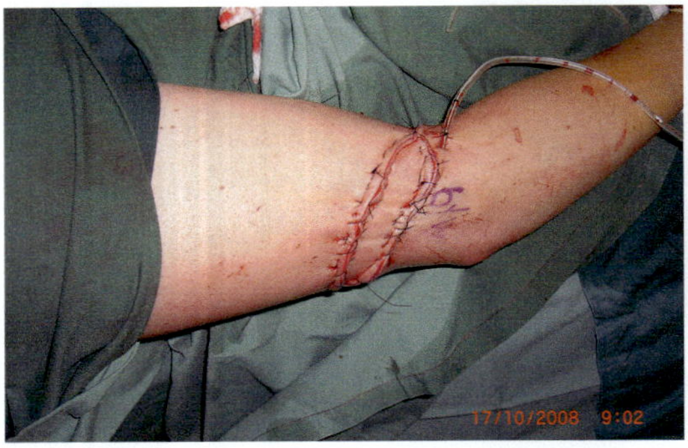

Fig. 4.24 The elbow had to be partially flexed to achieve closure intraoperatively and gradually brought into full extension as healing became stabilised. The 3-phase suture technique applies with these wounds closed under tension – locking mattress sutures along the convex and concave sides of the Keystone and further mattress for wound apposition and then a continuous nylon for epidermal seal. The 7, 14 and 21 day sequence is the wound dressing format for suture removal

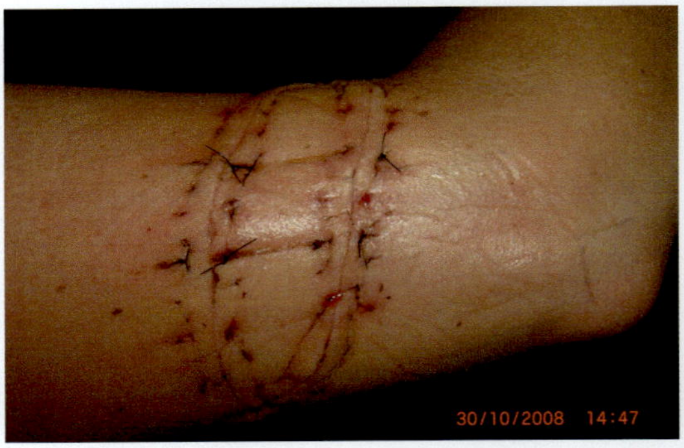

Fig. 4.25 The appearance at 2 weeks and the lines of tension are still evident because of the disorientation of the biopsy specimen. No necrosis evident

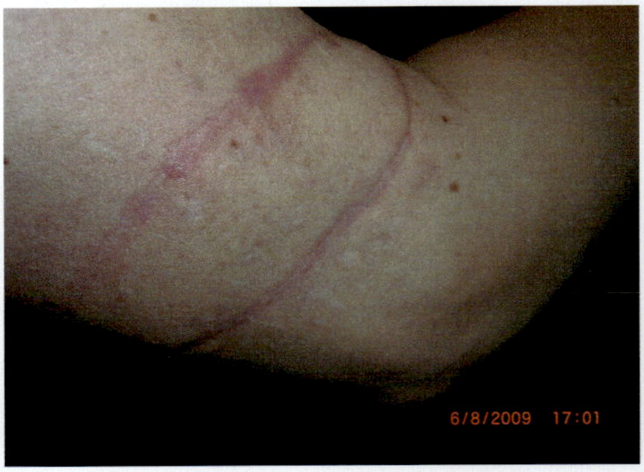

Fig. 4.26 Appearance at 10 months. The mildly hypertrophic scar reflects the closure under tension but acceptable to the patient and I repeat the P.A.C.E.S. acronym were all evident and such wound dressings should be done at the major clinic rather than left to an outside source

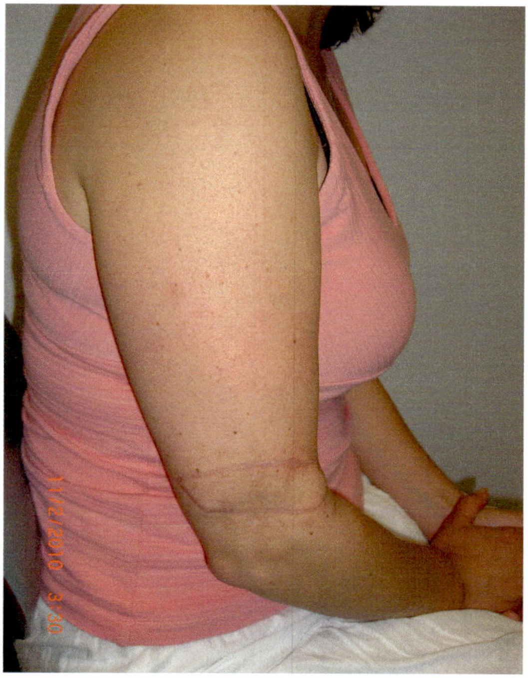

Fig. 4.27 Tumour-free interval 16 months

4.2.3 Case 43: Complicated Dorsum of the Hand Reconstruction – Poor Biopsy Orientation Again

Melanoma on the dorsum of the R hand at the base of the 2nd metacarpal. The biopsy Clark Level IV – 3 mm thick in a farmer's wife. The misorientation of the biopsy is the reason for a

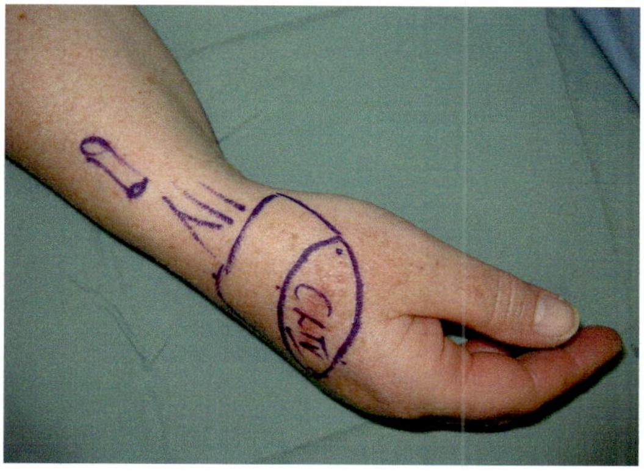

Fig. 4.28 The re-excisional mark out and the proximal Keystone sitting over the R anatomical snuff box. The neurovascular support of the radial cutaneous nerve and perforators through the anatomical snuff box are the basis for the random perforator support. Surgical caution around the radial cutaneous nerve will obviate any postoperative post traumatic sympathetic dystrophy if this nerve is damaged

difficult Keystone reconstruction (see Figs. 4.28, 4.29, 4.30, 4.31, 4.32, 4.32, 4.33, and 4.34).

Again, in summary, this biopsy orientation case which is circumferentially aligned at the wrist crease has been resolved by ensuring the integrity of loco-regional perforators, but more importantly in watching the cutaneous input from the radial cutaneous nerve which is always a source of chronic regional pain syndrome if damaged inadvertently.

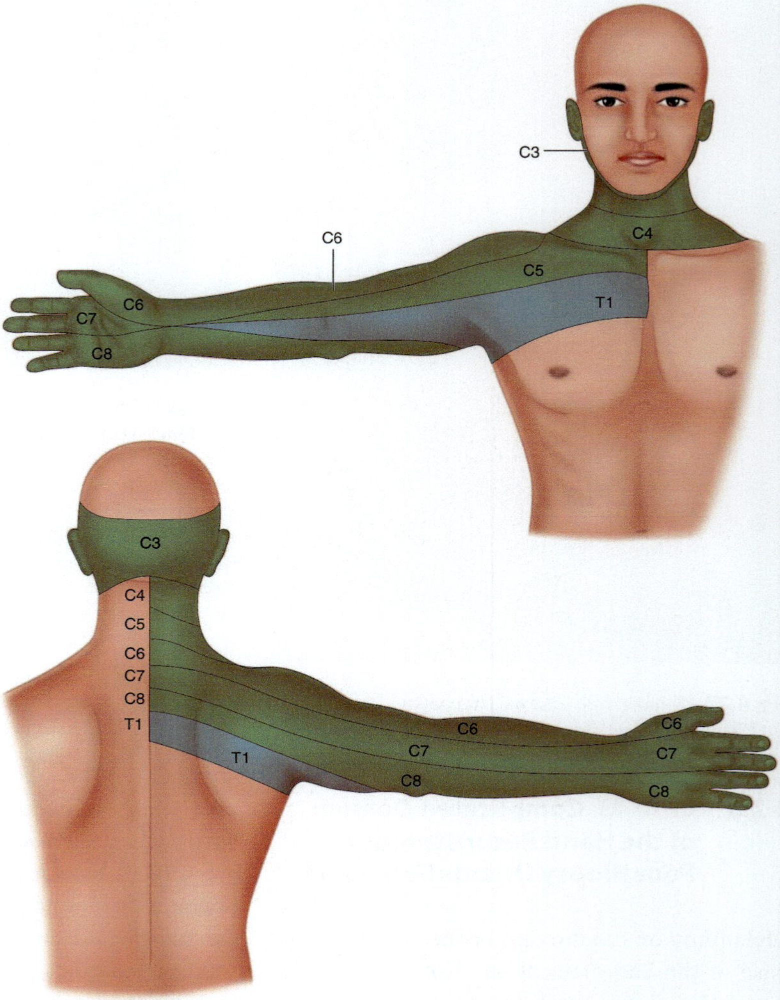

Fig. 4.29 The dermatomal mark out is the guide for the location of the random perforators coming through the fascia

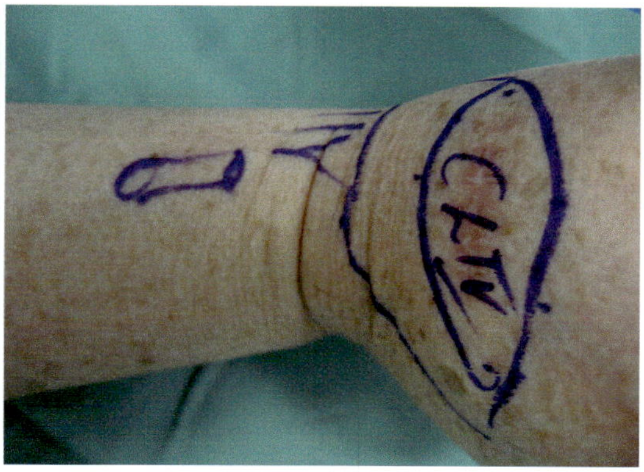

Fig. 4.30 The design of the circumferential Keystone is governed by the biopsy orientation. The wrist in extreme extension facilitates wound closure. The radial cutaneous nerve and the cephalic vein are part of the neurovascular support and the integrity of these structures must be maintained to avoid any chronic regional pain syndrome

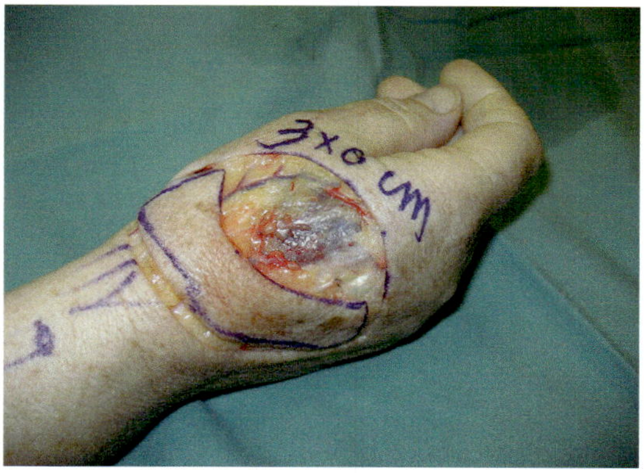

Fig. 4.31 The oncological defect 3 × 10 cm and the mark out of the proximal circumferential Keystone design to close the defect with exposure of the branches of the radial cutaneous nerve. Avoidance of neural damage is an absolute prerequisite in this closure under tension to avoid any potential chronic regional pain syndrome. The wrist in extension with radial deviation is the only method of achieving wound closure

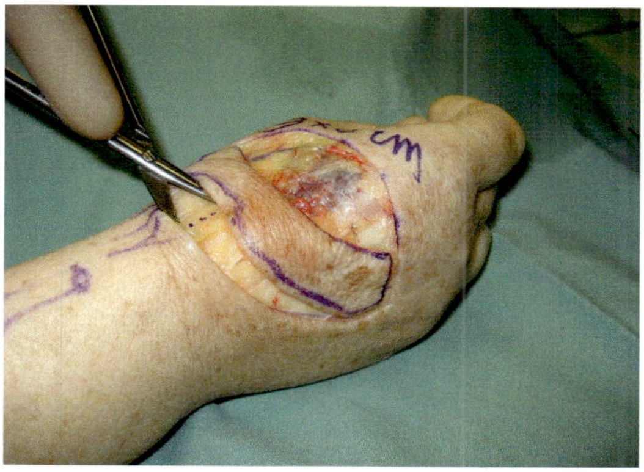

Fig. 4.32 The blunt dissection technique to help mobilisation of the Keystone, again avoiding neural damage. This technique loosens the subcutaneous communications without undermining using the open scissors to detach the underlying structures longitudinally and this facilitates closure

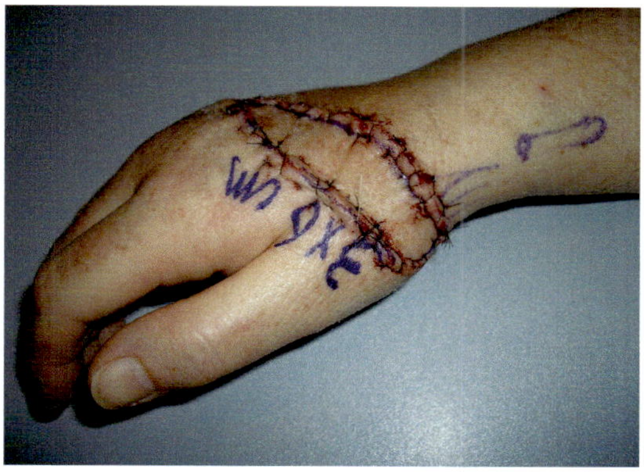

Fig. 4.33 The appearance at 7 days. The hyperaemic flare is evident and settling. The swelling of the thumb and hand is resolving and the patient is totally pain free

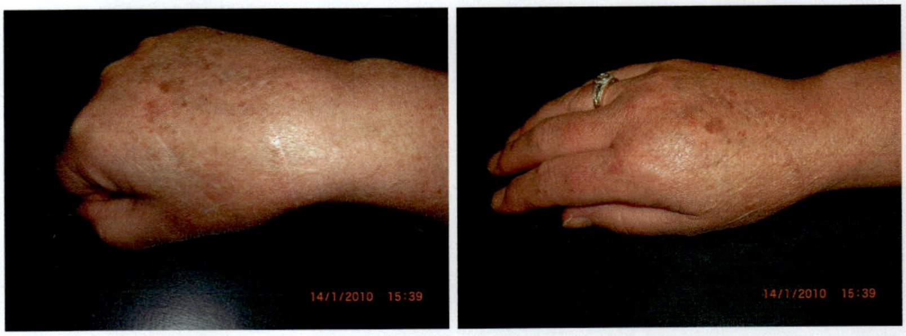

Fig. 4.34 Tumour-free interval is 3.5 years at the time of this image. There is a full range of normal pain free movement of the R wrist in this farmer's wife who was still milking cows. The P.A.C.E.S. characteristics were all exemplified

4.2.4 Case 44: Palmar Melanoma at the Wrist Crease

Clark Level II 0.4 mm melanoma of the ulnar side of the R palm wrist crease area in a 35 year old (see Figs. 4.35, 4.36, 4.37, 4.38, and 4.39).

In summary, a simple method of closing defects of the palmar tissue basically using the laxity of tissue in the wrist crease area.

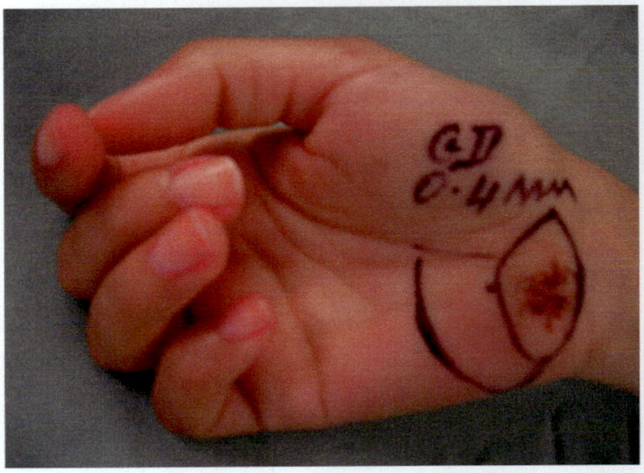

Fig. 4.35 The excisional defect is marked out at the ulnar border with the distally based Keystone based on random perforators in the base of the hypo thenar eminence

4.2.5 Case 45: Digital Sub-Ungual Melanoma

Sub-ungual melanoma of the L thumb on the cleft side (medial) over the distal phalanx closed

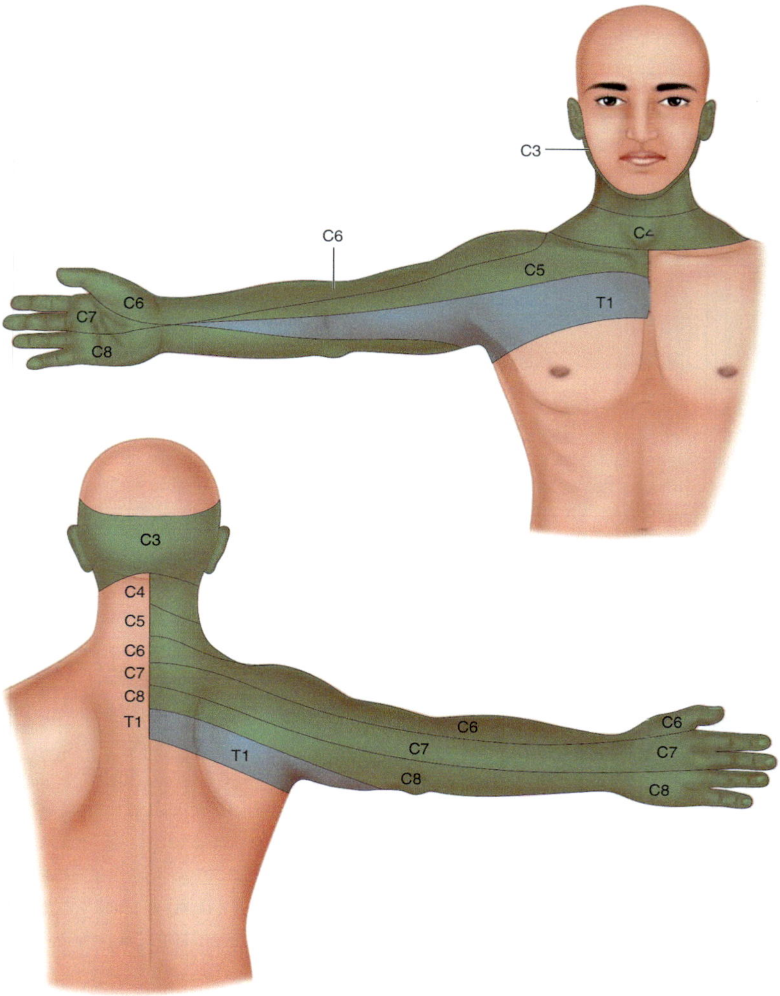

Fig. 4.36 The dermatomal mark out is the guide for the location of the random perforators coming through the fascia

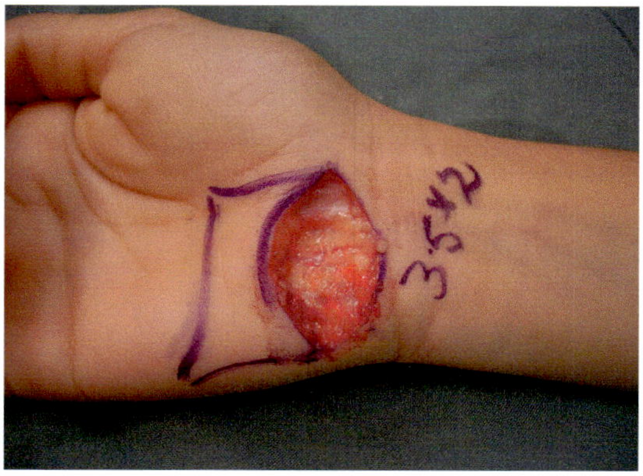

Fig. 4.37 The excisional defect 3.5 × 2 cm with the mark out of the distally based Keystone in the vicinity of the mid palmar crease to the ulnar border overlying the hypo thenar muscular elements, the source of blood supply

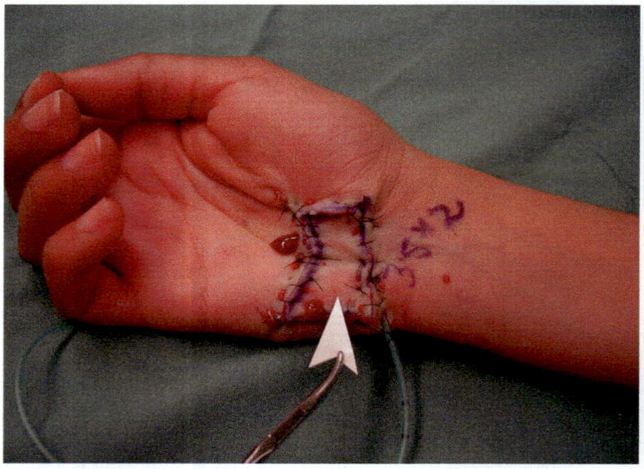

Fig. 4.38 Note the clinical findings with closure. The forearm integument has stretched down and there is only one longitudenal line of tension. Note the differential of vascular return on release of torniquet with the arrow indicating the increased vascular perfusion in the region of the ulnar styloid and this hyperaemic effect is more noticeable than that of the radial aspect of the Keystone. However, all flow reverts to normal within 24 h

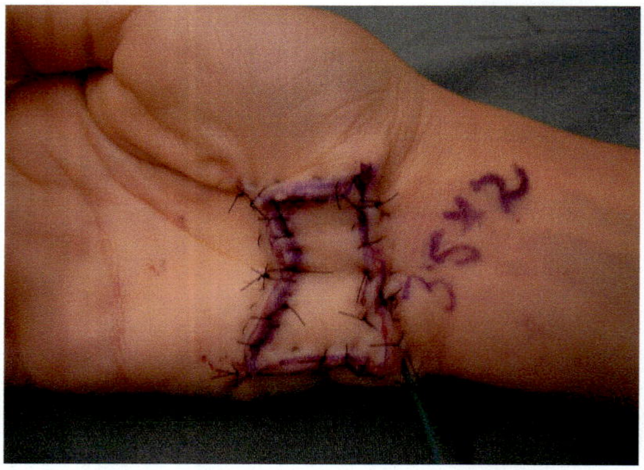

Fig. 4.39 The appearance days later confirming all the P.A.C.E.S. characteristics. The alternative of a skin graft defect here and weeks of dressings and the inconvenience of other biological social necessities are all eliminated by the Keystone technique, particularly pain free initially before somatic sensation occurs as in all surgical wounds

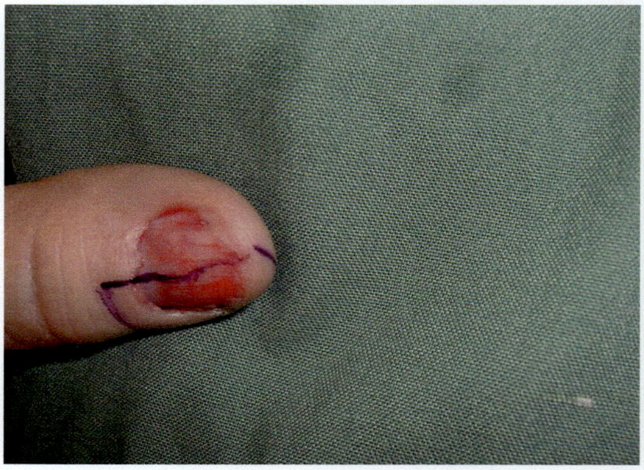

Fig. 4.40 The surgical excision of the radial side of the distal phalanx of the L thumb including the subcutaneous tissue proximally to the germinal matrix down to bone of the distal phalanx

with a neurovascular Littler island flap based on palmar digital circulation. Tensional closure of Keystones in the vicinity of any digit is totally contraindicted. Thus, grafting the secondary defect is an absolute prerequisite. This is because any tensional closure of Keystone alignment may cause complicated digital vessel perfusion and ultimately necrosis unless a graft is used in the secondary defect. In this case here, the Littler [1] neurovascular island flap is an excellent reconstructive tool hence the reason for its inclusion (see Figs. 4.40, 4.41, 4.42, 4.43, 4.44, 4.45, 4.46, and 4.47).

In summary, this is an acceptable aesthetic outcome. The smooth skin outline and functional normality in the use of the thumb which we know relates to 40% of the function of the hand. After 40 years of hand surgery and fingertip reconstruction, this is the basic prinicple used for easy surgical closure without delayed skin grafting.

Fig. 4.41 The dermatomal mark out is the guide for the location of the random perforators coming through the fascia

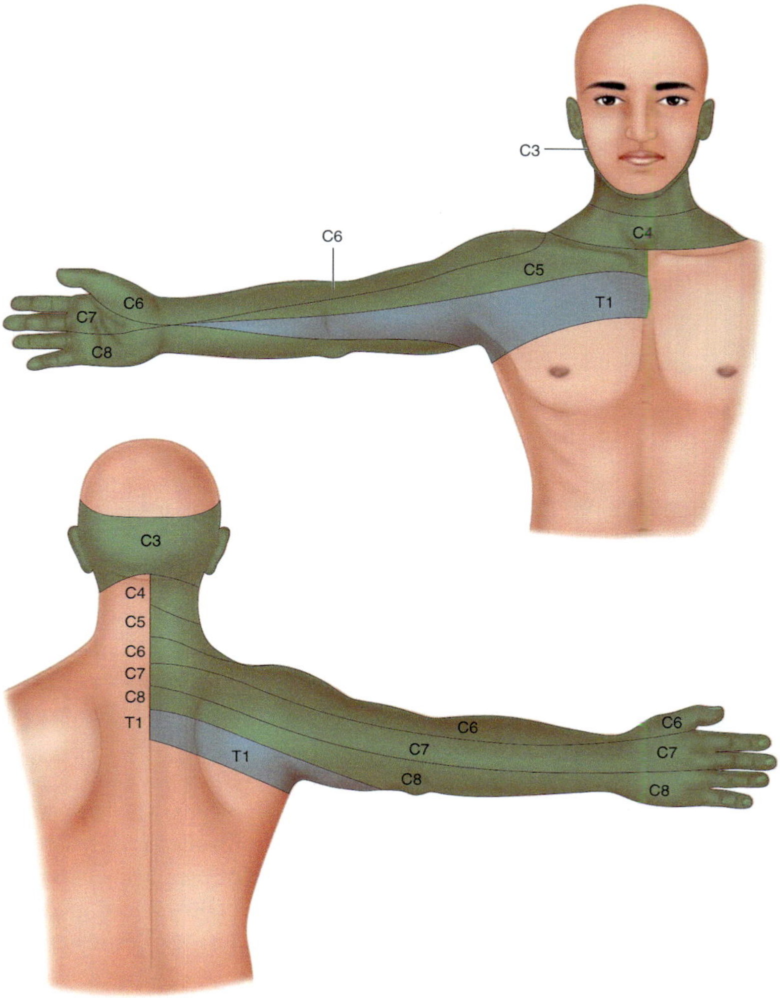

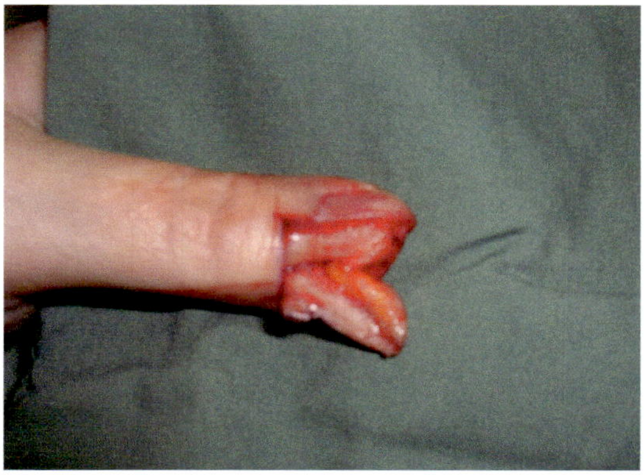

Fig. 4.42 The surgical site and the radial neurovascular Littler island flap transposed dorsally after the division of Cleelands and Graysons ligaments to allow release and dorsal alignment and insertion

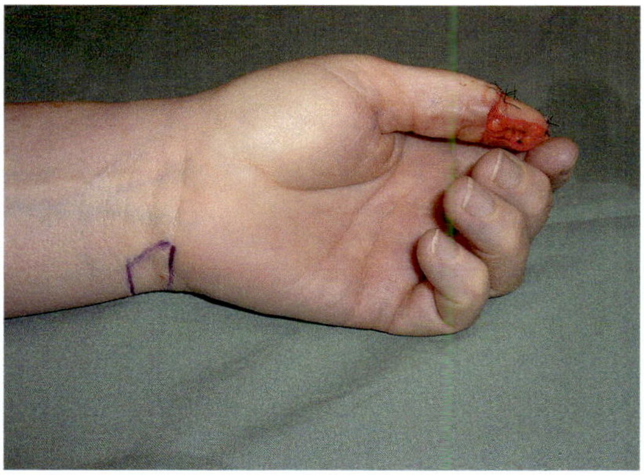

Fig. 4.43 A handy site for skin graft for hand reconstruction is the lax tissue of the wrist crease. A rhomboid full thickness graft which is fenestrated is an excellent means of harvesting to achieve repair provided fenestrating holes are inserted and the need for a tie over dressing for the graft is eliminated, again avoiding tension

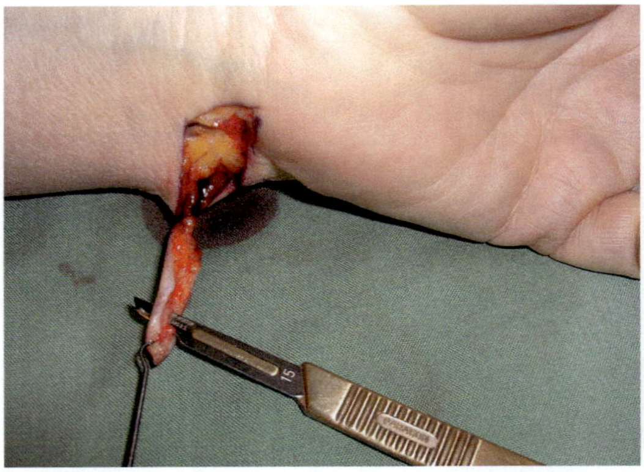

Fig. 4.44 Fenestrated full thickness graft using a number 15 blade

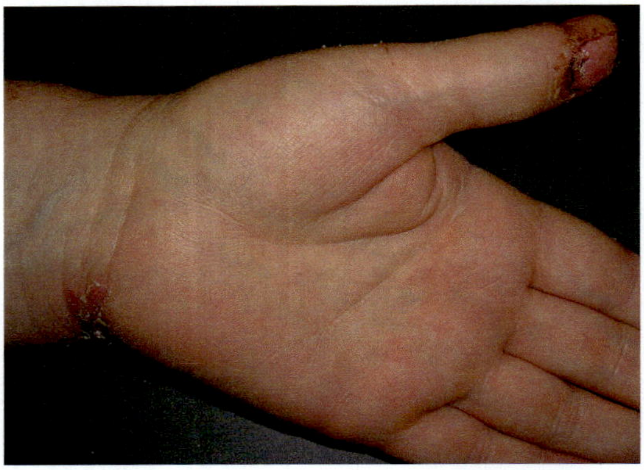

Fig. 4.45 The healed donor site and the healed thumb. Scars are indiscernible

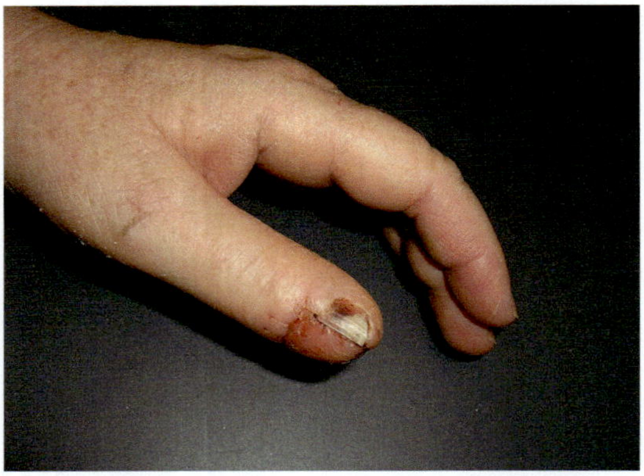

Fig. 4.46 The healed thumb and an acceptable aesthetic outcome

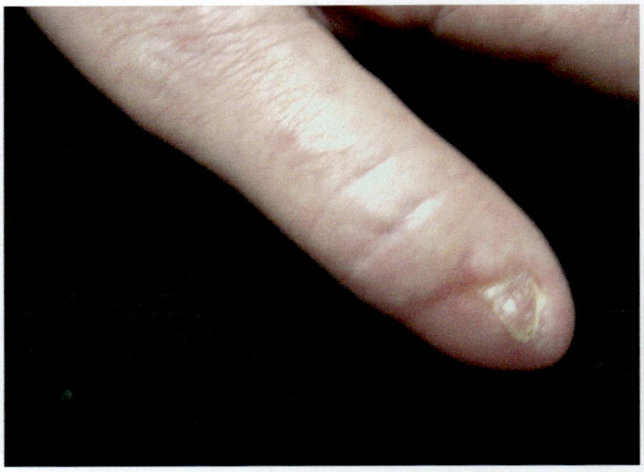

Fig. 4.47 A postoperative appearance of a successful neurovascular island flap (Littler) based on the radial neurovascular bundle and advanced over the tip covering the bone. This follows oncological excision and produces a sensate flap along the radial side to advance to the tip with the secondary defect over the interphalangeal joint closed with a fenestrated full thickness graft

4.3 Is Pregnancy a Contraindication?

Clark level IV 4.5 mm melanoma of the inner biceps. This Keystone repair site above the elbow resulted in a hypertrophic scar reflecting her state of pregnancy at 6 months. Consequently, the use of Keystones in pregnancy where tensional closure applies is best avoided (see Fig. 4.48).

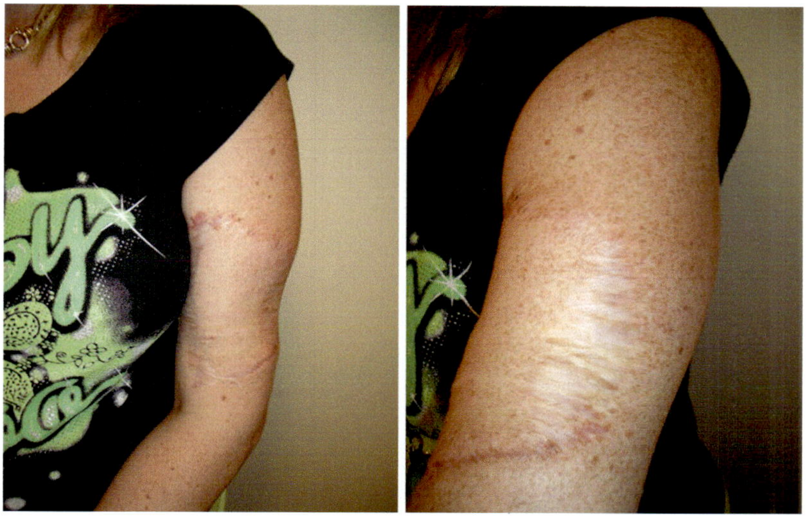

Fig. 4.48 The closure under tension in the medial bicipital region left stretch marks in this pregnant patient. The patient subsequently died of terminal malignancy. Where or not the pregnancy had an effect of dissemination of the melanoma remains indeterminate

4.4 Keystone Flap to Salvage a Wound Breakdown by Another Unit

Clark level IV deltoid melanoma in a 65 year old excised and closed directly by another unit leading to wound breakdown. Primary Keystone salvage repair (see Figs. 4.49 and 4.50).

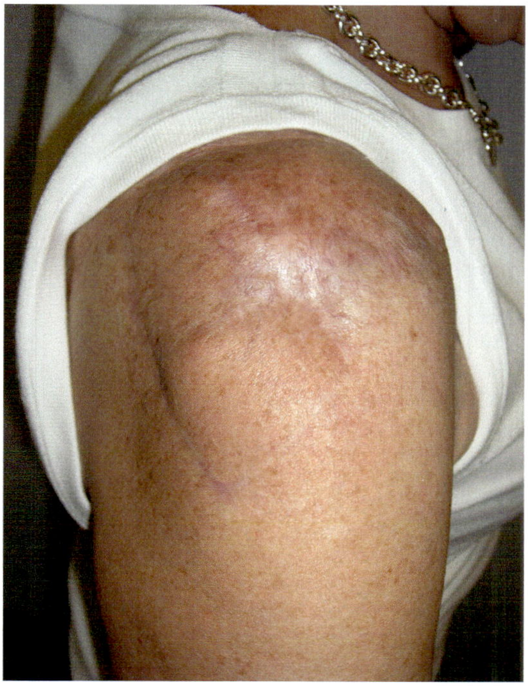

Fig. 4.49 Finally healed after reconstruction with the Keystone producing a satisfactory outccme eventually

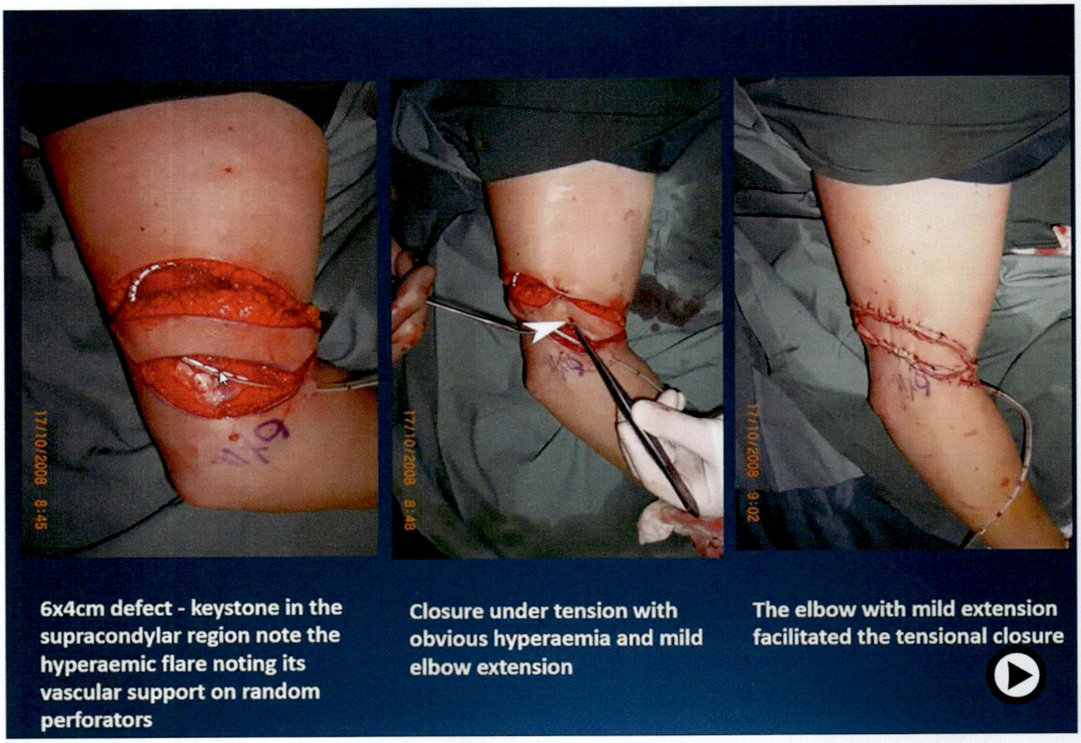

Fig. 4.50 Upper limb Atlas (▶ https://doi.org/10.1007/000-b5w)

Reference

1. Littler JW. The neurovascular pedicle method of digital transposition for reconstruction of the thumb. Plast Reconstr Surg. 1946;12:303–19.

Lower Limb Defects Using the Keystone Technique

5

Contents

Supplementary Information The online version contains supplementary material available at https://doi.org/10.1007/978-3-031-39868-1_5. The videos can be accessed individually by clicking the DOI link in the accompanying figure caption or by scanning this link with the SN More Media App.

F. Behan, *Atlas of Keystone Reconstructive Technique in Melanoma Management*,
https://doi.org/10.1007/978-3-031-39868-1_5

5.1 Case Presentations

5.1.1 Case 46 : Hutchinson's Melanotic Freckle L Calf Below the Hemline – The Ultimate Aesthetic Outcome with Oncological Clearance

Clark Level I, defect 5 × 8 cm. This is a prime example of an aesthetic closure and oncological clearnace for an Hutchinson's melanotic freckle/ melanoma of the L calf (see Figs. 5.1, 5.2, 5.3, 5.4, 5.5, 5.6, 5.7, 5.8, and 5.9).

In summary, an excellent outcome for a classic Keystone repair of the lateral calf illustrating all the P.A.C.E.S. characteristics.

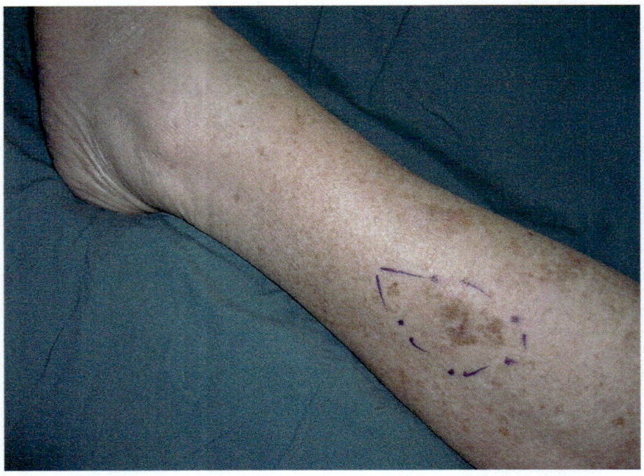

Fig. 5.1 The mark out of the L calf lesion

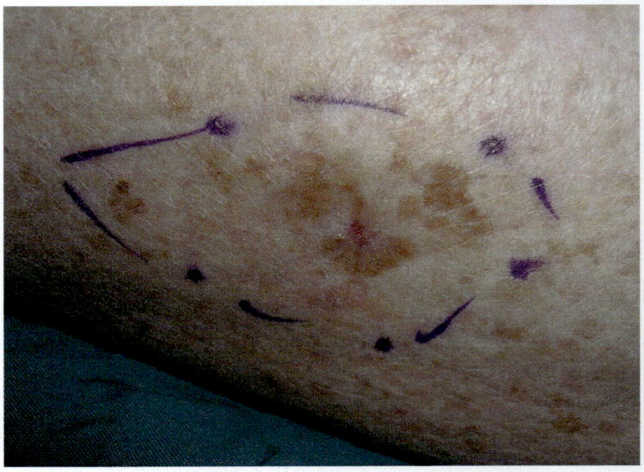

Fig. 5.2 Close-up of the Hutchinson's melanotic freckle/ L1 melanoma

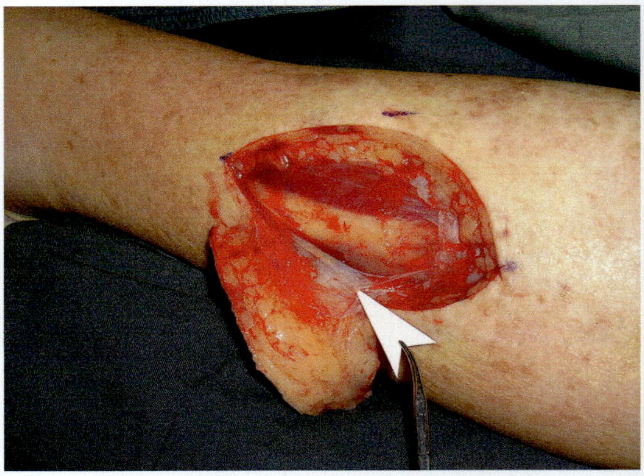

Fig. 5.3 Excision in progress including the deep fascia (arrowed) and muscles of the peroneal compartment are evident in the depths of the wound

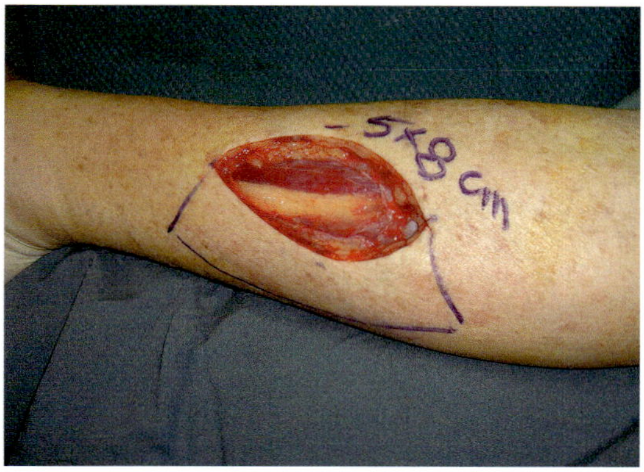

Fig. 5.4 The melanotic defect and the laterally based Keystone sited over the soft muscles of the lateral calf. Whereas to do a Keystone along the medial side encroaches on the anterior tibial tissues and the laxity for closure is not possible and may lead to adverse outcomes. Here the number of random perforators would certainly be sparse, and the softness of the muscles of the calf and compressibility when based laterally facilitates appositional closure, even under tension

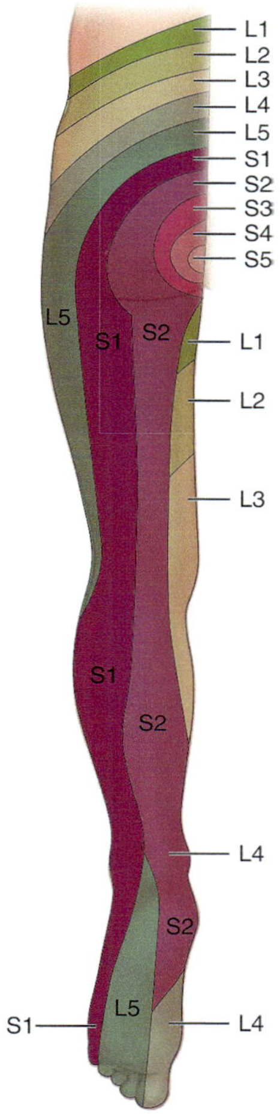

Fig. 5.5 The dermatomal mark out is the guide for the location of the random perforators coming through the fascia

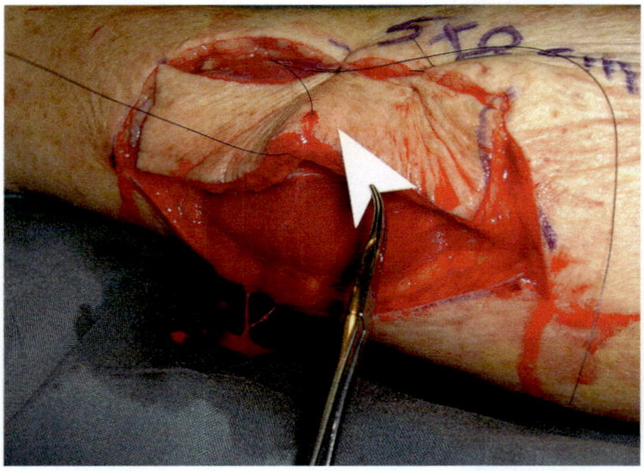

Fig. 5.6 Using the 3-phase single layer closure technique using locking mattress sutures × 3 per side placed intermittently along the concave and the convex sides of the flap

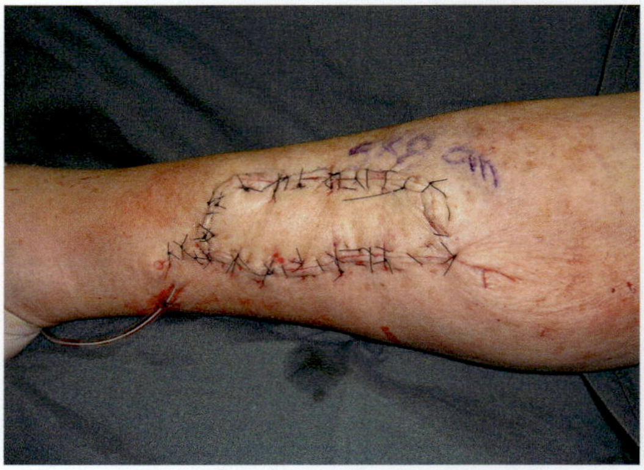

Fig. 5.7 On completion using the 3-phase nylon suture technique of closure. The vascular dynamics show the hyperaemic flare and the aesthetic contour has been retained in the calf. All wounds are Redi-vac drained with a single tubing in a u-shaped manner to drain both sites

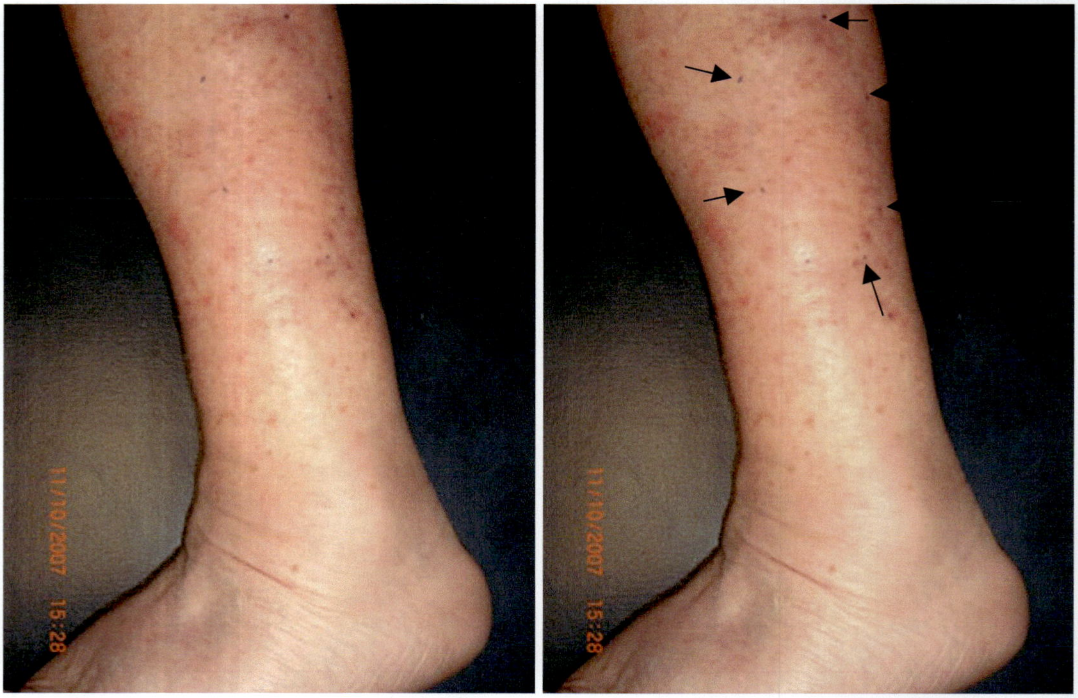

Fig. 5.8 The indiscernible scarring of the calf in spite of closing under tension if this 3-phase suture technique is adopted for insertion and removal. There are no cross-hatch marks and the outcome has the added bonus in the female that the options of clothing are not restrictive

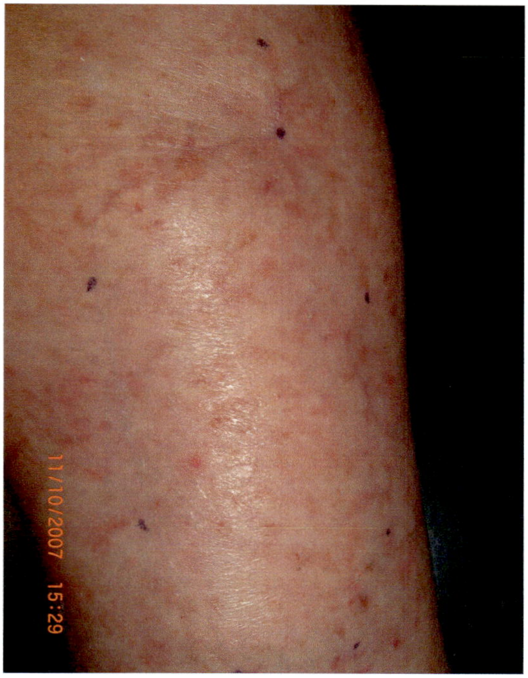

Fig. 5.9 A close-up view of the satisfactory outcome of the indiscernible scar line defined. Blue dots around the limit have had to be added to confirm its integrity and aesthetic outcome

5.1.2 Case 47: Postoperative Appearance of the R Lateral Calf

Melanoma Clark Level II 0.6 mm of the R lateral calf. A 14-year postoperative appearance in a 47-year-old female golfer (see Fig. 5.10).

In summary, this same patient wanted the same aesthetic outcome for her cheek which we achieved in her calf using the Keystone principle. The closure using the 3-phase suture technique and the 3 week removal of sutures has achieved an excellent match compared with the excision defect on her calf [1].

5.1.3 Case 48: Postoperative Appearance of the L Cheek

See Figs. 5.11 and 5.12

All the P.A.C.E.S. characteristics were exemplified.

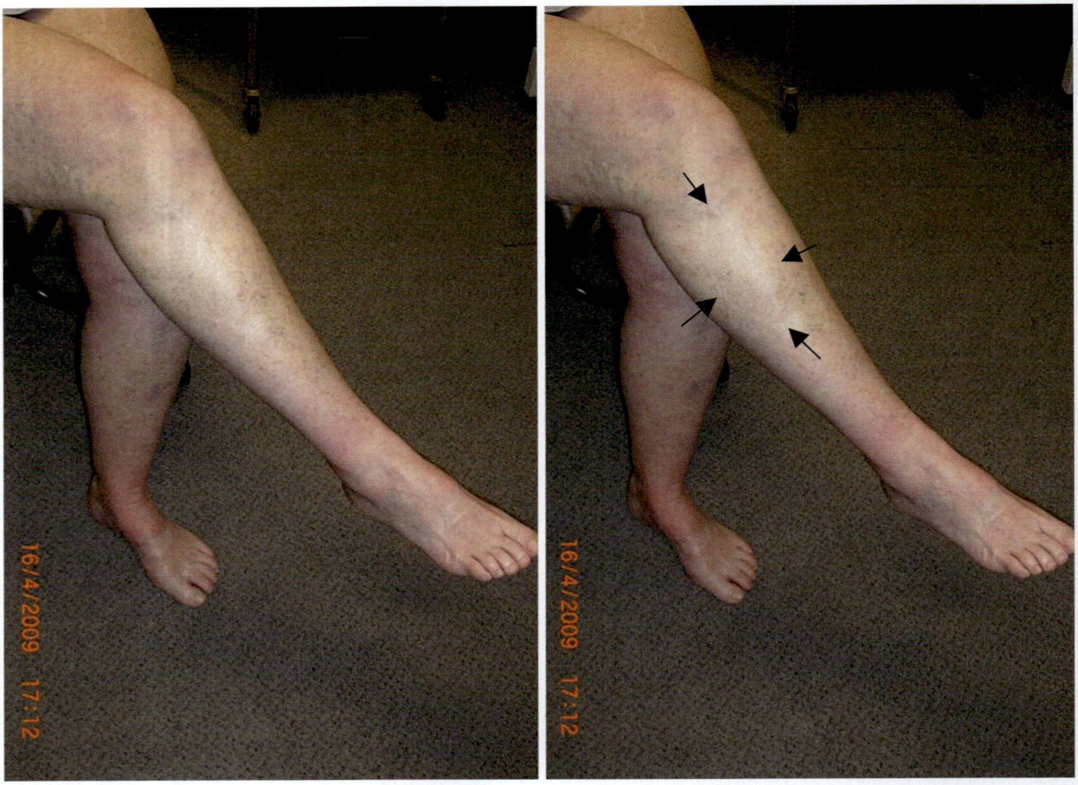

Fig. 5.10 The scars are indiscernible. The single layer 3-phase closure technique is used throughout and there are no restrictions on the type of clothing she chooses to wear – a social relief. The patient was so grateful for the Keystone results on her face in case 48 indicating how she appreciated the refinements of the Keystone technique

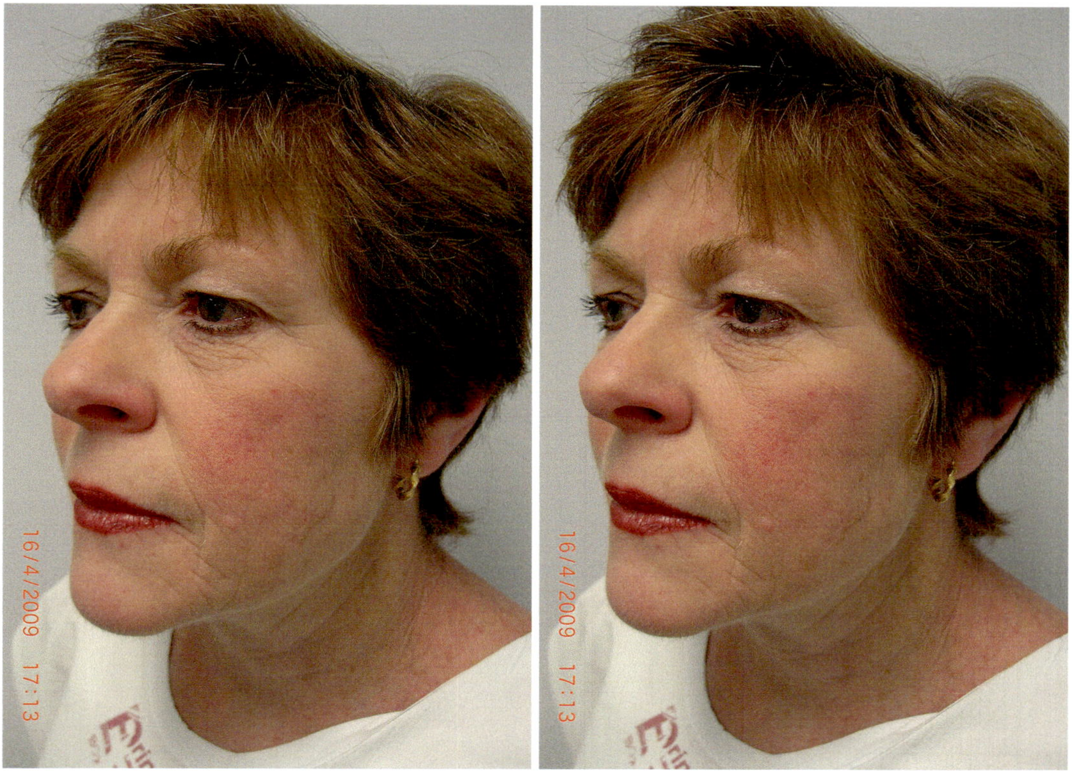

Fig. 5.11 Melanoma L cheek in a Hutchinson's melanotic freckle. Clark Level II with a Keystone closure

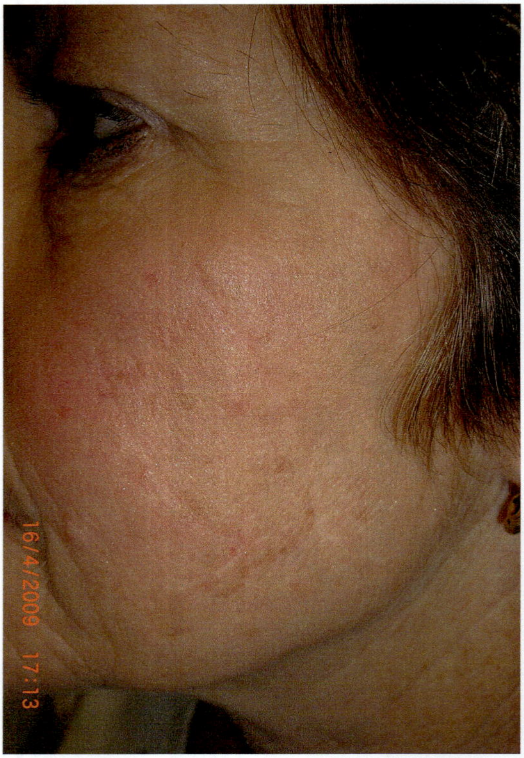

Fig. 5.12 Aesthetic outcome

5.1.4 Case 49: a Difficult Site for Reconstruction over the Tendo Achilles

Melanoma tendo achilles Clark Level IV 0.86 mm depth with a superficial spreading component (see Figs. 5.13, 5.14, 5.15, 5.16, 5.17, 5.18, 5.19, and 5.20).

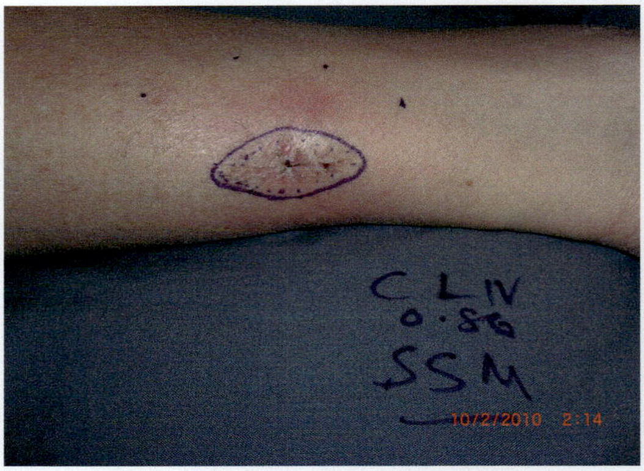

Fig. 5.13 The excisional defect marked out

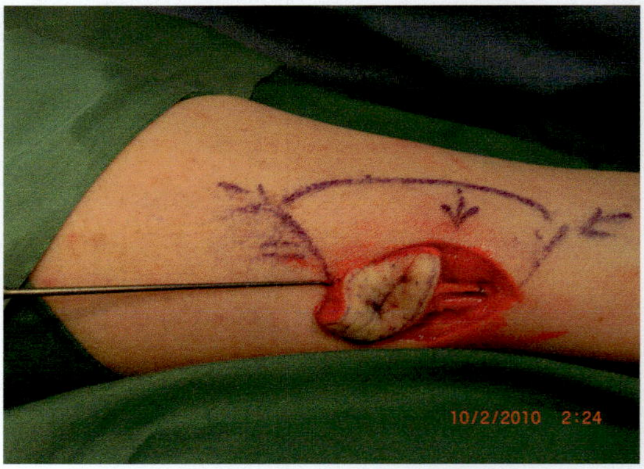

Fig. 5.14 Staged excision of the lesion. The Keystone mark out from the loose tissue side (peroneal compartment of the lower calf)

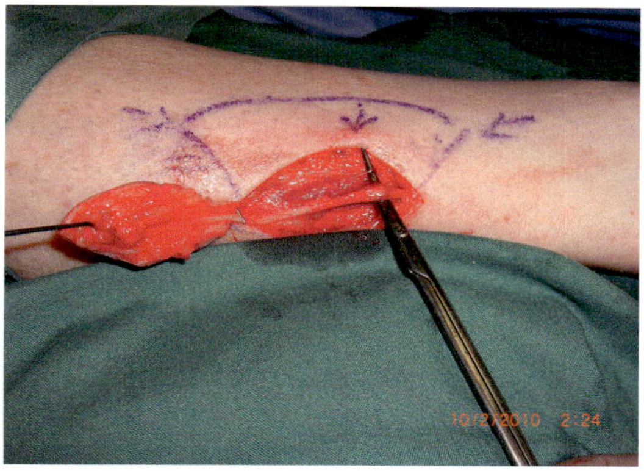

Fig. 5.15 Preserving the integrity of the neurovascular structures – sural nerve retracted

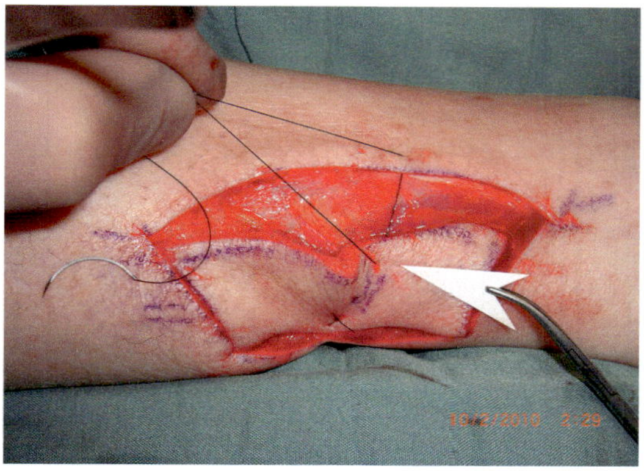

Fig. 5.16 Staged reconstruction and the use of locking mattress suture technique at the center of the convex and concave arcs

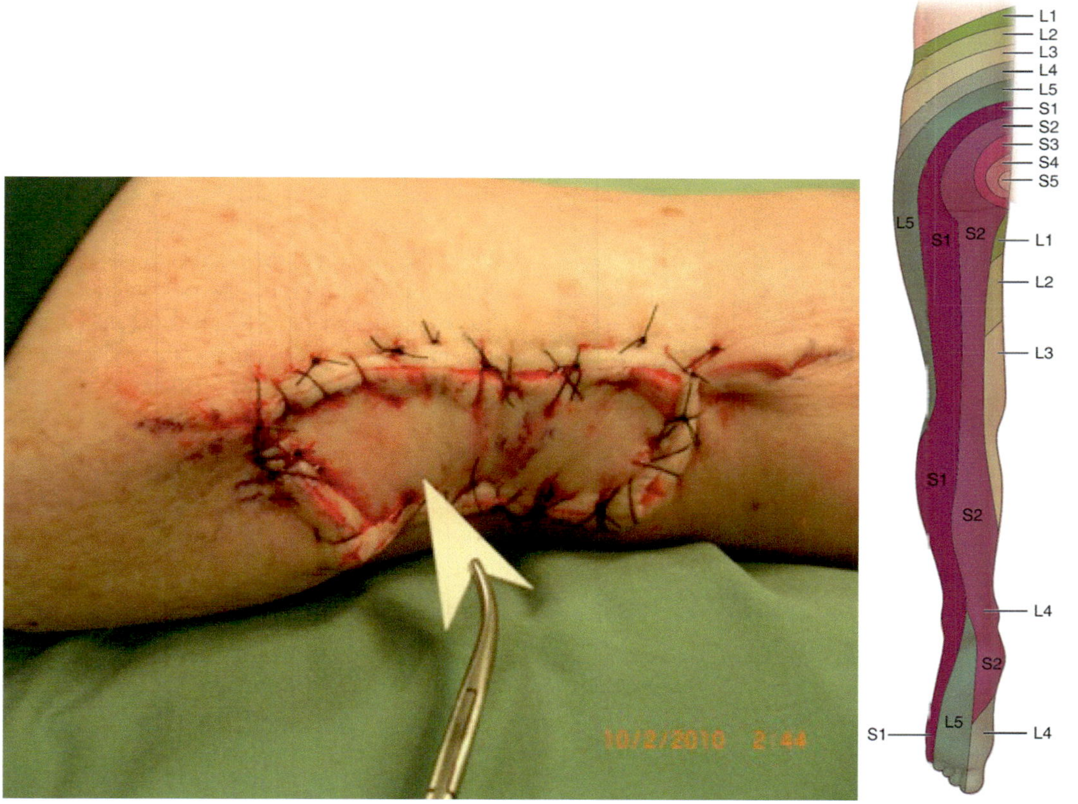

Fig. 5.17 On the release of torniquet and the hyperaemia is noted in the inferior aspect of the Keystone wound preferentially superior to that of the other aspects of the Keystone aligned along the S1, S2 dermatomes before the Keystone becomes universalised and hyperaemic

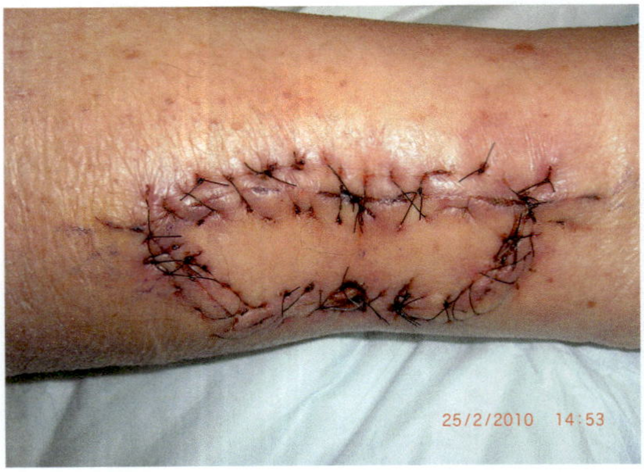

Fig. 5.18 The somewhat grotesque appearance settles down over the next 2–3 weeks. This image taken at approximately 2 weeks before wound dressing starts which consists of cutting the continuous loop and leave in situ, take out some of the mattress sutures that do not cause any bleeding and the tension locking sutures stay in 3 weeks plus

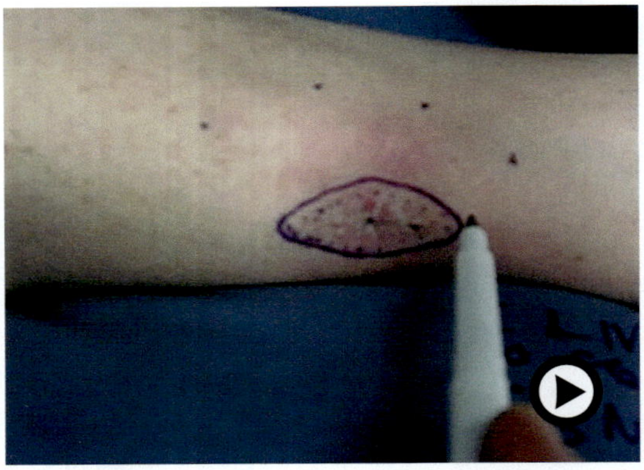

Fig. 5.19 Operative sequence (▶ https://doi.org/10.1007/000-b6a)

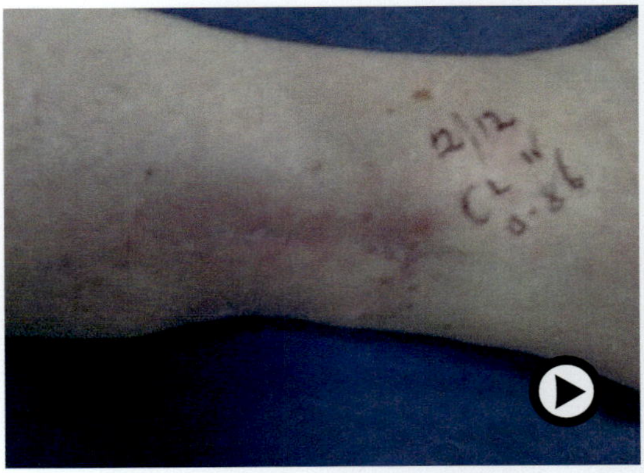

Fig. 5.20 Postoperative 2 months – patient perspective (▶ https://doi.org/10.1007/000-b5y)

5.1.5 Case 50: Lateral Lower Limb Melanoma in an 88 Year Old with a 6 × 6 cm Defect

Melanoma R antero-lateral tibial region Clark level IV 0.6 mm in an 88-year-old female (see Figs. 5.21, 5.22, 5.23, 5.24, 5.25, and 5.26).

In summary, a standard rotation advancement island flap that is two thirds undermined, fascial lined in the proximal one third is the site of deep attachment. Grafting of the secondary defect achieved an acceptable aesthetic outcome. This is too tight an area to do direct closure hence the need for insertional graft manouevre because there is no soft tissue of muscle bellies to compress just above the ankle.

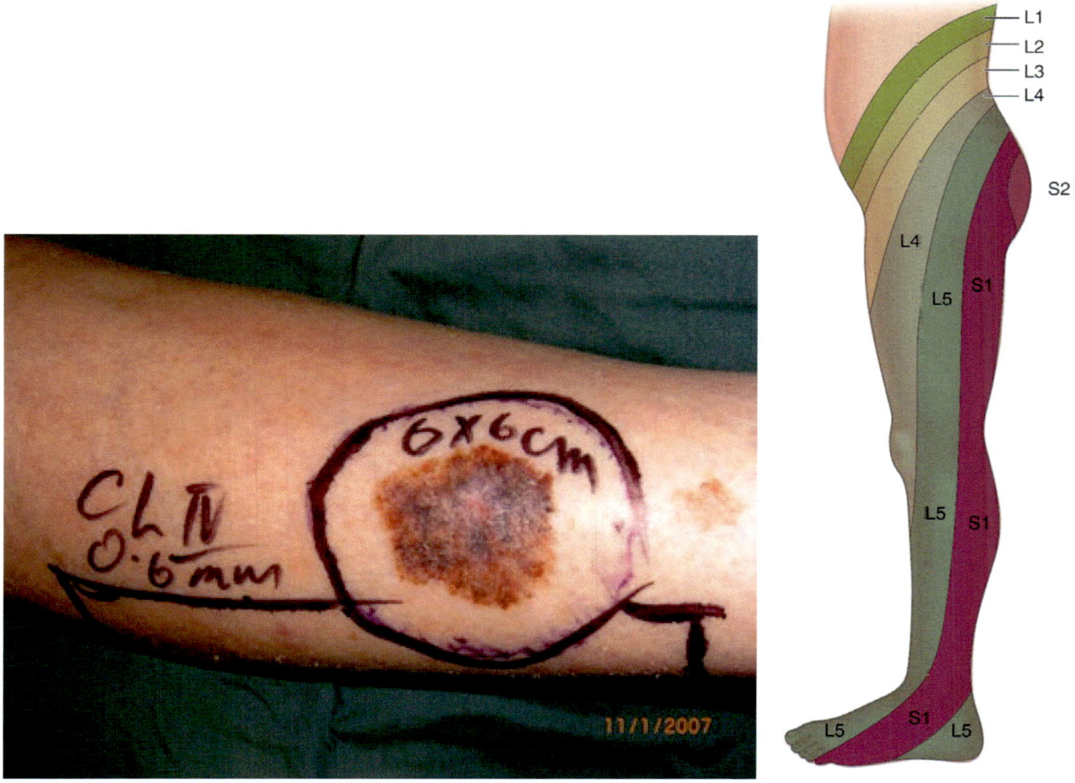

Fig. 5.21 The Keystone mark out overlies the S1 dermatome to incorporate random perforators in the lateral aspect lower third of the R lower limb with a 2 cm macro clearance

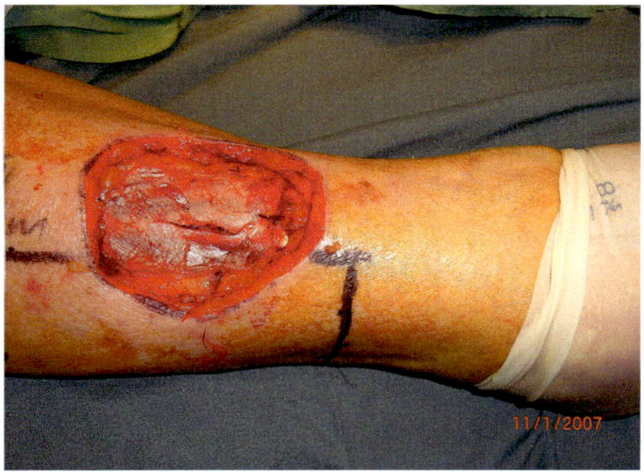

Fig. 5.22 The excisional defect and the mark out of the S1 dermatome Keystone. I bring to your attention a simple technique of a sterile glove over the foot as an attempt to optimise wound sterility in an area hard to prep. When I was in France showing them the Keystone principles with Jack Baudet's unit in Bordeaux, they were totally unaware of this simple manoeuvre

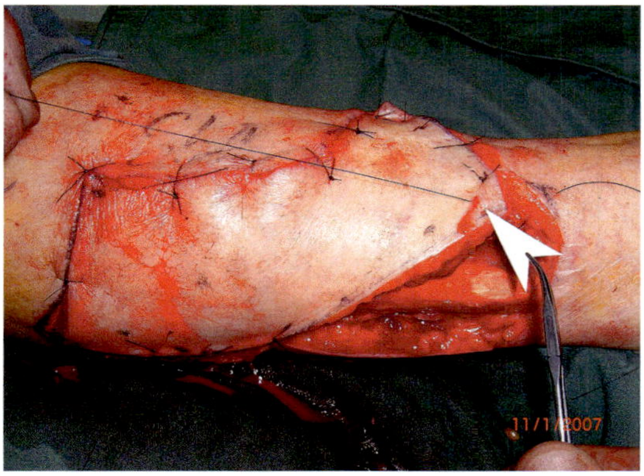

Fig. 5.23 The advancement, rotation and transposition of the Keystone flap. The arrow indicates the Red Dot Sign, a reflection of the hyperaemia throughout the flap which is hypothesised as being possibly a sympathectomy effect from cutting the dermis with an element of hydrostatic restriction of the subdermal plexus due to the island incisional mark out

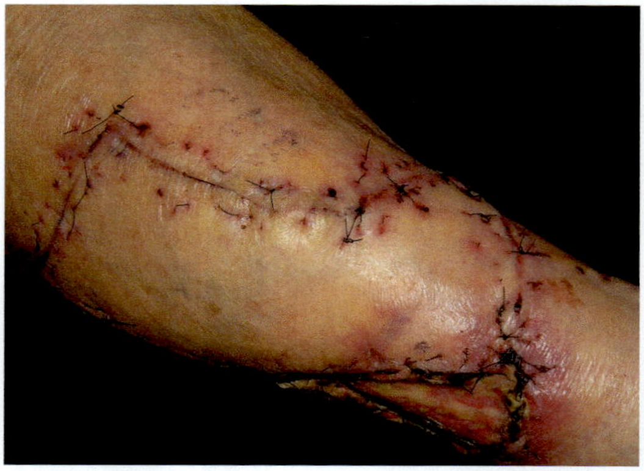

Fig. 5.24 Progress healing at 3 weeks. The 3-phase suture technique has been applied with some removal completed and the healing skin graft avoided any tensional apposition

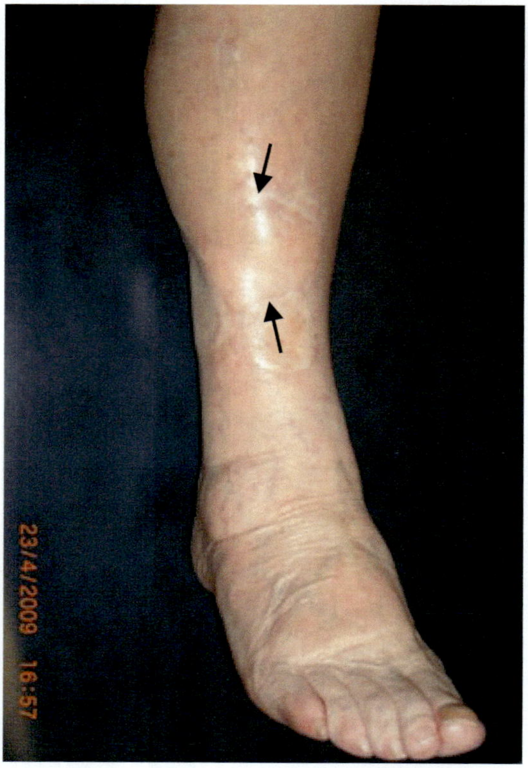

Fig. 5.25 The surgical appearance and outcome after 2 years confirming the P.A.C.E.S. characteristics again. The arrows indicate the surgical margins of the Keystone and the excellent wound healing by this everting nylon suture which puts the dermis in apposition and aligns the epidermis. An aesthetic outcome – the basis of a good wound appearance

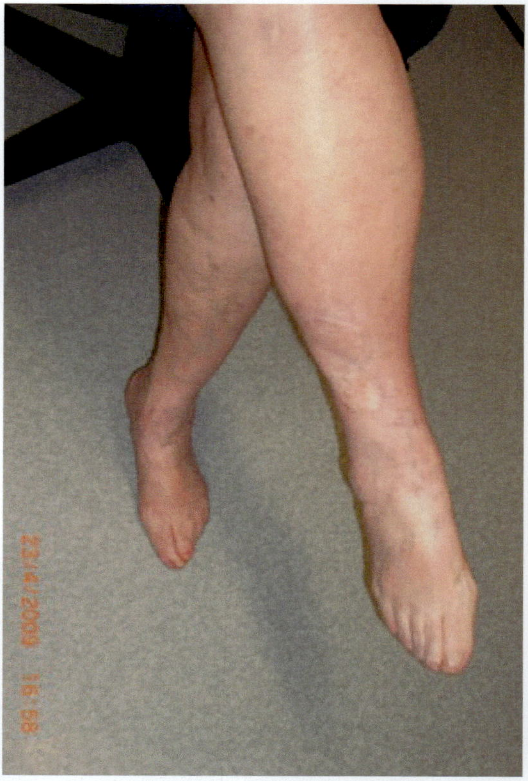

Fig. 5.26 Tumour-free interval of 2 years

5.1.6 Case 51: Melanoma Tendo Achilles Site

Melanoma L tendo achilles Clark level IV 1 mm depth (see Figs. 5.27, 5.28, 5.29, 5.30, 5.31, 5.32).

In summary, once one goes beyond the soft muscle complex of the calf muscles, closure of the secondary defect under tension must be done

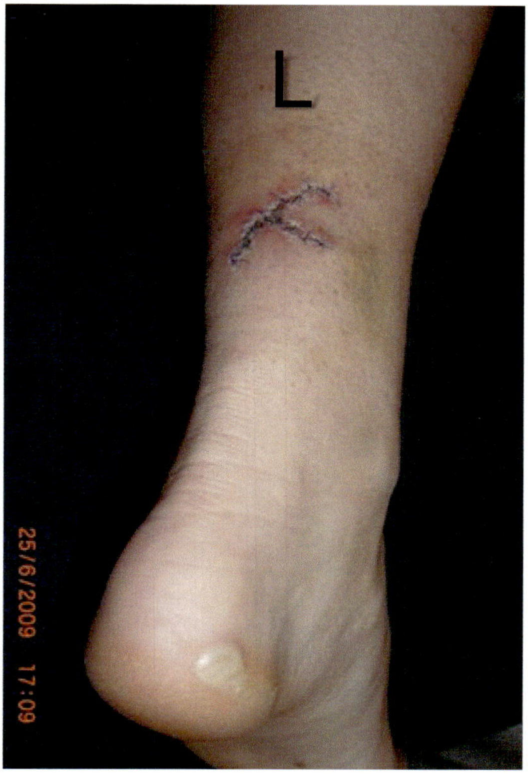

Fig. 5.27 Showing the biopsy site

in association with split skin grafting because tendons are not compressible and will lead to subclinical necrosis, particularly in the diabetic. All P.A.C.E.S. characteristics were all exemplified and the most painful site was the donor site for the skin graft from the contralateral thigh – why – all melanoma skin grafts must be taken from the contralateral thigh as it has been recorded clinically in the past that diseminating melanoma has been known to occur and pepper the donor site on the ipsilateral leg and that is why it is necessary to always use the contralateral thigh – written up in the British Journal of Plastic Surgery [2].

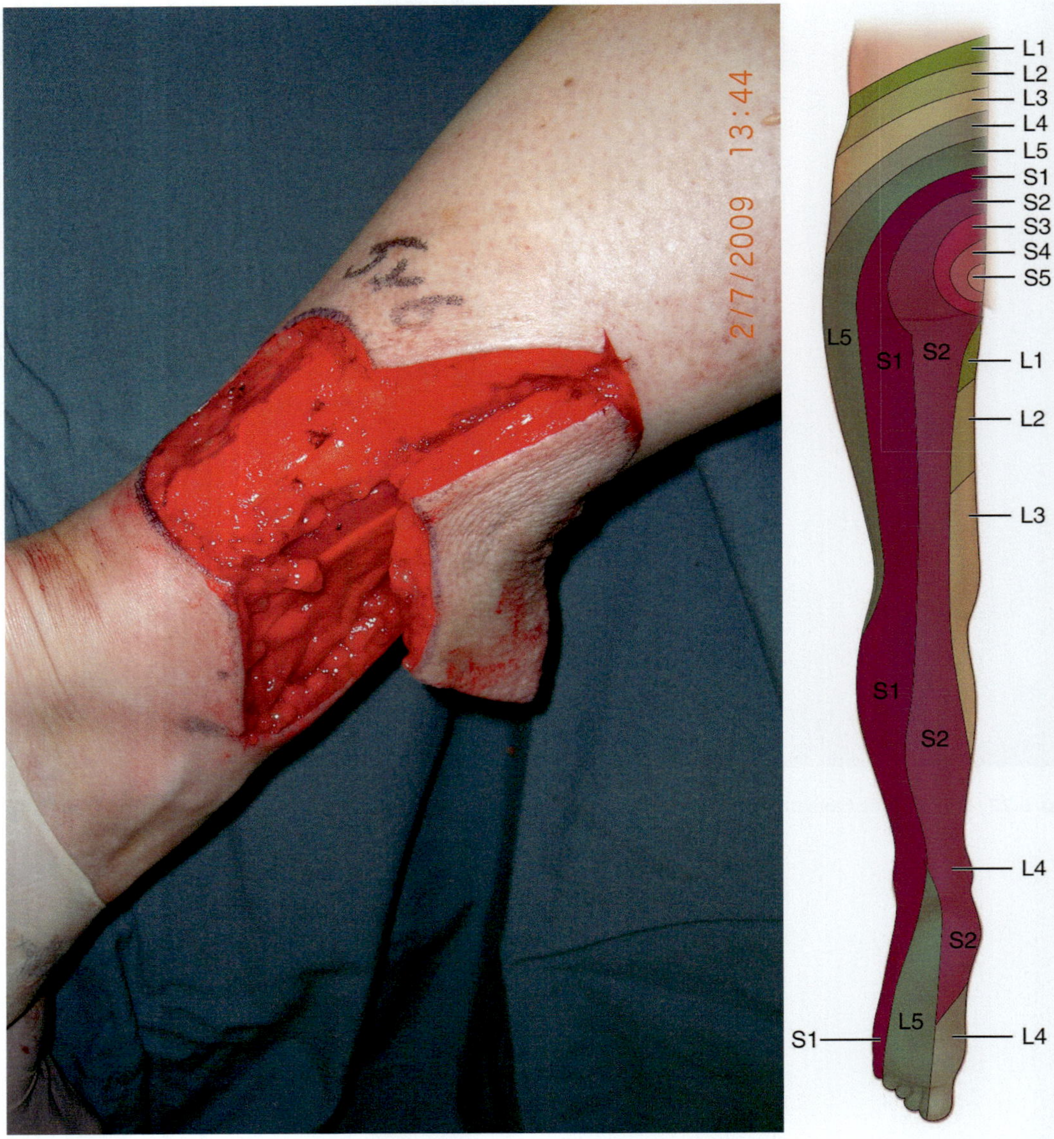

Fig. 5.28 The 5 × 6 cm surgical defect site is closed with the Keystone along the S2 dermatome based on random perforators relying on a fascial base

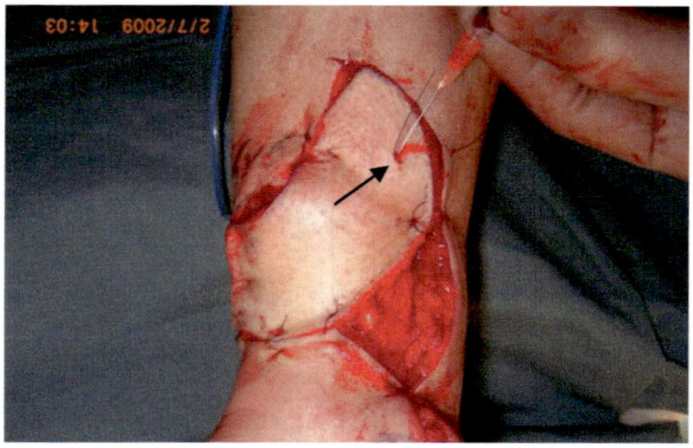

Fig. 5.29 The closure of the defect over the tendo achilles and the Red Dot Sign consistent with the hyperaemic development (arrowed) and the secondary defect is to be grafted because the tightness is too severe over tendons to attempt to achieve closure

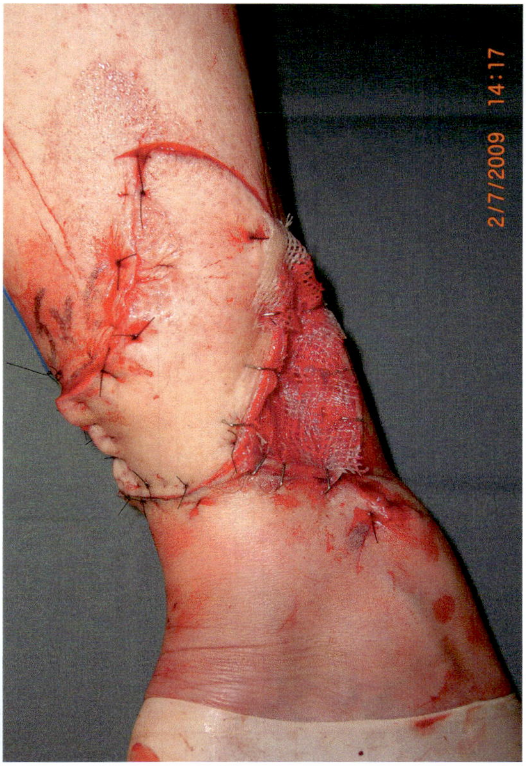

Fig. 5.30 The grafting of the secondary defect and the continued ooze in the Keystone flap indicating ongoing presence of Red Dot Sign and vascular hyperaemia. Procedure time record approximately 45 min

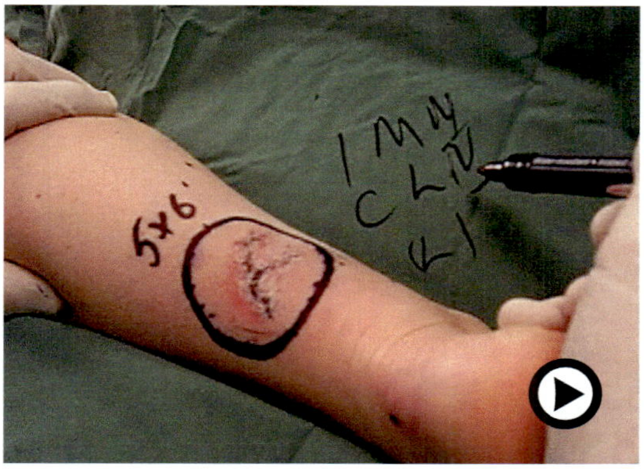

Fig. 5.31 Operative sequence (▶ https://doi.org/10.1007/000-b5z)

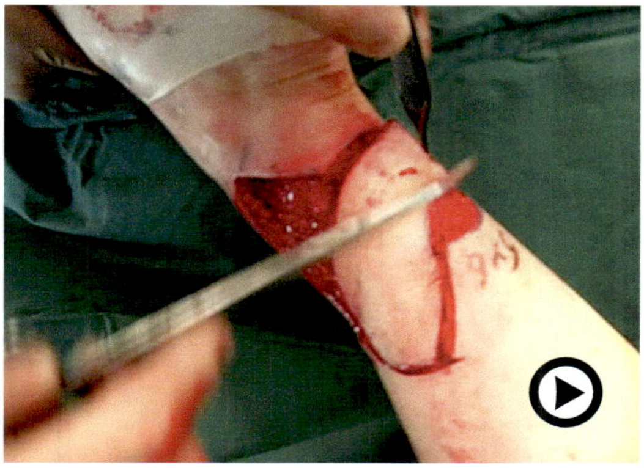

Fig. 5.32 Operative sequence (▶ https://doi.org/10.1007/000-b60)

5.1.7 Case 52: Antero-Lateral Leg

Clark level II 0.56 mm melanoma R antero-lateral leg. Tumour-free interval of 4 years (see Figs. 5.33 and 5.34).

In summary, what was particularly noteworthy is the aesthetic outcome. All P.A.C.E.S. characteristics were also exemplified.

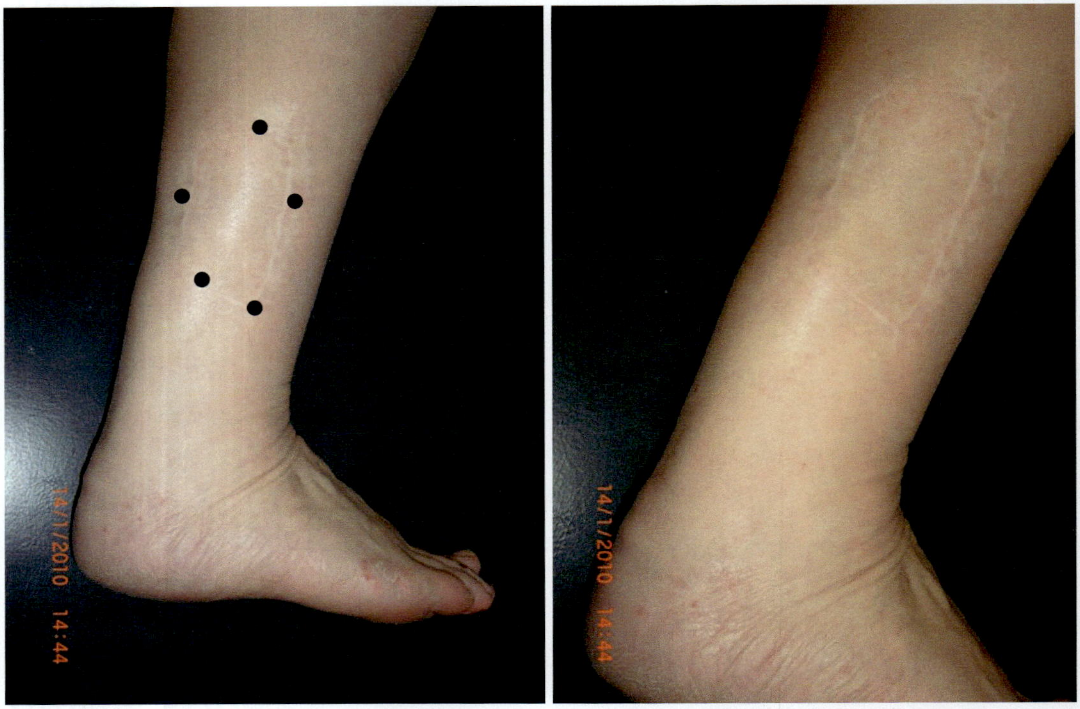

Fig. 5.33 This the lower limit for direct closure avoiding any grafting

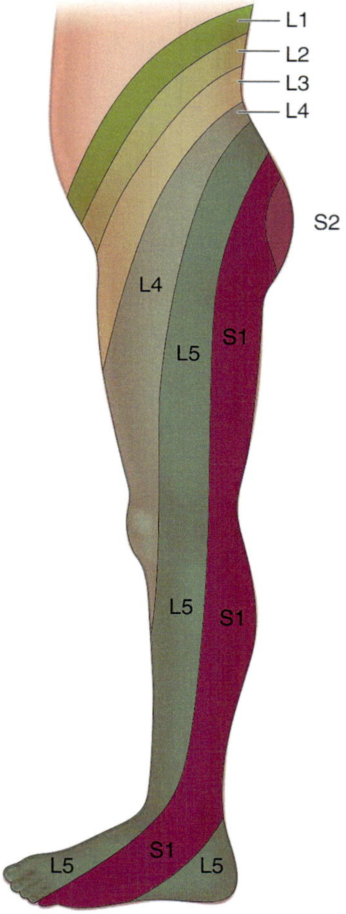

Fig. 5.34 The dermatomal mark out is the guide for the location of the random perforators coming through the fascia

5.1.8 Case 53: Anterior Shin Melanoma in an 84-Year-Old Female

Melanoma lower limb – Delayed Reconstruction After Pathology Evaluation (DRAPE) procedure in this 84-year-old female.

The Keystone in the peroneal area of the L5 dermatome is raised leaving one third proximal attachment and transferred over the anterior tibial bony defect creating the Omega variant (see Figs. 5.35, 5.36, 5.37, 5.38, 5.39, 5.40, 5.41, 5.42, 5.43, 5.44, and 5.45).

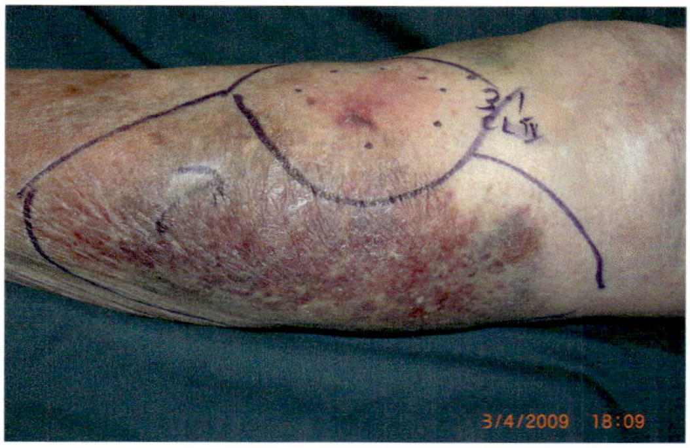

Fig. 5.35 The mark out of the lesion and the design of the Omega variant of the Keystone overlying the L5 dermatome, leaving one third proximal deep attachment

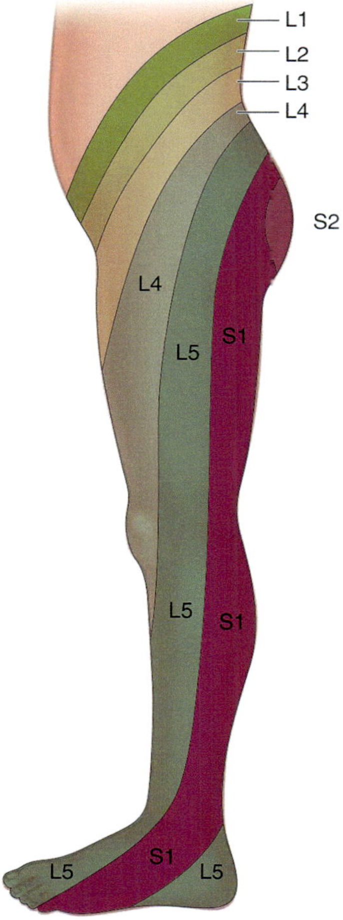

Fig. 5.36 The dermatomal mark out is the guide for the location of the random perforators coming through the fascia

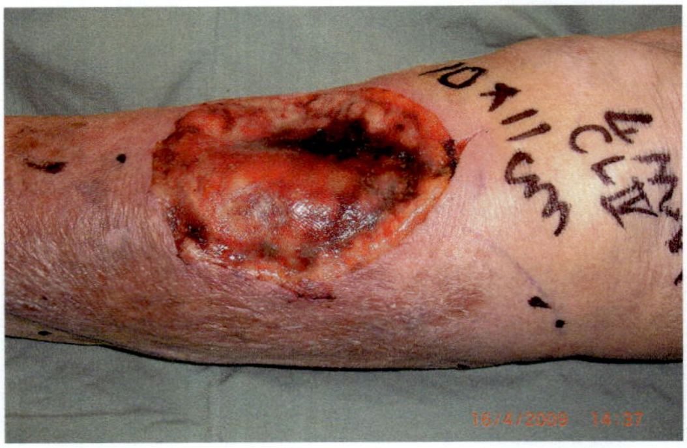

Fig. 5.37 The surgical defect 10 × 11 cm down to periosteum

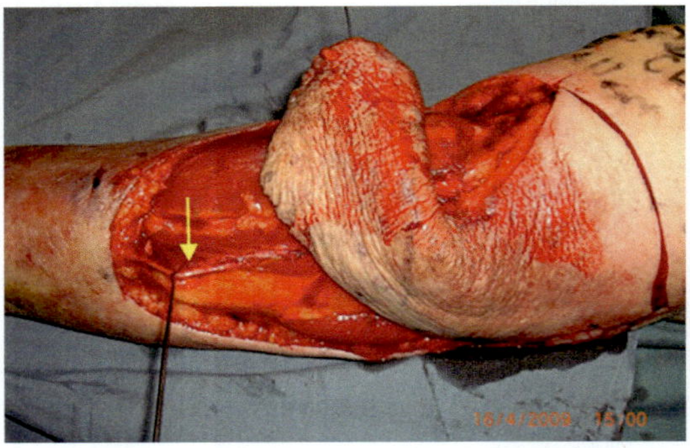

Fig. 5.38 The Omega variant is raised distally undermining two thirds leaving a fascial lined flap with one third proximal deep attachment, with the outline of the Keystone island at the dermal epidermal level in this proximal one third, preserving the superficial peroneal nerve (arrowed)

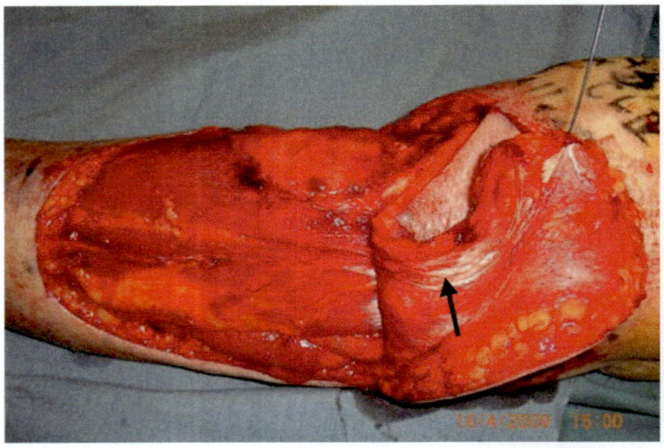

Fig. 5.39 The fascial lined base Keystone (arrowed) undermined two thirds and this fascial lining is the guarantee of its circulatory integrity. The superficial peroneal nerve is noted in the depths and left in situ. It is preserved to ensure distal innervation. The Keystone is rotated anteriorly to close the melanotic site and grafting the secondary defect – the Omega variant is this design concept of the Keystone

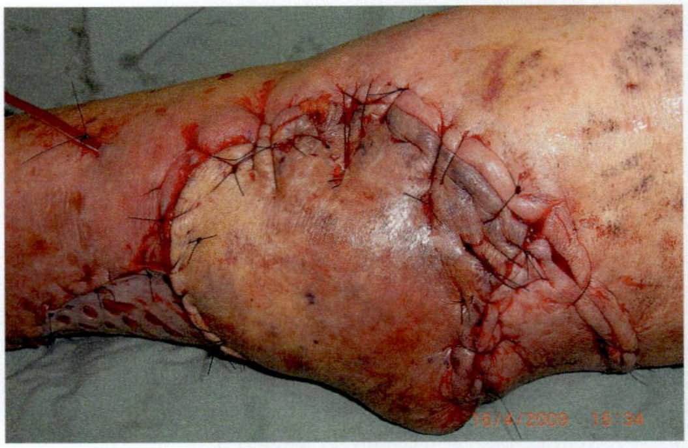

Fig. 5.40 The flap in situ without any evidence of vascular impedance using the 3-phase single layer appositional nylon suture technique

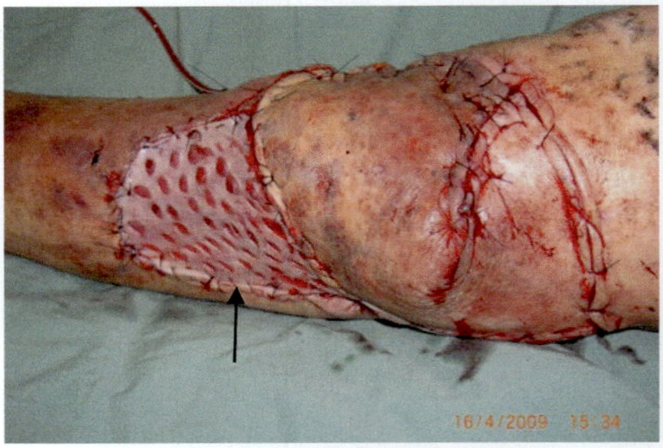

Fig. 5.41 The secondary defect (arrowed) is a fenestrated full-thickness graft harvested from the contralateral R groin [3]

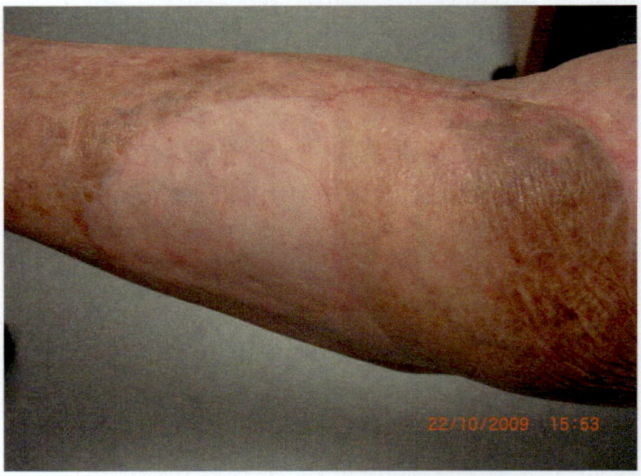

Fig. 5.42 Postoperative appearance at 6 months. Subsequently tumour-free interval of 2 years has been recorded clinically

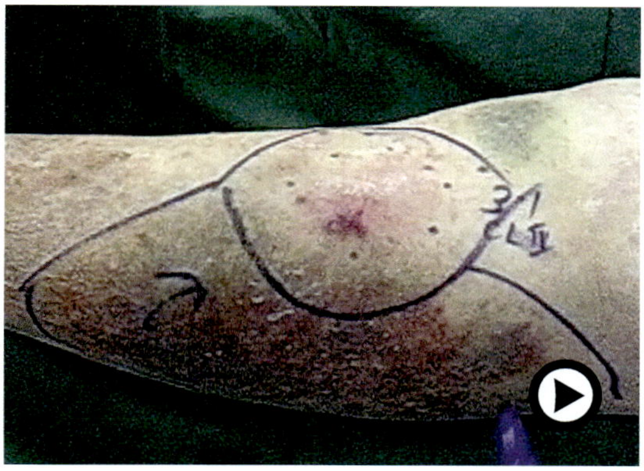

Fig. 5.43 Operative plan (▶ https://doi.org/10.1007/000-b61)

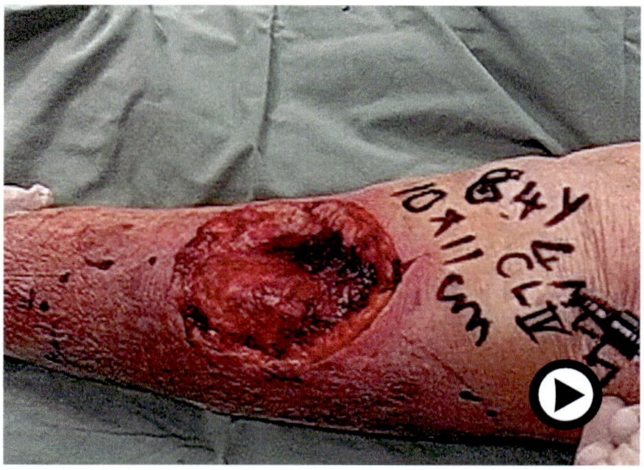

Fig. 5.44 Operative plan (▶ https://doi.org/10.1007/000-b62)

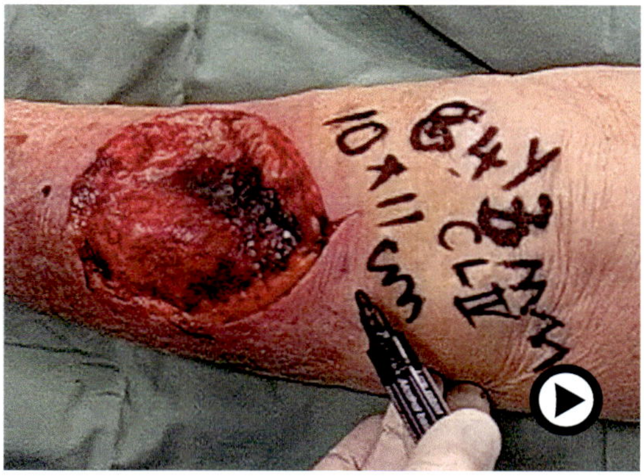

Fig. 5.45 Operative plan (▶ https://doi.org/10.1007/000-b63)

In summary, the P.A.C.E.S. characteristics of the Keystone were all exemplified and repeated.

5.1.9 Case 54: Intransit Metastasis – A Keystone Solution for This Problem of Spreading Disease in a Person That Might Have a Limited Lifespan. An Expeditious Surgical Manoeuvre Is Essential and the Keystone Fulfils Requirements Here

Lower lateral thigh Keystone for intransit metastasis (see Figs. 5.46, 5.47, 5.48, 5.49, 5.50, and 5.51).

In summary, the P.A.C.E.S. characteristics of the Keystone have all been exemplified and the patient with possible pre-terminal disease can now enjoy her life again

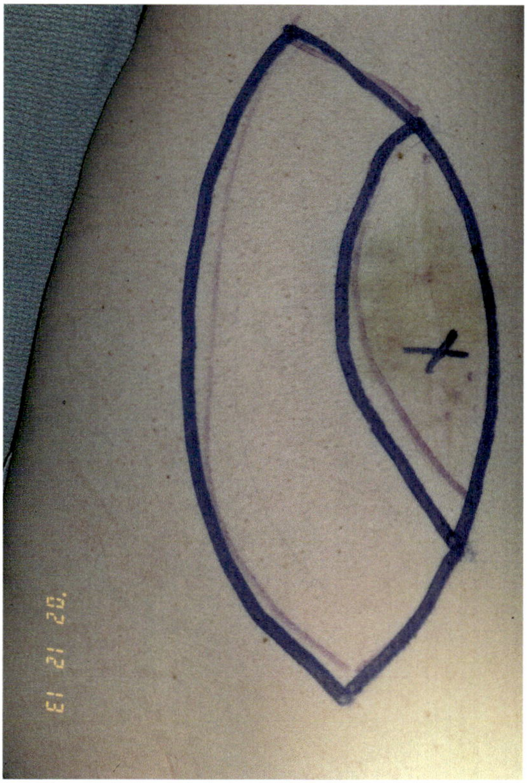

Fig. 5.46 Excision of the tumour recurrence as marked out and a Keystone closure of the thigh in a young female

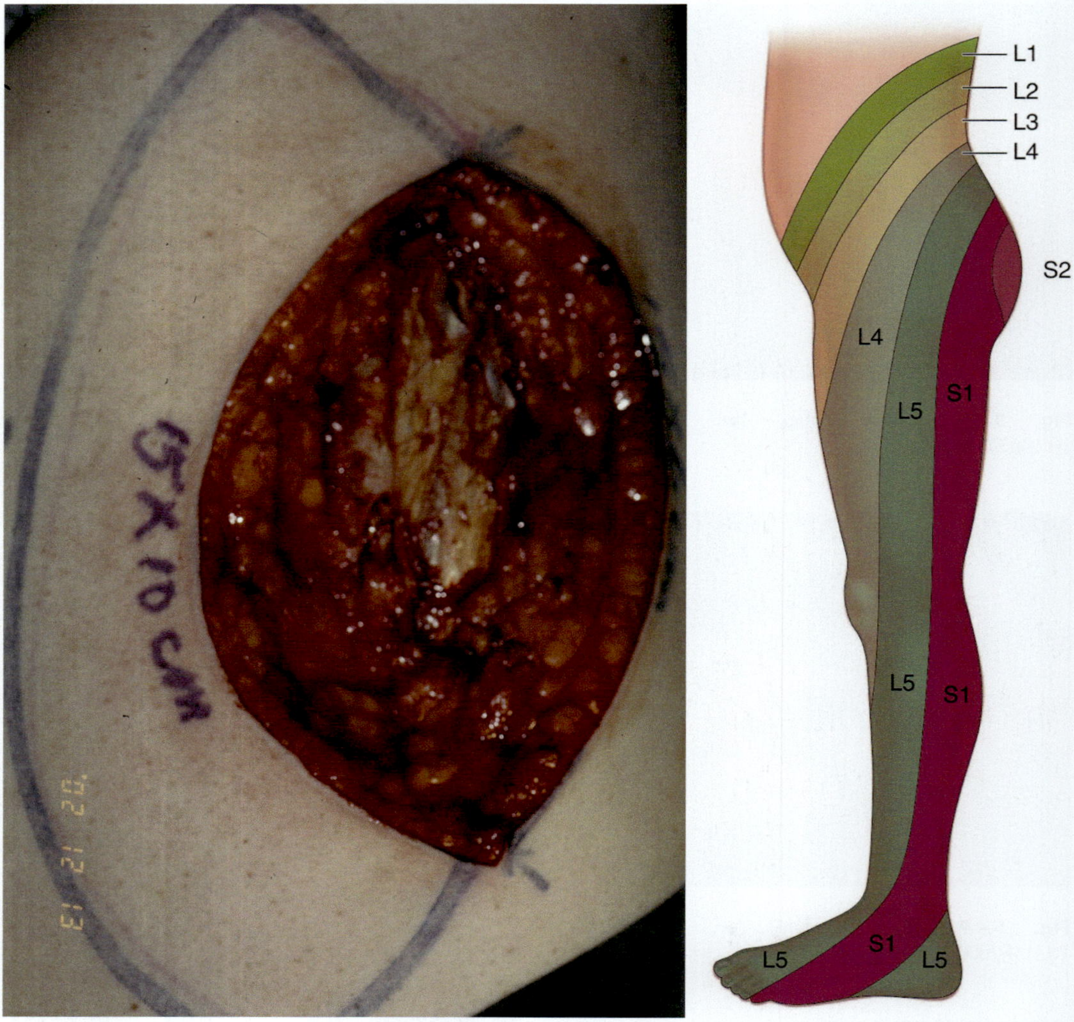

Fig. 5.47 The 15 × 10 cm defect of the thigh in the L5 dermatome

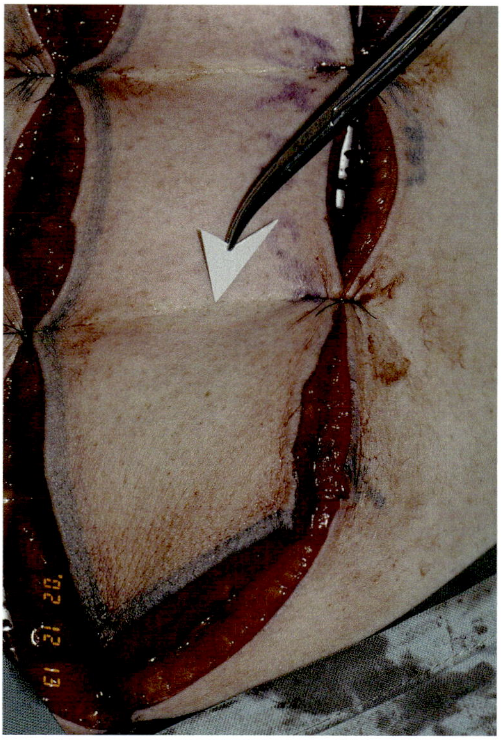

Fig. 5.48 Partially closed with lines of tension which disappear on completion of the closure

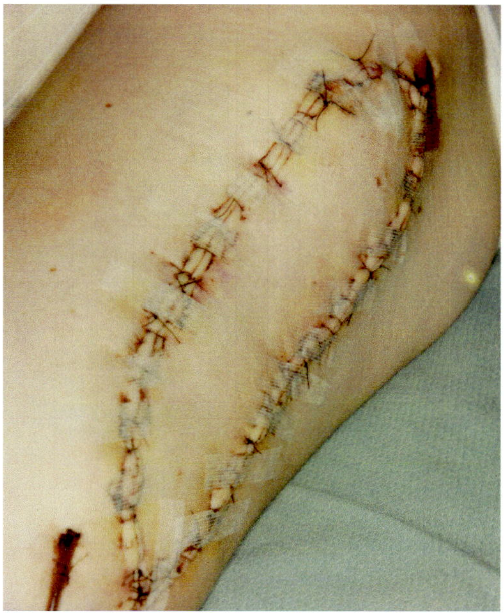

Fig. 5.49 Appearance at 24 h and the Redi-vac tubing inserted in a u-shape design so one tube can drain two surgical sites and this helps avoid any haematoma formation

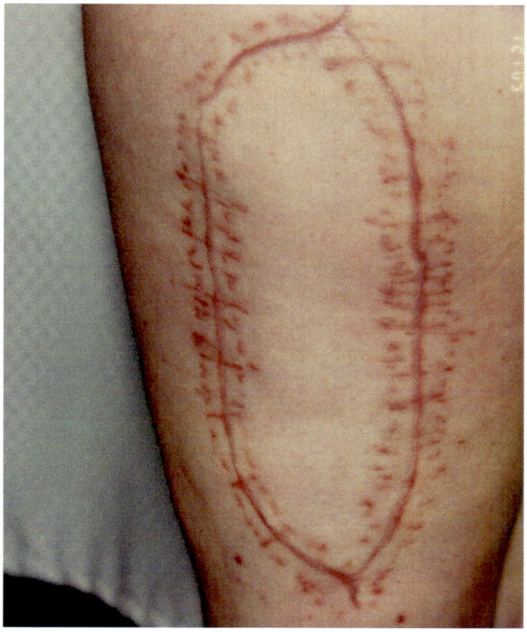

Fig. 5.50 Appearance at 3 weeks on completion of wound dressing

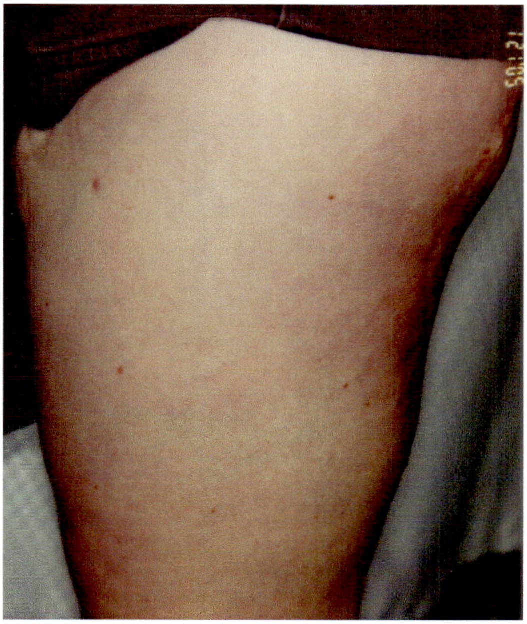

Fig. 5.51 Appearance at 4 months enjoying her social wellbeing with no limitations on clothing preferences

5.1.10 Case 55: Intransit Metastases Lower Thigh

Intransit metastases in the lower third lateral L thigh as in Case 54.

Postoperative appearance at 3 months using the Keystone technique (Fig. 5.52).

In summary, the P.A.C.E.S. characteristics of the Keystone were all exemplified.

5.1.11 Case 56: Intransit Metastases Lower Thigh

Another acceptable outcome (see Figs. 5.53, 5.54, and 5.55).

In summary, intransit metastases are a testing problem for grafting procedures in a person which might be in the preterminal phase of life. The Keystone provides a solution with an aesthetic outcome, and in summary, the P.A.C.E.S. characteristics of the Keystone offer some consolation in what could be a pre-terminal phase of life.

5.1.12 Case 57: Intransit Metastases Over the Medial Malleolus Towards the Groin

Tumour-free interval of 5 years for melanoma of the L groin following a superficial acral lentiginous melanoma (ALM) of the big toe.

Intransit metastasis (excised and grafted) was followed by a groin dissemination needing excisional treatment for Stage III disease. The groin mass was excised with a lymphadenectomy and closed with a quadrangular shaped Keystone overlying the quadriceps muslces in the L2, L3, L4 dermatomes (see Figs. 5.56, 5.57, 5.58, 5.59, 5.60, 5.61, 5.62, 5.63, and 5.64).

In summary, the P.A.C.E.S. characteristics of the Keystone were all exemplified.

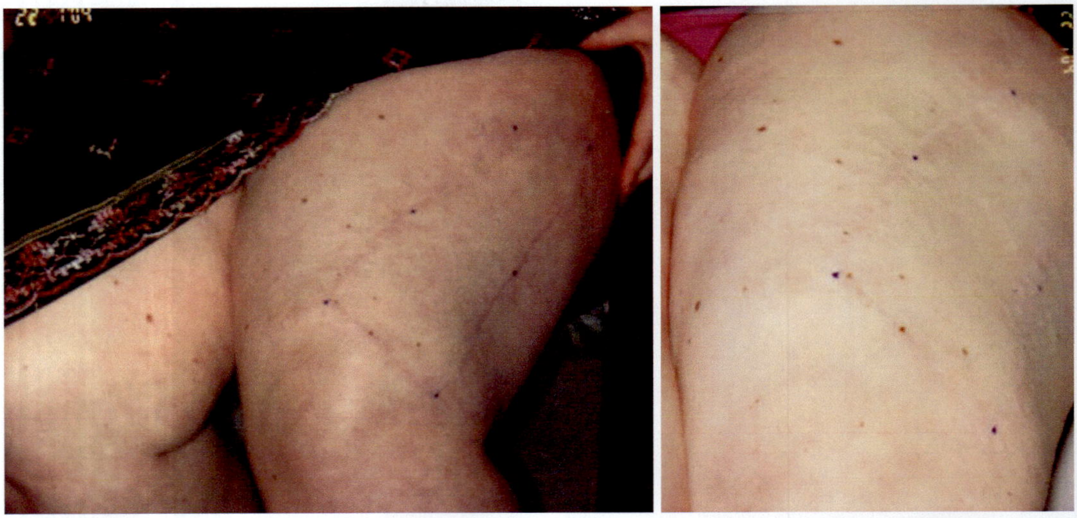

Fig. 5.52 The dimensions of the Keystone are outlined to close a large excisional defect. Postoperative appearance at 3 months following the Keystone closure for intransit metastases – an aesthetically acceptable outcome without limitations on clothing preferences

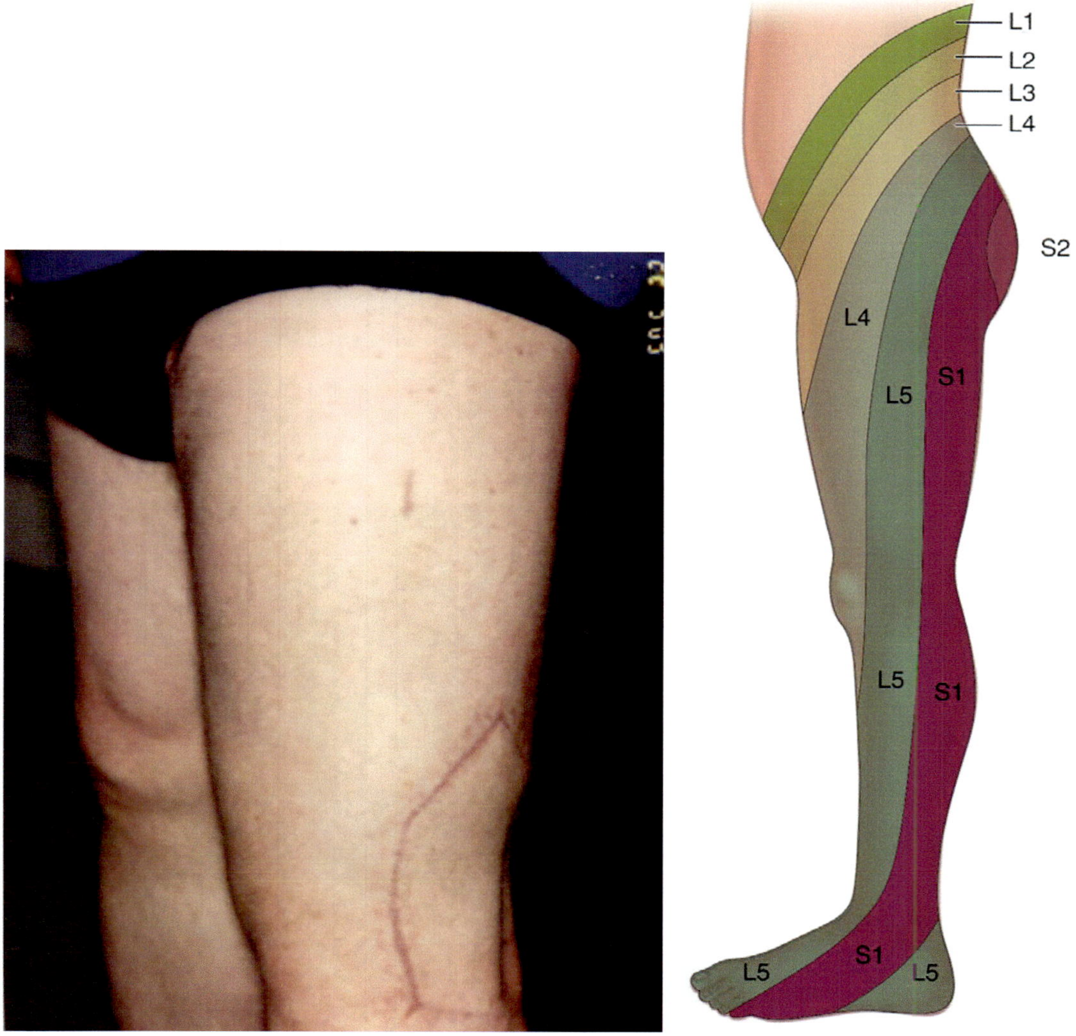

Fig. 5.53 The postoperative appearance of a Keystone closure, lateral to the knee joint using L5, S1 dermatomes for random perforators adjacent to the joint

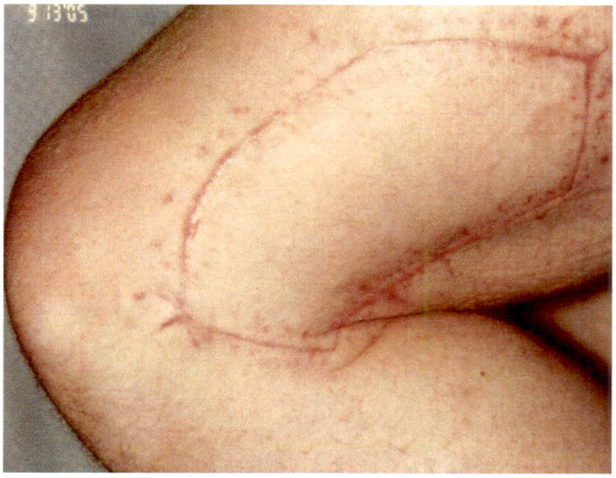

Fig. 5.54 No restriction of knee joint movement and pain free

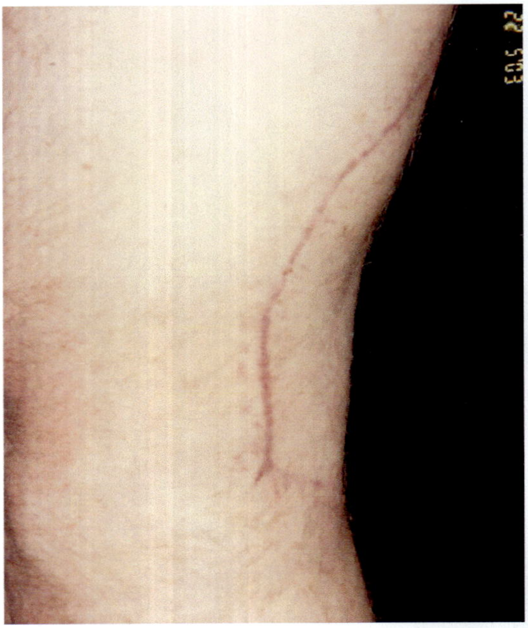

Fig. 5.55 A close-up view of the aesthetic outcome. The vertical scar across the knee joint area has not become hypertrophic

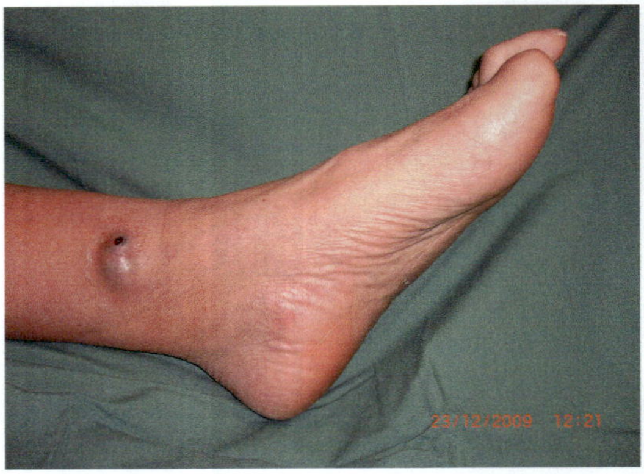

Fig. 5.56 Intransit metastases over the medial malleolus excised and grafted

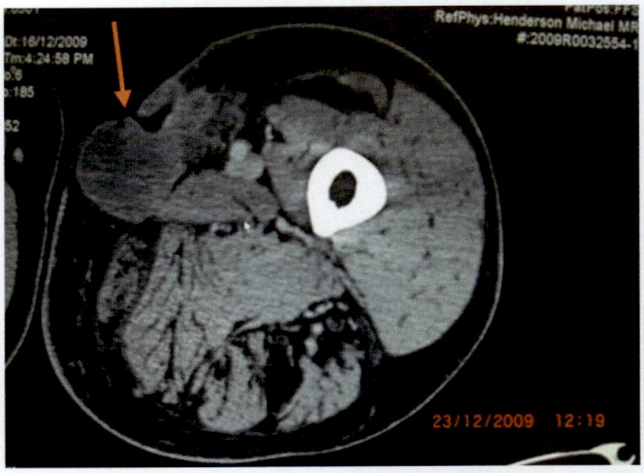

Fig. 5.57 CT verification of the melanotic groin mass with external protrusion

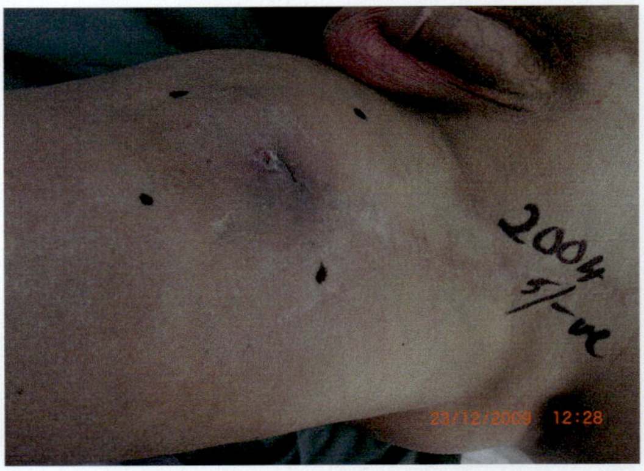

Fig. 5.58 The subcutaneous presence of the nodal recurrence extending up the L groin

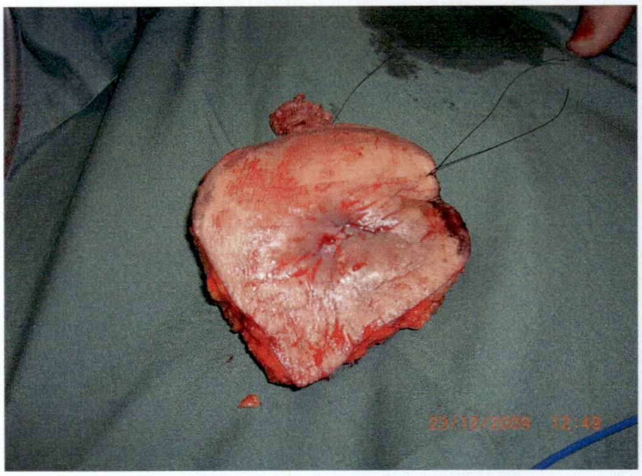

Fig. 5.59 The tumour mass after excision from the L groin

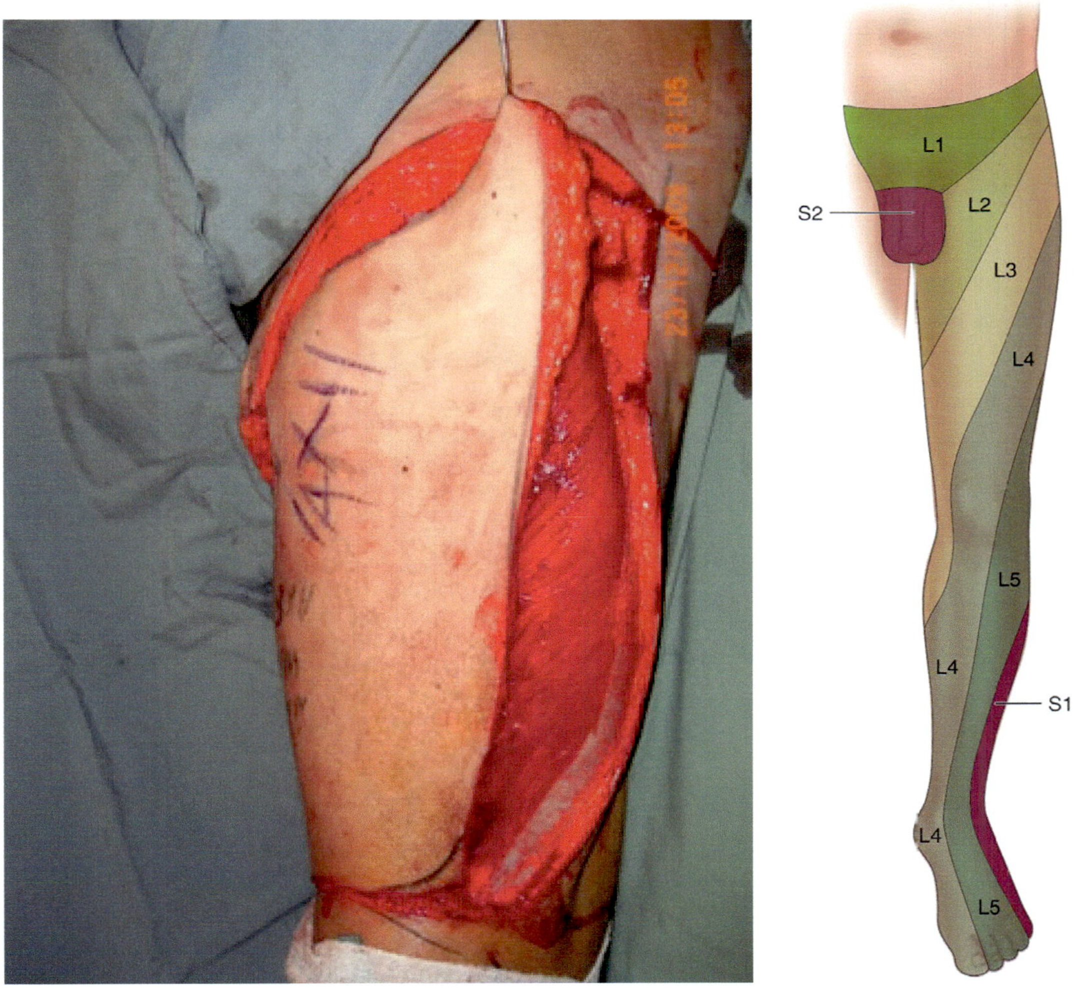

Fig. 5.60 The quadriceps complex site and the Keystone design over the L2, L3, L4 dermatomes showing the division of the deep fascia along tensor fascia lata (arrowed) and the transverse skin incision across the suprapatellar pouch region to complete the island design concept. This incision is only at the skin epidermal dermal level and it is closed directly after incision and must be supported with Redi-vac drainage as haematomas can occur

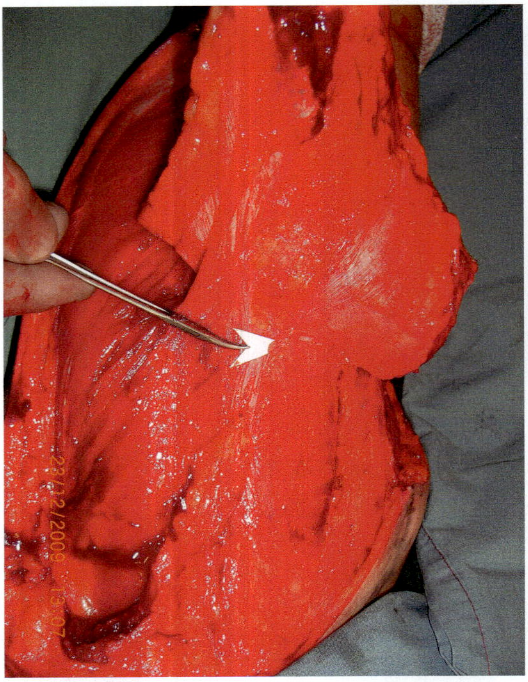

Fig. 5.61 The fascia is turned down the thigh as part of the groin dissection incision so the long saphenous nerve vein can be safely ligated. The reason for the extra length in the quadriceps Keystone is because all the proximal random perforator supports may have been sacrificed in the groin dissection and the Keystone is living on distal perforators in the L4 dermatome (arrowed) in the distal third

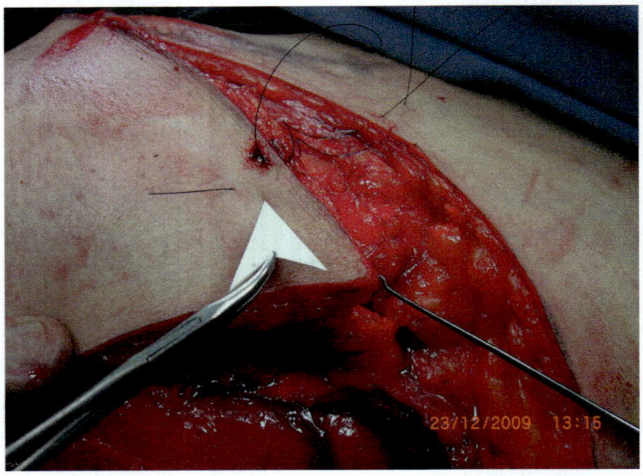

Fig. 5.62 Closure – The Red Dot Sign on the flap at the point of surgical mattress locking suture. This confirms the hyperaemic flare where the suture point bleeds more than that at the site of flap attachment and this vascular reliability ensures sound healing with a single layered closure

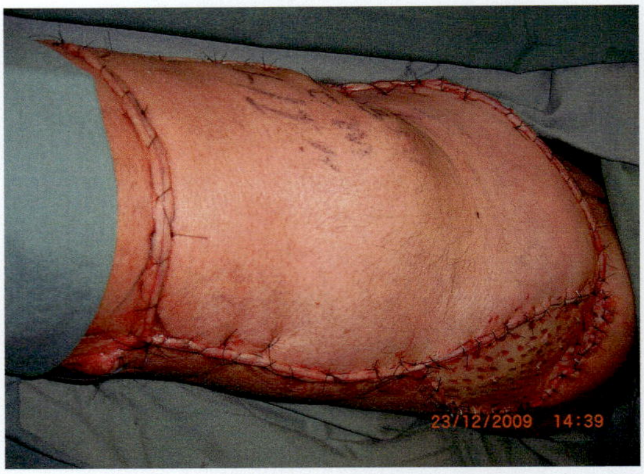

Fig. 5.63 Appearance on completion using the 3-phase suturing technique of tension closure using locking mattress sutures at the tension points, further locking mattress sutures to recreate tissue alignment and finally the continuous nylon for dermal seal with epidermal apposition and the suprapatellar wound (part of the island design) is just closed directly. Note the hypervascularised flare in the flap that is 50% undermined. This is a guarantee for full vascular perfusion from random perforators distally based. There is no cyanotic element nor any indication of impending vascular embarrassment without any definition of pedicle support. A fenestrated graft in the inferior limits of the repair was installed to avoid tension

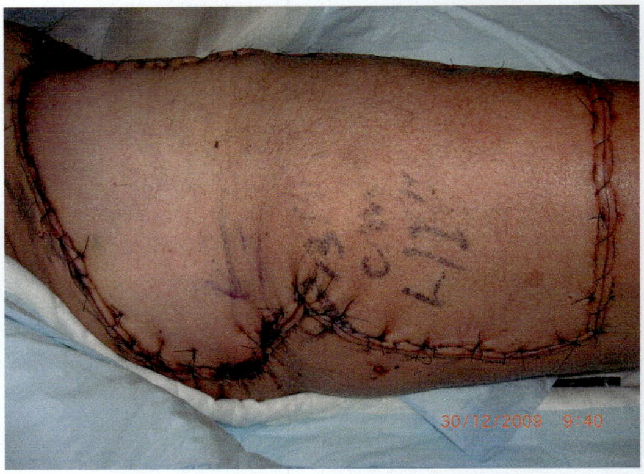

Fig. 5.64 Appearance at 1 week with no sign of vascular necrosis and a satisfactory wound healing

5.1.13 Case 58: Groin Secondary Melanoma from an Acral Lentiginous Melanoma of the Plantar Surface of the Foot

Secondary melanoma in the groin in a 48-year-old male with an acral lentiginous melanoma (ALM) over the metatarsel head of T1 of the L foot.

ALM Stage III disease and L groin dissection. Six-year history before groin reccurrence (see Figs. 5.65, 5.66, 5.67, 5.68, 5.69, and 5.70).

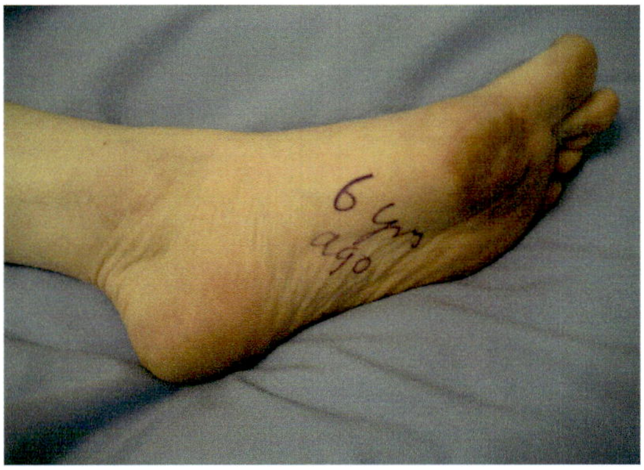

Fig. 5.65 Original presentation. No sign of local recurrence of the ALM of the plantar surface of the L foot over the 1st metatarso-phalangeal joint

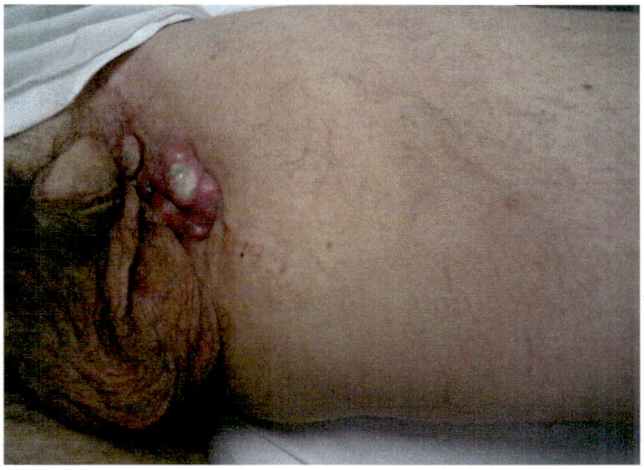

Fig. 5.66 Suppurating cutaneous nodal mass of the L groin with a mitotic mass measuring 10 × 15 cm

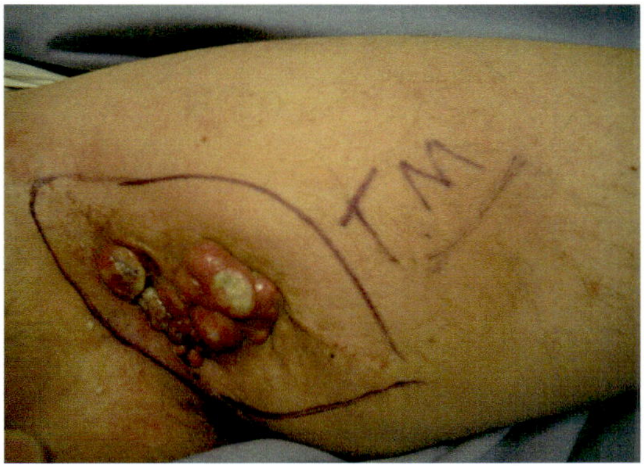

Fig. 5.67 L groin dissection including cutaneous clearance of the L inguinal tumour mass approximately 10 × 15 cm

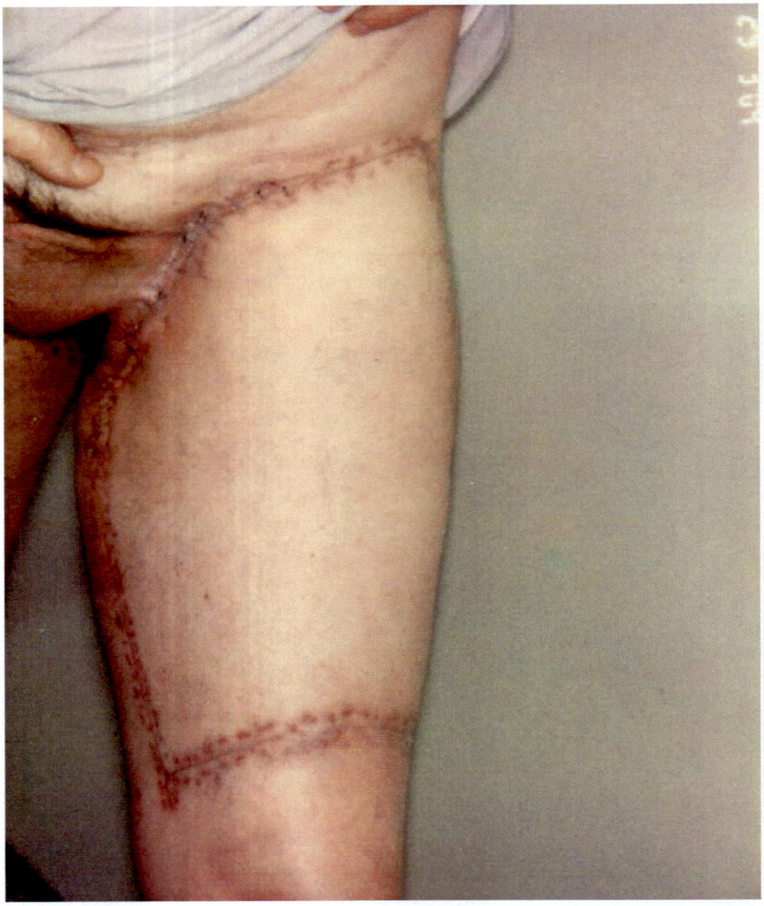

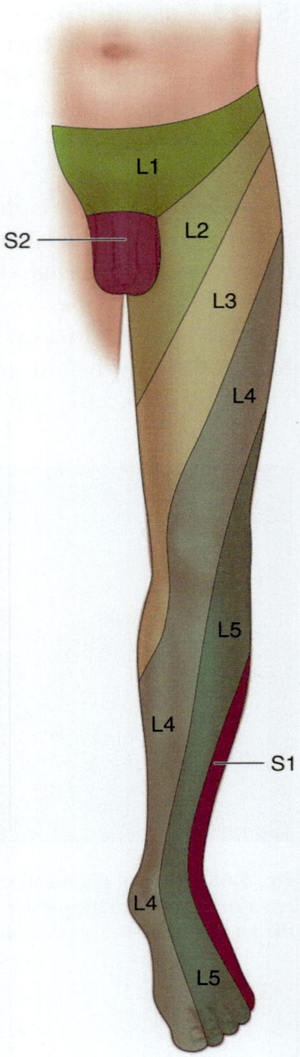

Fig. 5.68 The appearance of the healed wound of the L2, L3, L4 groin dermatome for this Keystone groin flap technique Technique: The Keystone, almost quadrangular in design, extends from the line of the inguinal excision at the upper level of L2 and is outlined. The operative technique consists of a lateral incision along and dividing the tensor fascia lata laterally then transversely across the suprapatellar region and then subsequently ascending medially up the inner thigh still dividing the deep fascia. This creates an umbrella of tissue based on random perforators straddling L2, L3, L4 dermatomes and movement facilitates the closure of large groin oncological defects

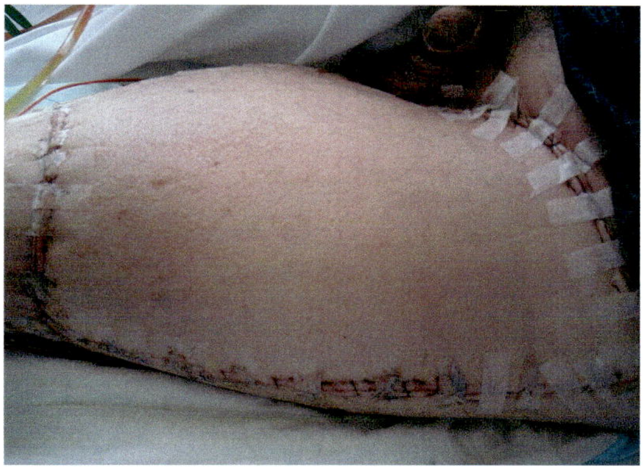

Fig. 5.69 The inferior wound of skin and epidermis is just closed directly and the rest of the wound is closed by the 3-phase suture technique. This immediate postoperative appearance shows the reactive hyperaemia, an important background for sound healing

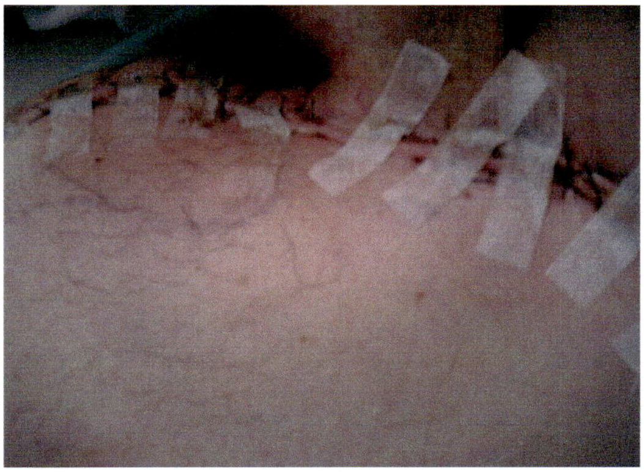

Fig. 5.70 A close-up over the oncological defect without any vascular impedance. The patient lived 12 months following surgery with a comfortable lifestyle. The mild inflammatory reaction along the suture line settled with antibiotic cover reflecting its earlier inflammatory episode

In summary, the P.A.C.E.S. characteristics of the Keystone were all exemplified contributing to the patient's wellbeing in that final life stage.

5.1.14 Case 59: Groin Melanoma Recurrence

Melanoma groin Stage III disease, anterior thigh Keystone and seroma as a complication of the groin dissection (see Figs. 5.71, 5.72, and 5.73).

In summary, the P.A.C.E.S. characteristics of the Keystone were all exemplified.

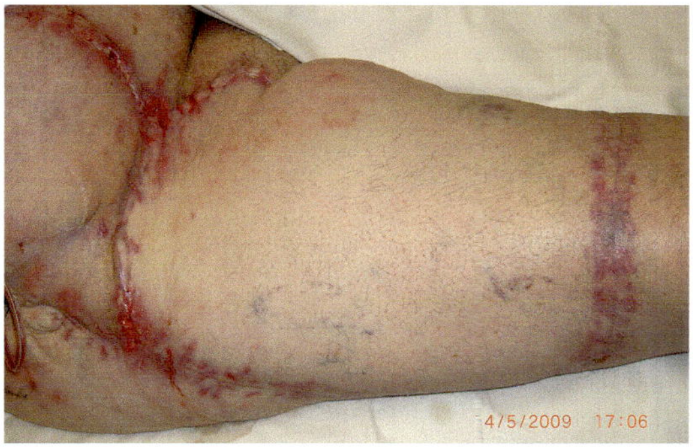

Fig. 5.71 Well-healed quadriceps Keystone. No sign of necrosis

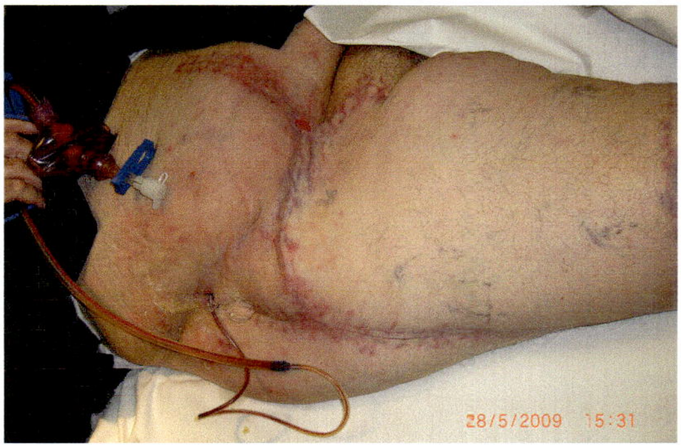

Fig. 5.72 Well healed wound following a groin dissection for cutaneous recurrence

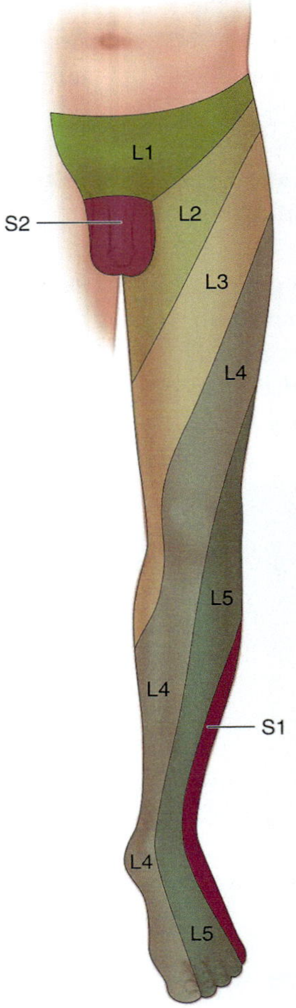

Fig. 5.73 The dermatomal mark out is the guide for the location of the random perforators coming through the fascia

5.1.15 Case 60: Groin Metastases

Melanoma of the R lower limb. Nodal metastases into the R groin.

A surgical excisional defect 20 × 8 cm for the groin resection.

Closure with anterior thigh Keystone (see Figs. 5.74, 5.75, 5.76, and 5.77).

In summary, large defects of the groin are not a contraindication for anterior thigh Keystone cover.

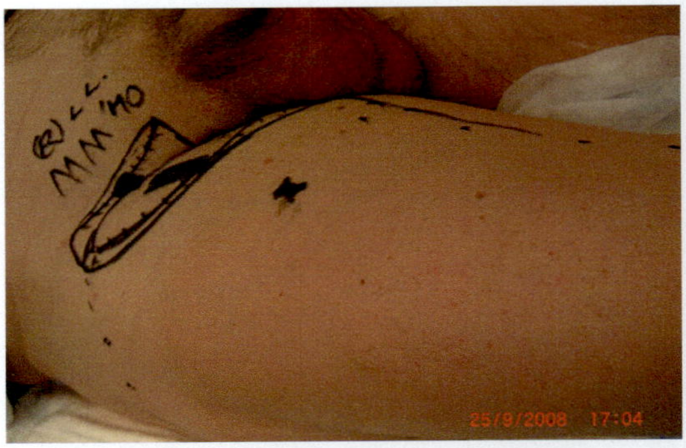

Fig. 5.74 The mark out of the nodal mass of the R groin including the subcutaneous plane

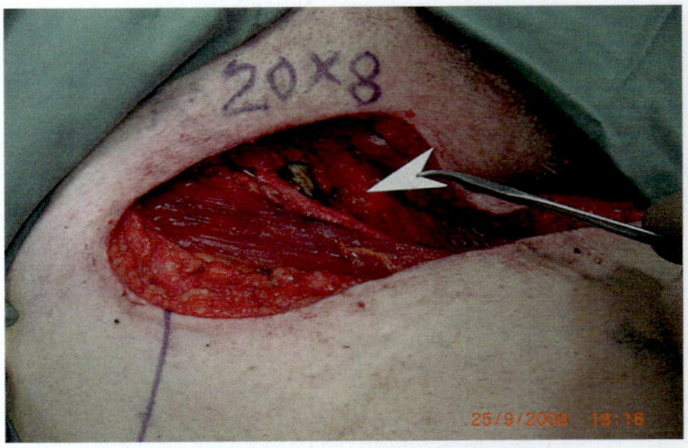

Fig. 5.75 The 20 × 8 cm surgical groin defect after removal of nodes and integument. The vital structures in the depths of the wound, the femoral neurovascular complex (arrowed) which must be covered with the anterior thigh Keystone

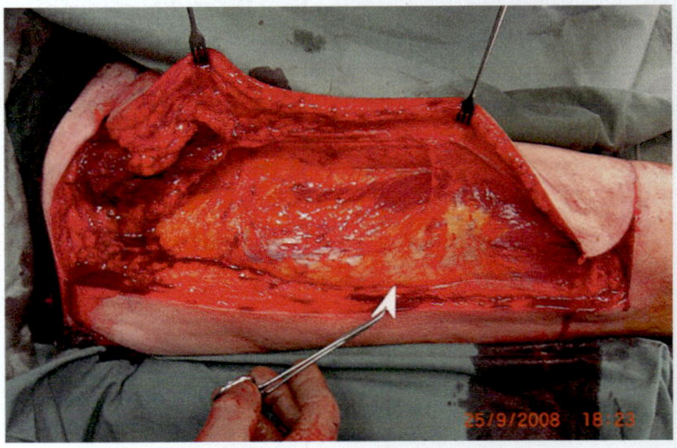

Fig. 5.76 The division of the lateral tensor fascia lata (arrowed) to facilitate upward and medial movement slide to cover large groin defects and the underlying femoral structures. Note the multiple line up of perforators along the anterior thigh region

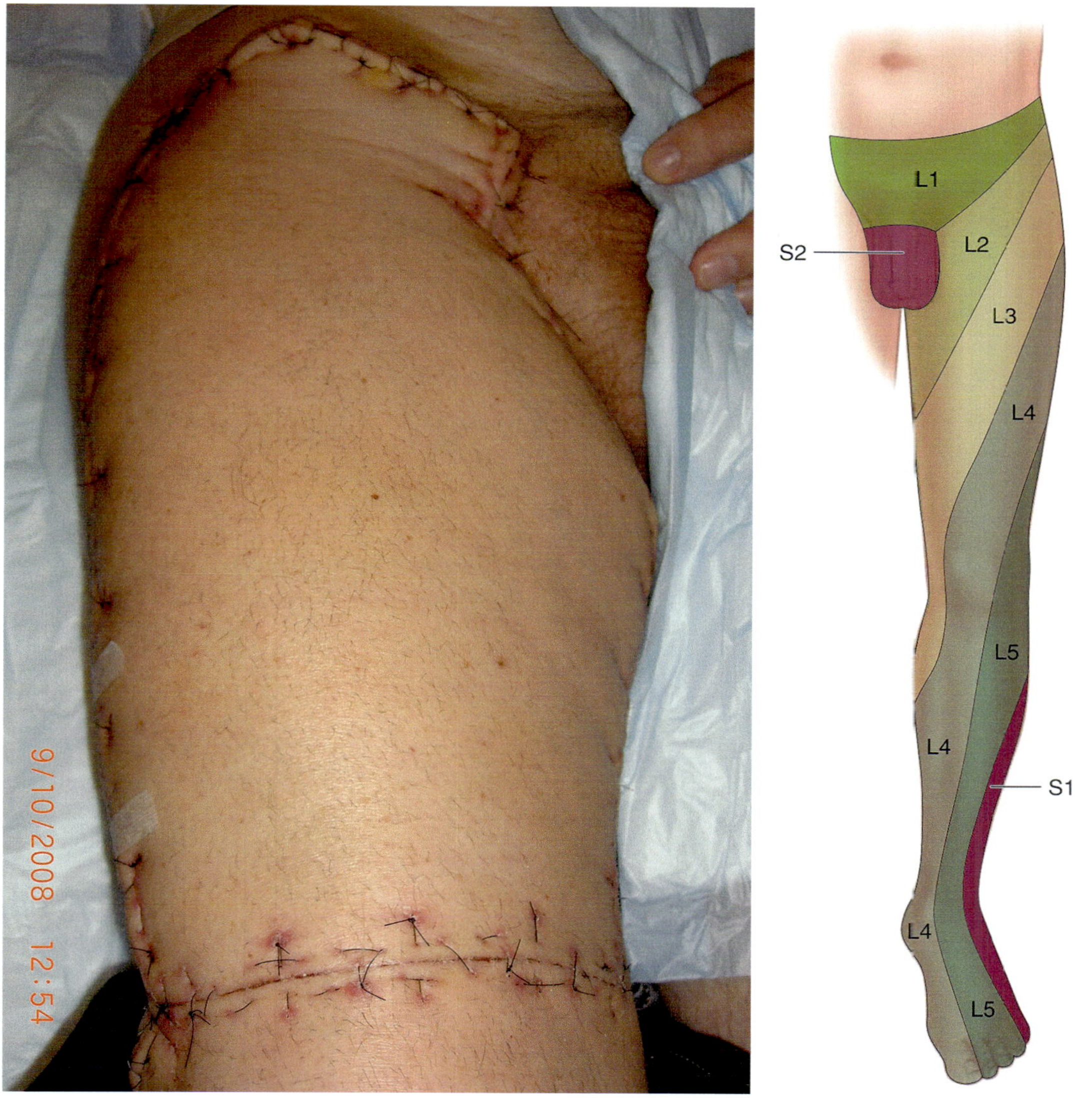

Fig. 5.77 Appearance at 2 weeks with serial removal of sutures in the wound using the 3-phase suture technique of insertion and removal. The anterior thigh Keystone of the R thigh overlying L2, L3, L4 dermatomes has been surgically delineated. The undermining of the proximal half of the flap as part of the R groin dissection. The random perforators in the lower half of the flap sit mainly on L3, L4 dermatomes from which the random perforators emerge to supply the total volume from one third distal deep attachment

5.1.16 Case 61: Groin

Melanoma mass of the R groin in a 26-year-old male. Excision of the groin defect 22 × 10 cm (see Figs. 5.78, 5.79, 5.80, and 5.81).

In summary, the islanding of the flap ensures the hyperaemic phase and therefore maximum perfusion to guarantee wound at the groin heals the inferior wound in the suprapatellar region is just excised and closed directly, preserving the longitudinal running sutures and blood supply.

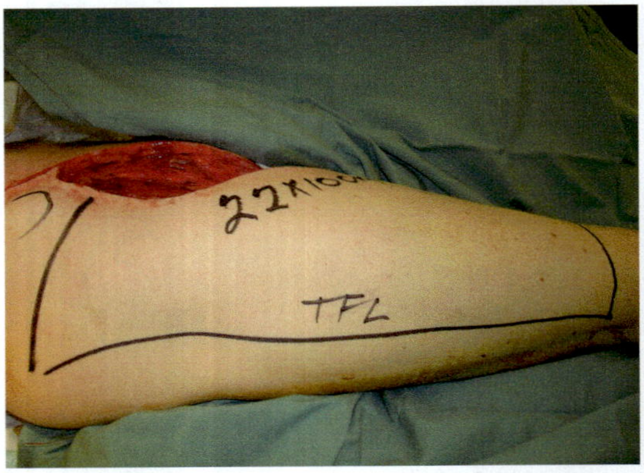

Fig. 5.78 The mark out for the anterior thigh Keystone is noted. It extends from the region of the greater trochanter vertically going down the line dividing tensor fascia lata. Then transversely in the suprapatellar region of skin subcutaneous tissues only, preserving longitudinally running neurovascular structures. Then ascend medially up the thigh to meet the inguinal nodal resection site. The groin defect measures 22 × 10 cm

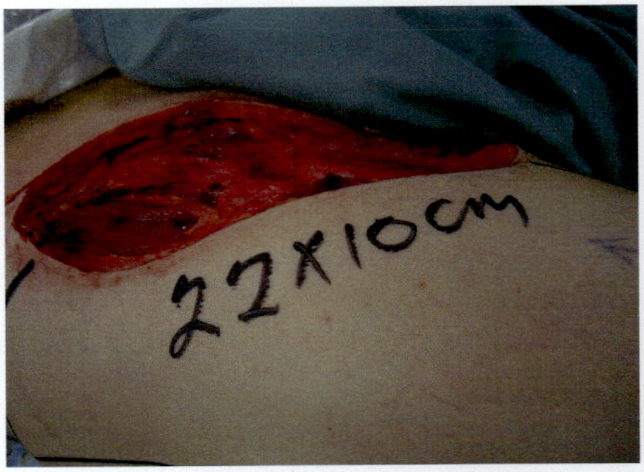

Fig. 5.79 Close-up of the surgical defect easily reconstituted using the anterior thigh Keystone technique, based on L2, L3, L4 dermatomes leaving the distal third attached for perforator support

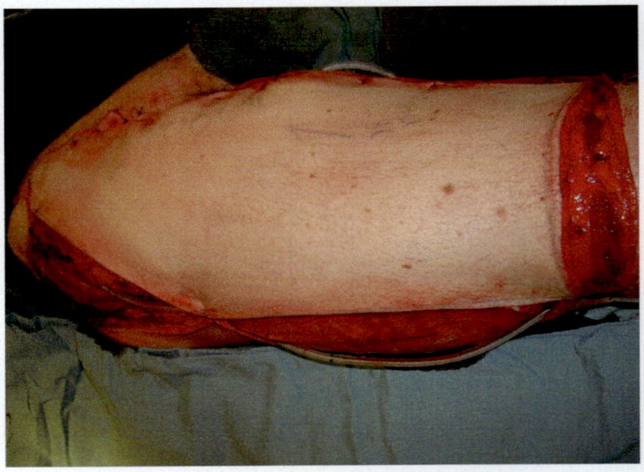

Fig. 5.80 Note the Redi-vac drainage along the medial wound and groin. Laterally a second drain tube along the tensor fascia lata wound ensures optimal healing. The lateral wound may bleed more extensively than the medial thigh wound and we have had one haematoma needing drainage from the lateral tensor fascia lata incision

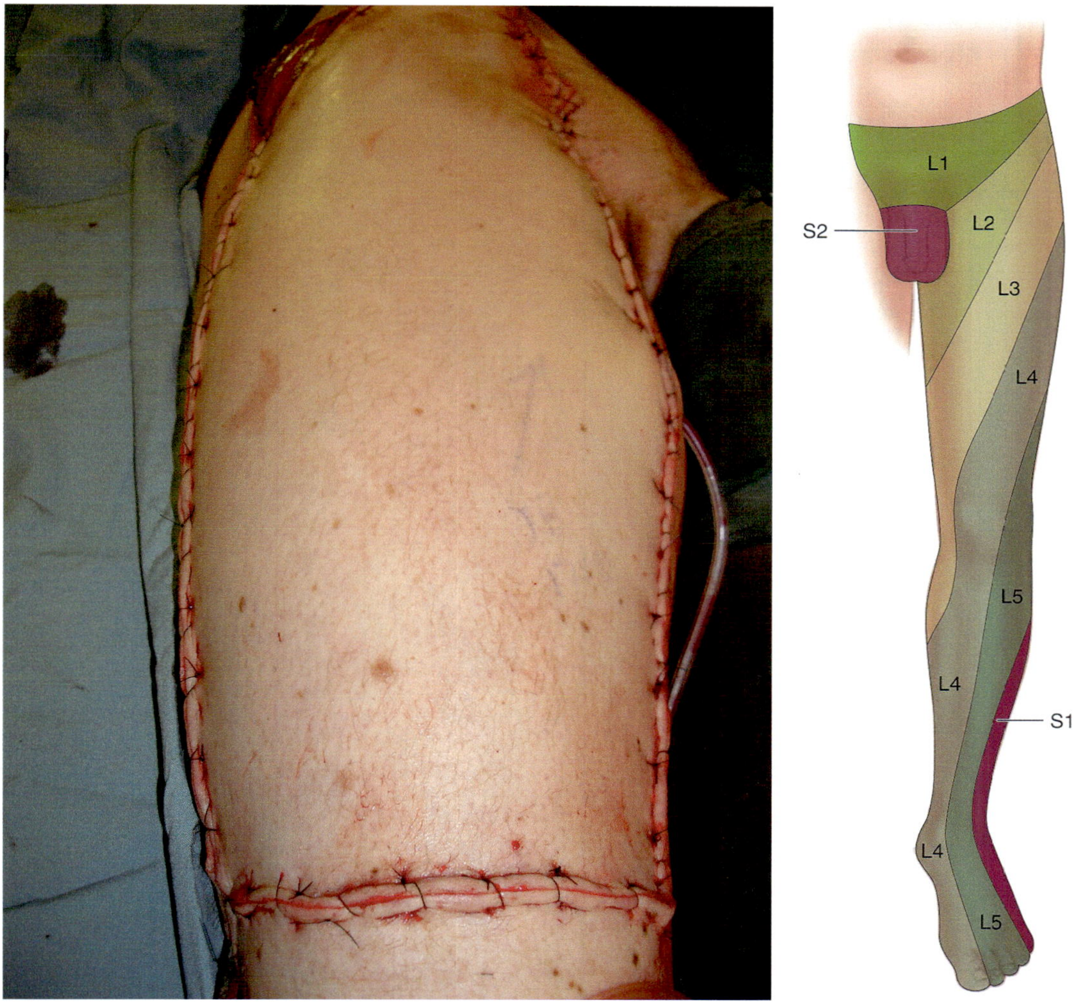

Fig. 5.81 The circulation for the flap reconstruction is mainly on the L3, L4 dermatome and the L2 section of the flap being undermined as part of the groin resection. Note the 3-phase suture technique in using locking mattress sutures at the tension point, further mattress sutures for wound apposition and security and finally a continuous nylon to achieve epidermal alignment and closure. The 1, 2 and 3 week timeframe described above must also apply for the wound dressing technique and serial removal as described above

5.1.17 Case 62: Groin Mass Recurrent Melanoma

Groin dissection and the same Keystone principles apply as above for this DUET procedure with Professor Michael Henderson for the oncological ressection and the easy closure with the Keystone (see Figs. 5.82, 5.83, 5.84, and 5.85).

In summary, the P.A.C.E.S. characteristics of the Keystone were all exemplified.

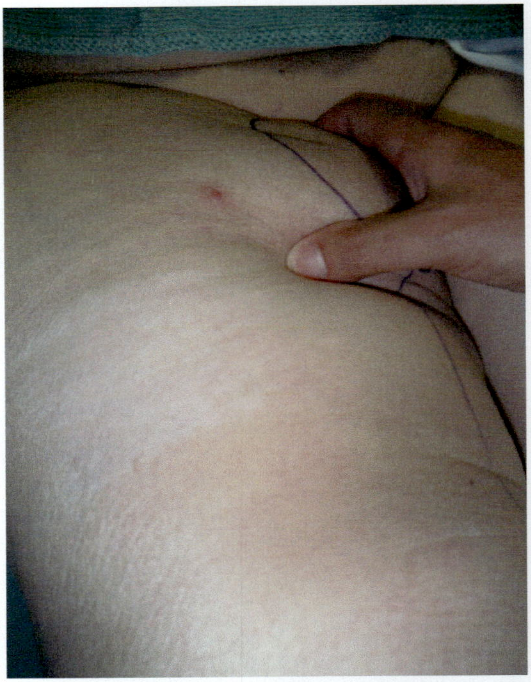

Fig. 5.82 Same principles apply as in earlier descriptions. In other words, the groin clearance is completed and the anterior thigh Keystone is marked out with the division of tensor fascia lata laterally, fascia on the medial side of the thigh and subcutaneous only across the suprapatellar region

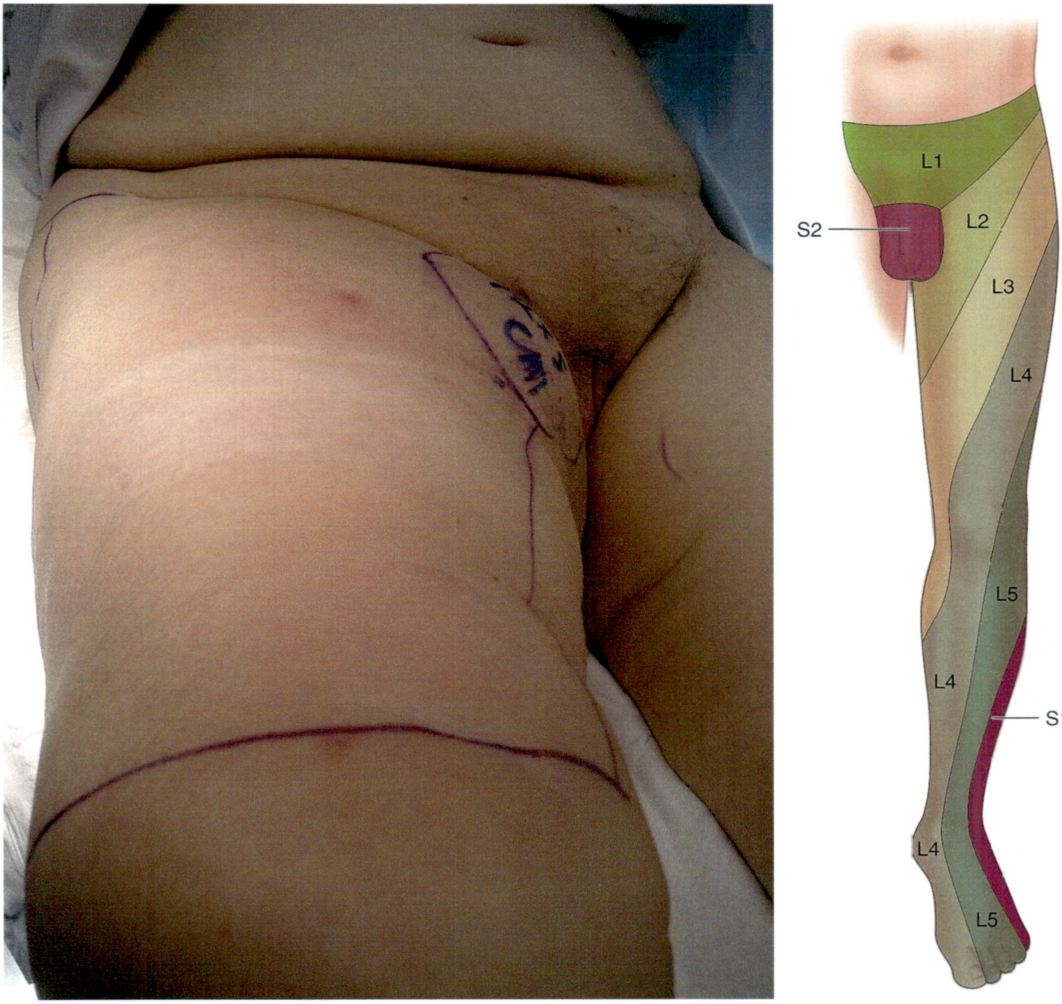

Fig. 5.83 The anterior thigh Keystone mark out. The dermatomal mark out is the guide for the location of the random perforators coming through the fascia

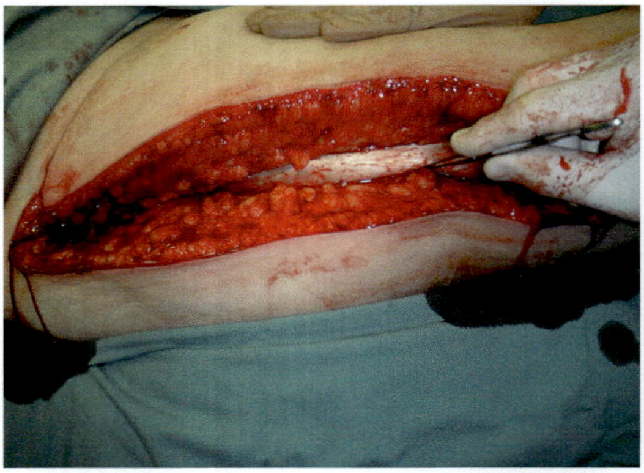

Fig. 5.84 The technique of division of tensor fascia lata – an essential prerequisite for this Keystone closure technique

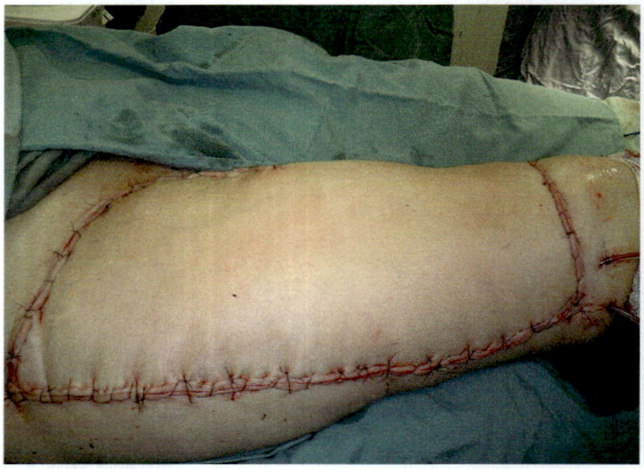

Fig. 5.85 Appearance on completion using the 3-phase suturing technique of tension closure using locking mattress sutures at the tension points, further locking mattress sutures to recreate tissue alignment and finally the continuous nylon for dermal seal with epidermal apposition

5.1.18 Case 63: Heel Recurrence

Melanoma of the L heel Clark level IV indepth recurrence after 4 years confirmed by the biopsy site (see Figs. 5.86, 5.87, 5.88, 5.89, 5.90, 5.91, 5.92, 5.93, 5.94, 5.95, 5.96, and 5.97).

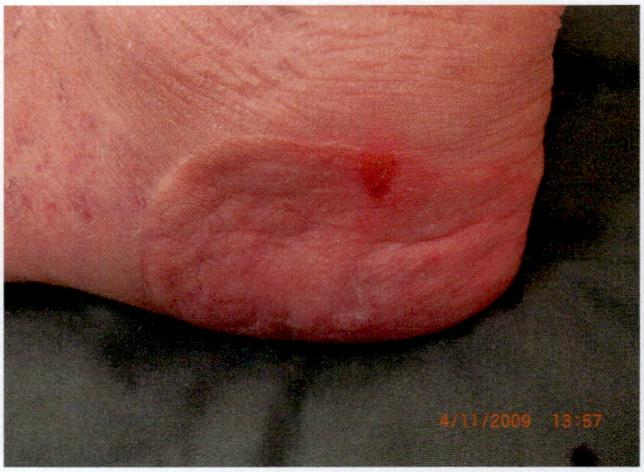

Fig. 5.86 On presentation

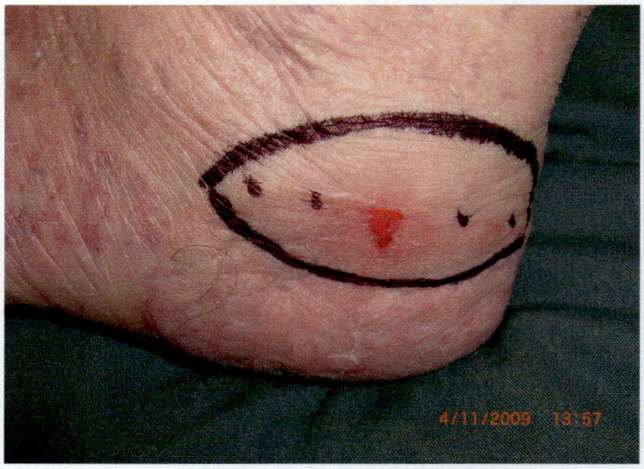

Fig. 5.87 The excisional mark out for removal of the confirmed biopsy recurrence

In summary, Keystones can be applied around the tendo achilles and heel areas; however, in type II diabetes, be wary of closure under tension and apply split skin grafts when granulating tissue is evident as a discreet alternative.

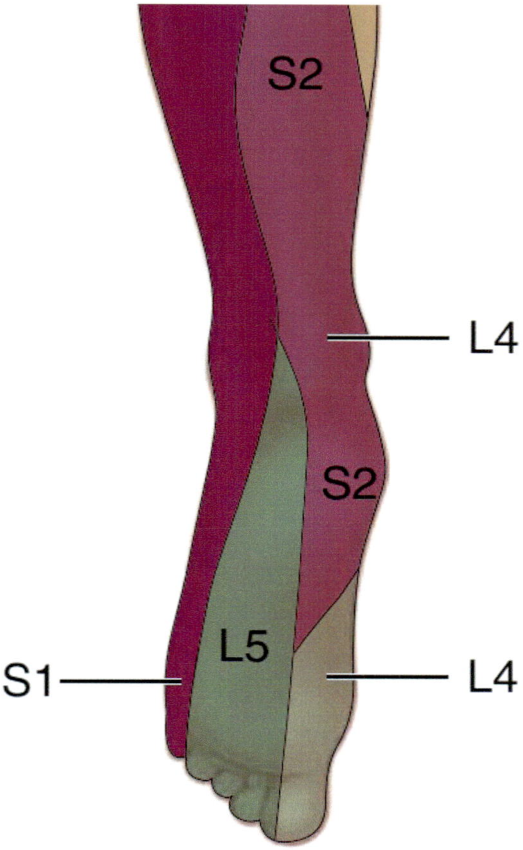

Fig. 5.88 The dermatomal mark out is the guide for the location of the random perforators coming through the fascia

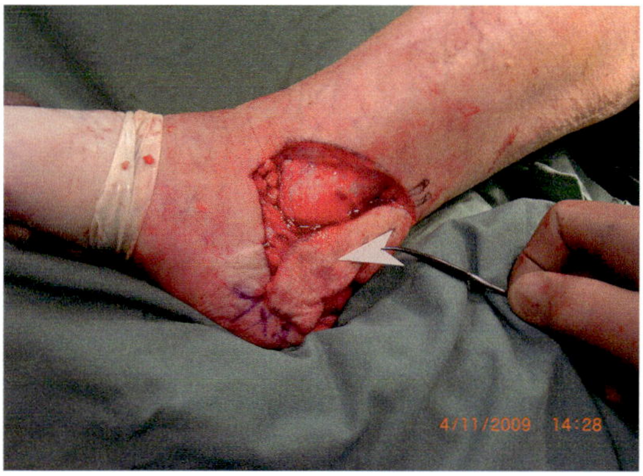

Fig. 5.89 The excisional defect 9 × 4 cm below the L lateral malleolus and the Keystone showing a hyperaemic phase (arrowed) and the Keystone has been raised to cover the area of the tendo-achilles insertion

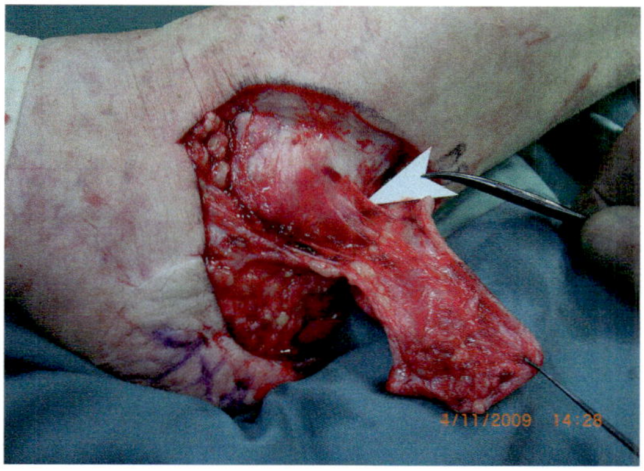

Fig. 5.90 Subdermal attachments from the lateral malleolus and sural nerve neurovascular supply (arrowed)

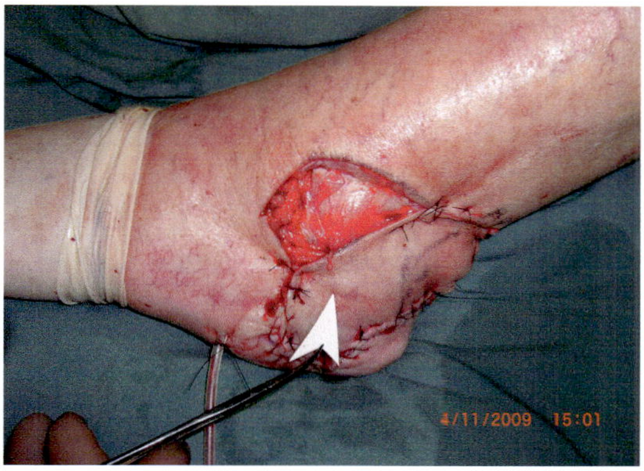

Fig. 5.91 Closure shows some cyanosis in view of the slight restriction of flow in the peripheral region of the lower limb commonly seen in diabetics

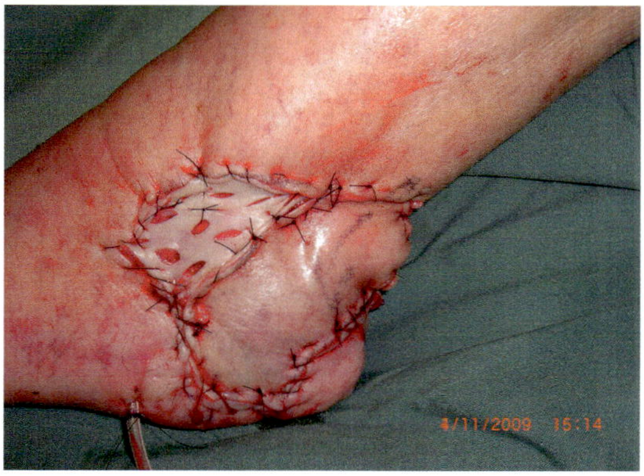

Fig. 5.92 The use of a fenestrated full thickness graft harvested from the groin to achieve wound closure and ensure healing.

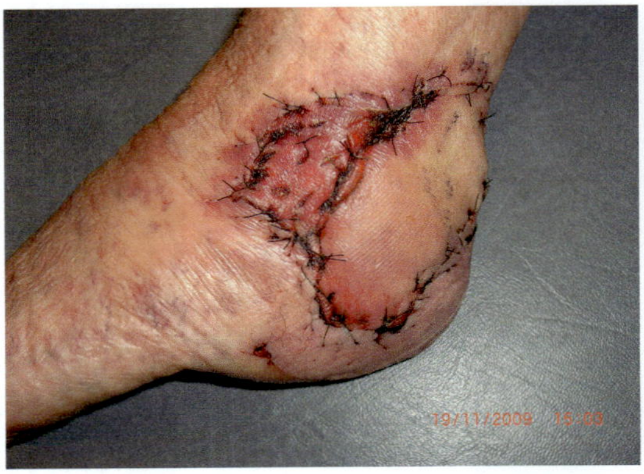

Fig. 5.93 Appearance at 2 weeks showing full viability in the flap and a successful full-thickness grafting. The 3-phase suture technique has been used and tie over dressings are avoided around Keystone flaps

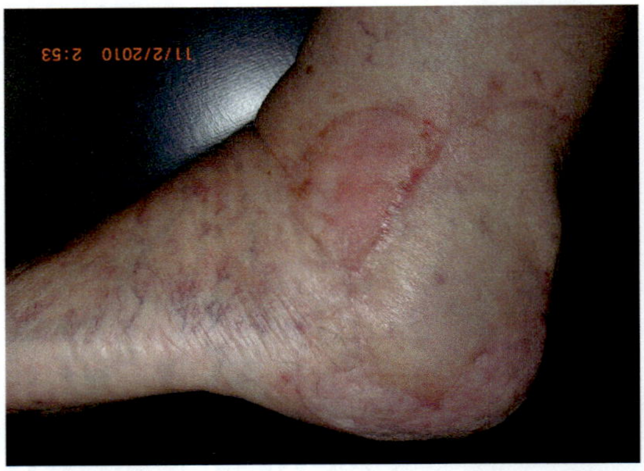

Fig. 5.94 Three months postoperative appearance with no sign of recurrence and can use footwear comfortably as the oedema resolves

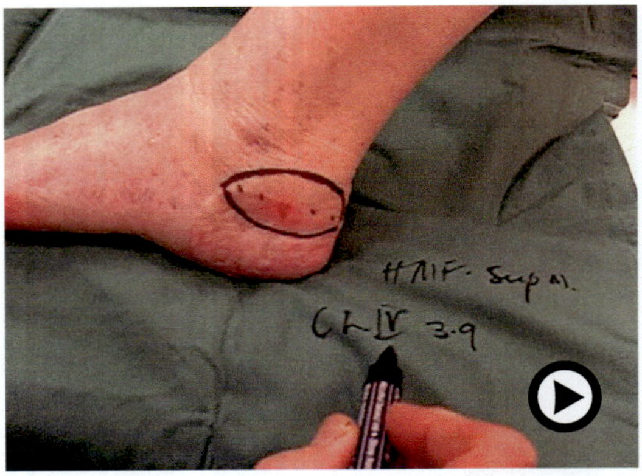

Fig. 5.95 Operative sequence (▶ https://doi.org/10.1007/000-b64)

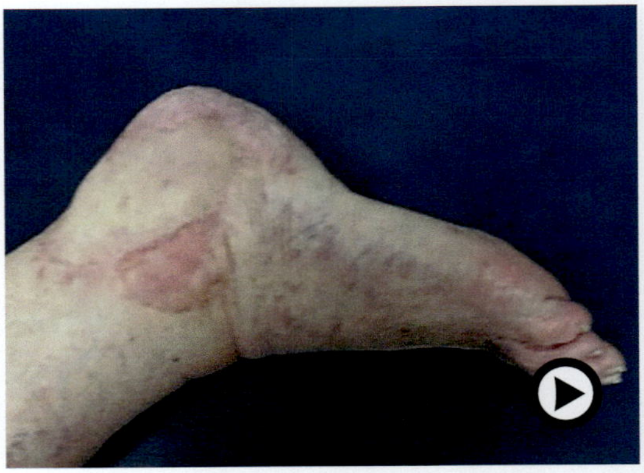

Fig. 5.96 Postoperative – patient perspective (▶ https://doi.org/10.1007/000-b65)

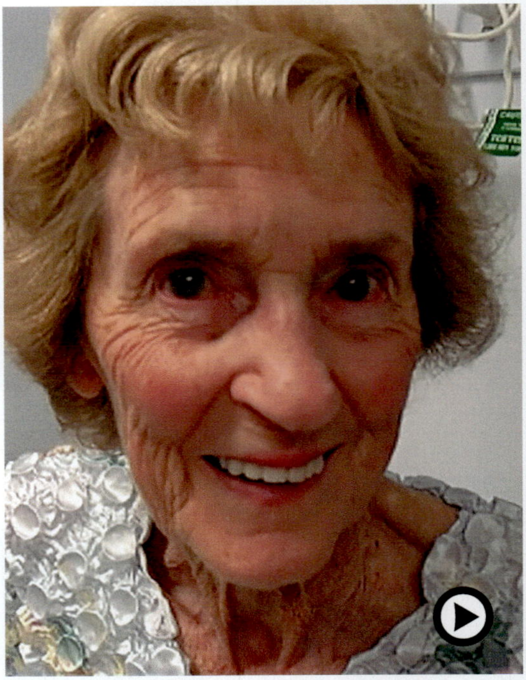

Fig. 5.97 Postoperative – patient perspective (▶ https://doi.org/10.1007/000-b66)

5.1.19 Case 64: Dorsum of Foot Over Metatarso Phalangeal Joints 4 and 5

Melanoma dorsum of L foot in a 54-year-old female. Pathology level I melanoma in a superficial naevus (see Figs. 5.98, 5.99, 5.100, 5.101, 5.102, 5.103, 5.104, 5.105, and 5.106).

In summary, the P.A.C.E.S. characteristics of the Keystone were all exemplified.

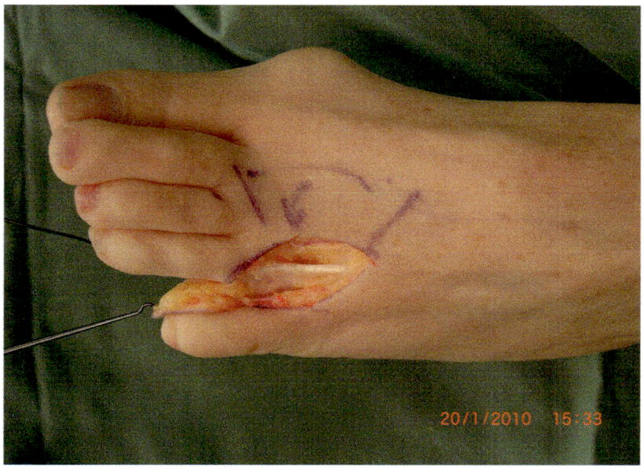

Fig. 5.98 The excision of the lesion at the head of the 4th and 5th metatarsals down to the paratenon of the extensor complex to the 4th toe

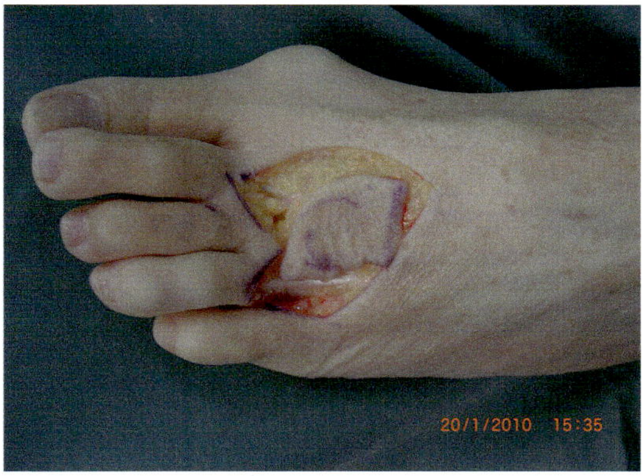

Fig. 5.99 The outline of the Keystone on random perforators in the vicinity of the 3rd and 4th metatarsal heads via the metatarso phalangeal joints from the lateral plantar supply

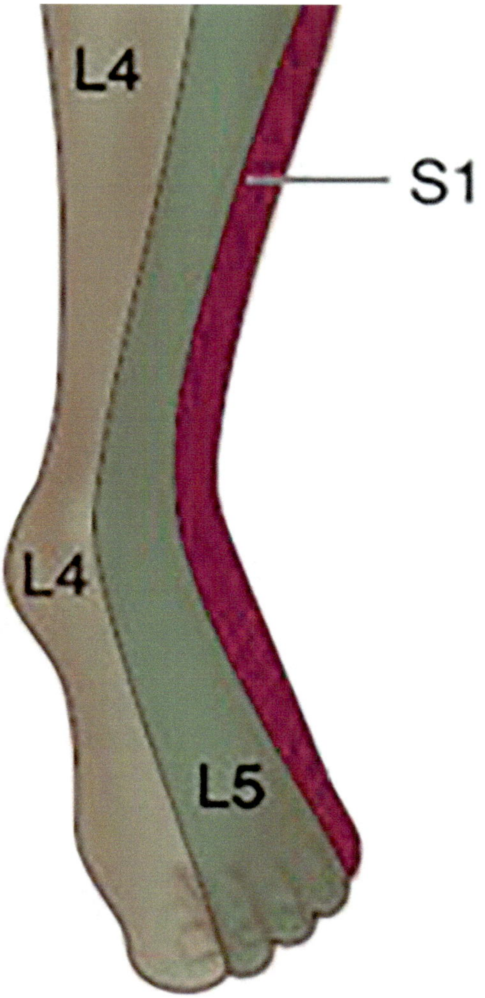

Fig. 5.100 The dermatomal mark out is the guide for the location of the random perforators coming through the fascia

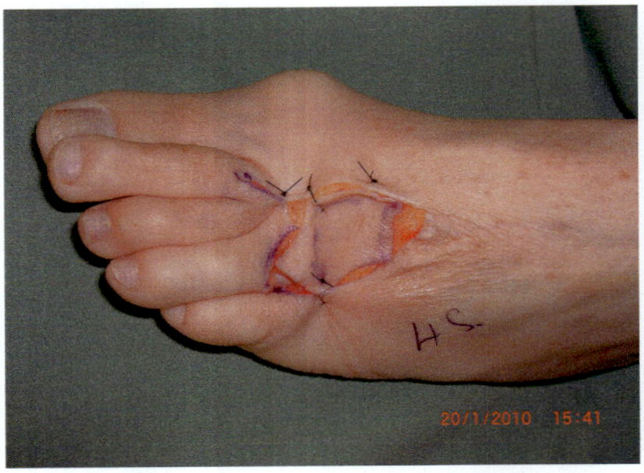

Fig. 5.101 Closure under tension and no embarrassment to the vascular supply which is all perforator based and not subdermal. No undermining of the subdermal complex just direct tensional closure over MTP 4 and 5

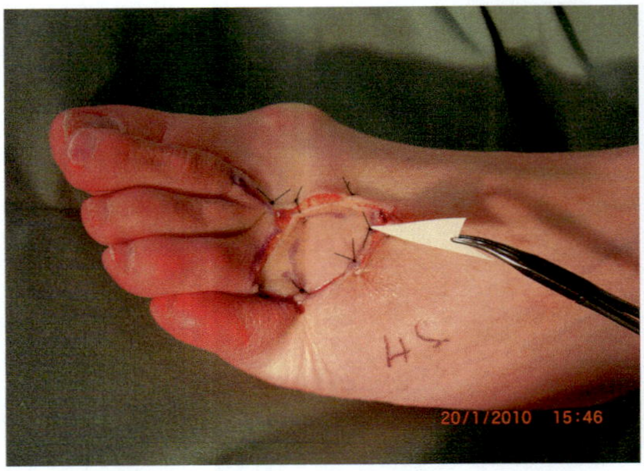

Fig. 5.102 Red Dot Sign in spite of epidermal closure under tension confirms full vascularity

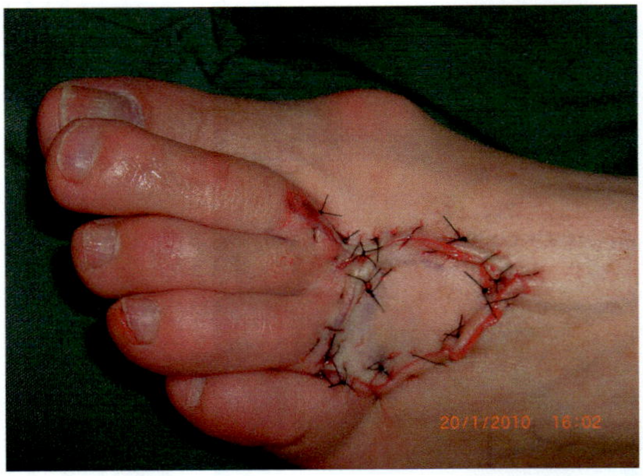

Fig. 5.103 Completed in an economic timeframe of 45 min and the 3-phase surgical suture technique is applied

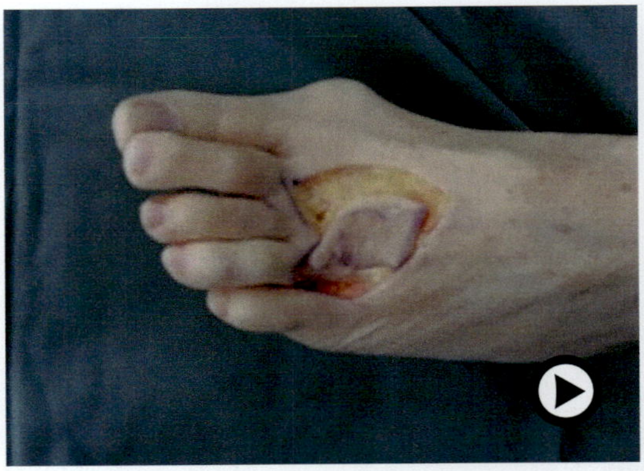

Fig. 5.104 Operative sequence (▶ https://doi.org/10.1007/000-b67)

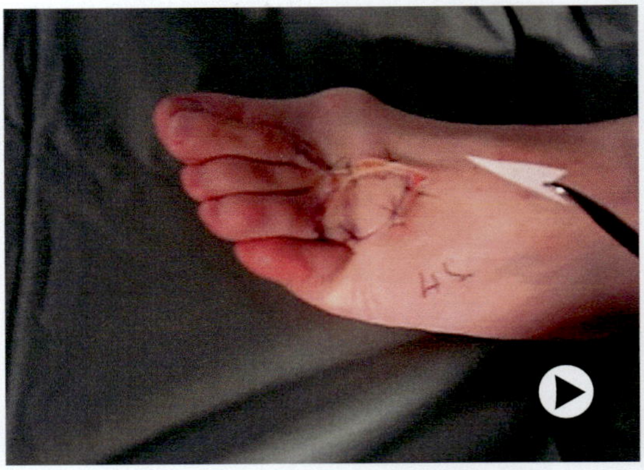

Fig. 5.105 Operative sequence (▶ https://doi.org/10.1007/000-b68)

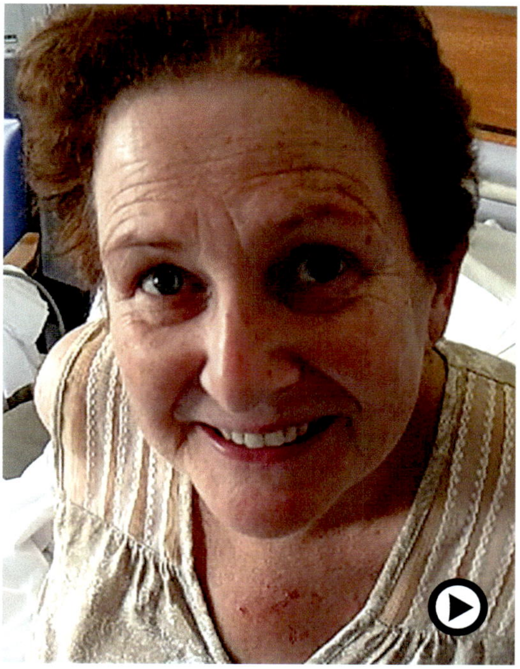

Fig. 5.106 Postoperative in hospital – patient perspective pain free (▶ https://doi.org/10.1007/000-b69)

5.1.20 Case 65: Keystone Dorsum of the Foot

Melanoma on dorsal surface of the L foot along the line of the 4th metacarpal. Clark Level IV 5.5 mm. Fixed pathology specimen 4.2 × 3 mm (see Figs. 5.107 and 5.108)

5.1.21 Case 66: Another Aesthetic Outcome in a Female

Clarke level II 0.55 mm melanoma, avoiding skin grafting on the foot. Pathology specimen 4 × 2 cm. This is particularly relevant in ladies with tight footwear (see Figs. 5.109 and 5.110).

5.1.22 Case 67: a Difficult Area for Reconstruction – Medial Malleolus

Clark level III 0.85 mm melanoma medial malleolus in a 75-year-old female (see Fig. 5.111).

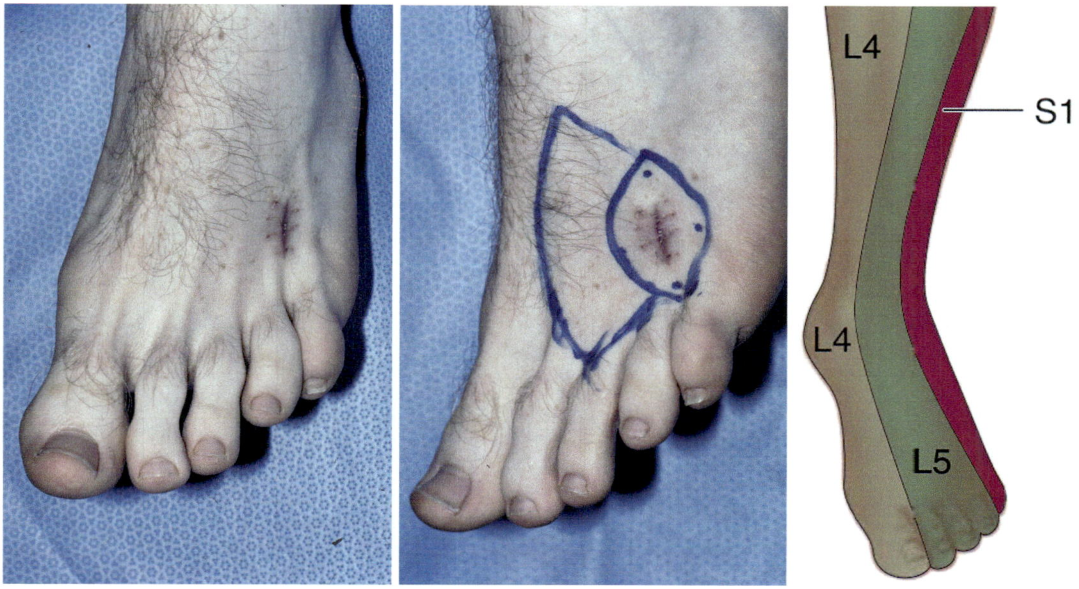

Fig. 5.107 Dorsum of the foot and the Keystone mark out in the S1 dermatome

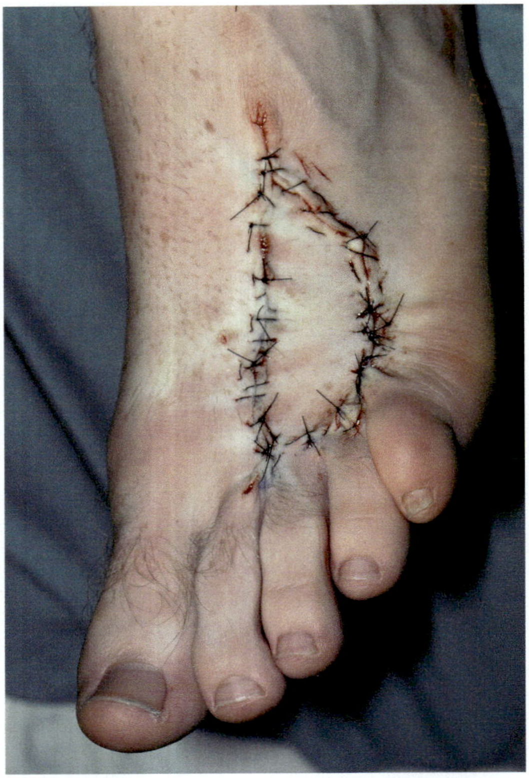

Fig. 5.108 The Keystone is on the medial side of the excisional defect because the lateral side did not have the laxity nor has the elastic movement to ensure direct closure as it borders on the plantar skin

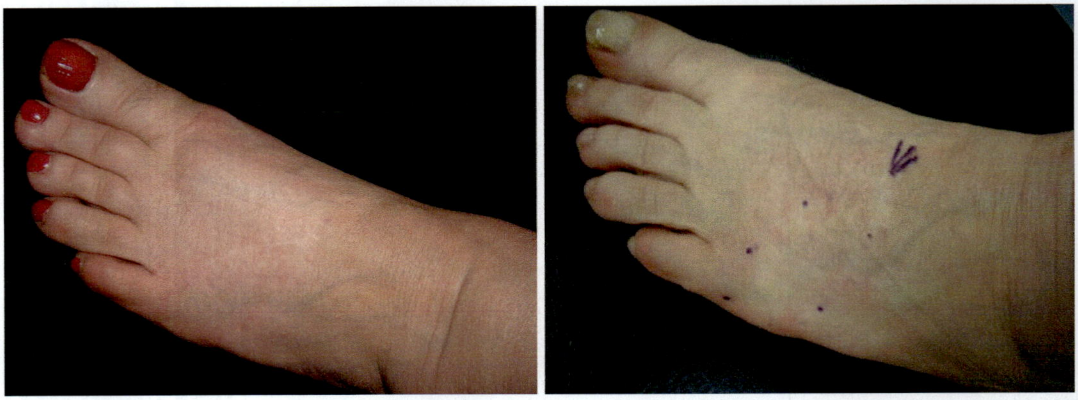

Fig. 5.109 The postoperative appearance of Keystone scars on the dorsum of the foot. This is barely discernible. The 3-phase single layer suture technique was used as well as the wound dressing technique for removal to achieve this aesthetic outcome. The wear and tear factor of normal sensate tissue has practical applications on this site, particularly when wearing tightly fitting footwear

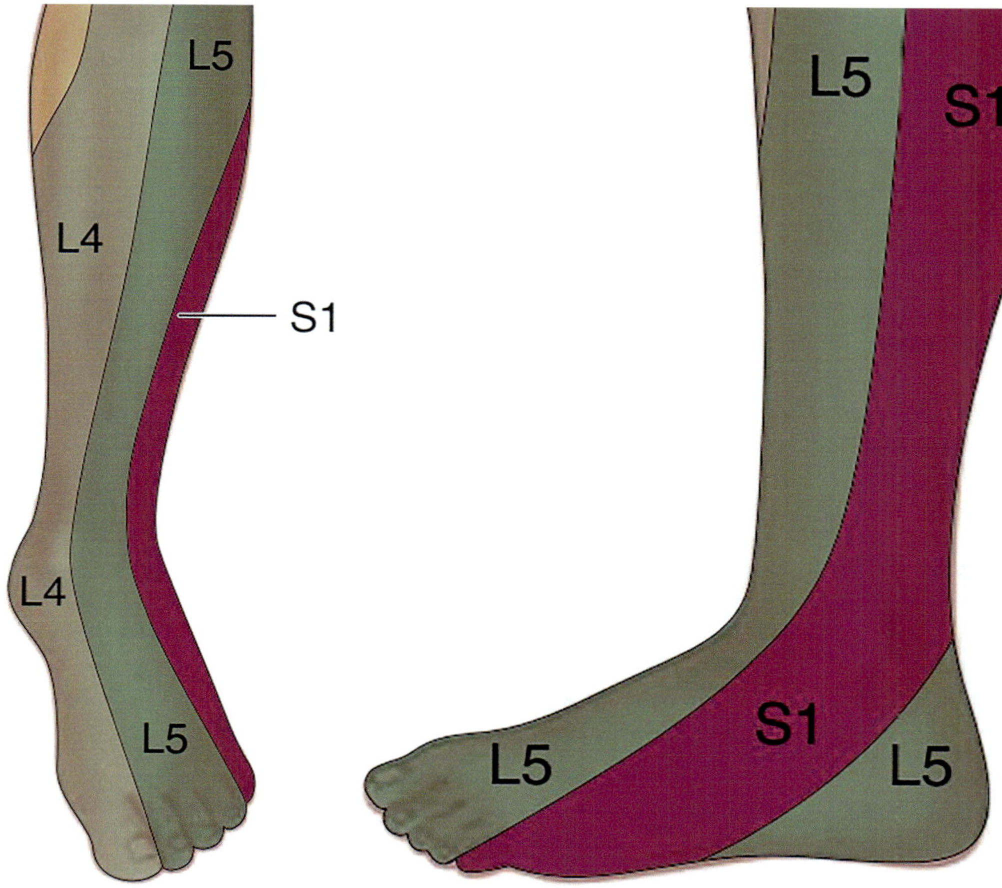

Fig. 5.110 The dermatomal mark out is the guide for the location of the random perforators coming through the fascia

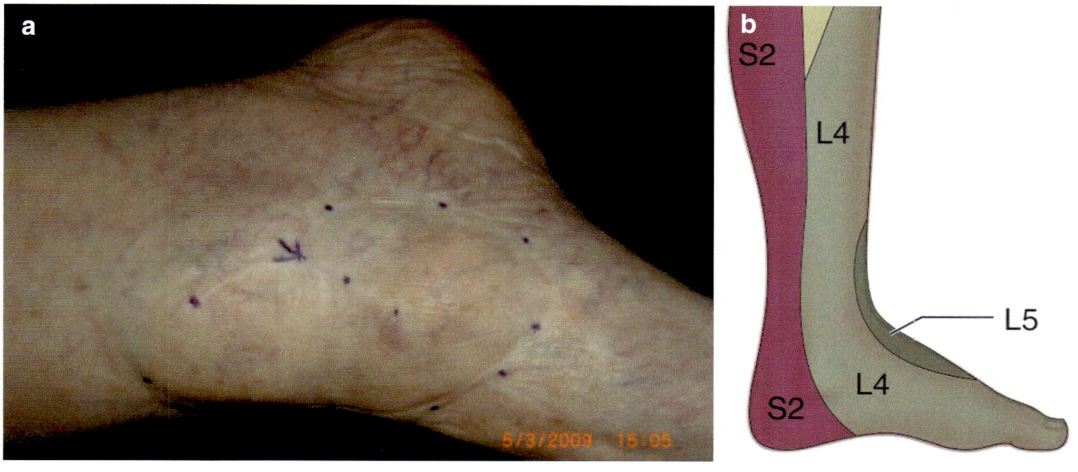

Fig. 5.111 Tumour-free interval 5.5 years. The aesthetic outcome is evident from the surgical mark out and is fully sensate

In summary, the P.A.C.E.S. characteristics of the Keystone were all exemplified particularly sensate tissue over the medial malleolus with a satisfactory aesthetic outcome and very functional from the point of view of wearing shoes in the elderly.

5.1.23 Case 68: Heel Acral Lentiginous Melanoma (ALM) Breslow Thickness 5.6 mm

Clark Level IV, 5.6 mm ALM in the weight bearing surface of the R heel in an 80-year-old patient (see Figs. 5.112, 5.113, 5.114, 5.115, 5.116, 5.117, 5.118, 5.119, and 5.120).

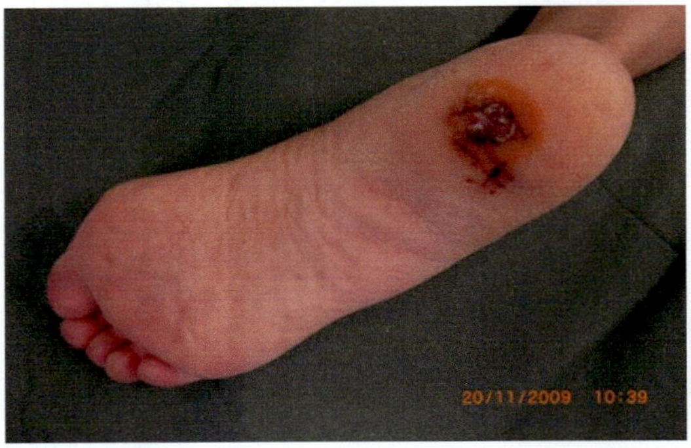

Fig. 5.112 The appearance in this elderly patient with a language barrier restricting communication. Her daughter did the translation

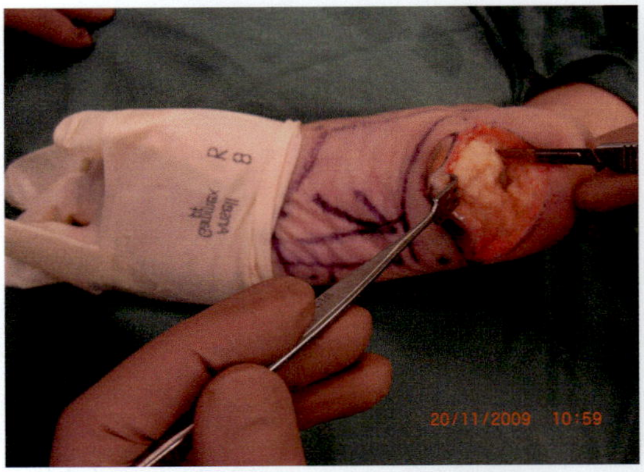

Fig. 5.113 Excision of the lesion down to and including periosteum of the calcaneum. The Keystone reconstruction of this weight bearing surface over the calcaneum is designed from the skin, fat and fascia of the plantar arch. Division of the medial and lateral sides allows rotation into the calcaneal defect. The plantar fascia renders support for this sensate, weight bearing surface. The surgical manoeuvre of enclosing the distal half of the foot within a sterile surgical glove goes some way towards ensuring sterile operative field

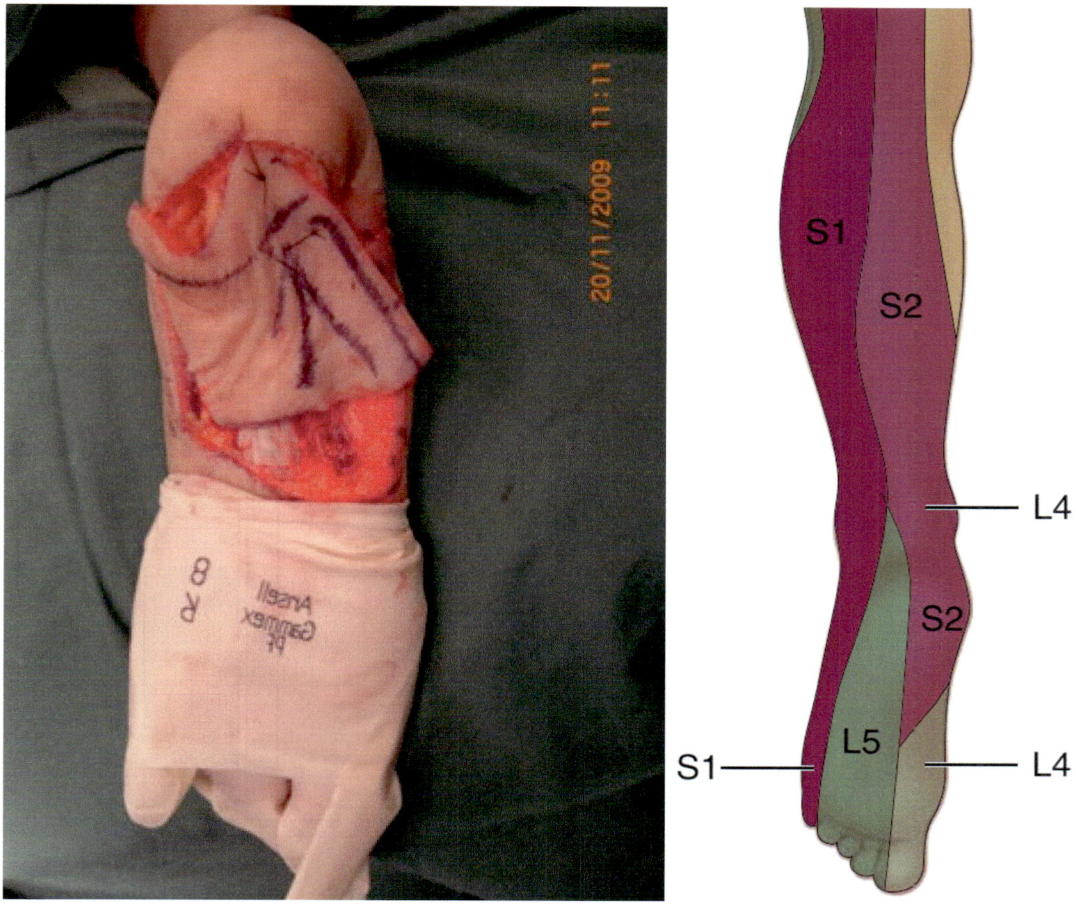

Fig. 5.114 The Keystone Island Flap is designed within the plantar arch. This is mainly overlying the L5 dermatome and is delineated around the periphery. The plantar fascia is released distally enough to ensure cover of the weight bearing surface of the heel

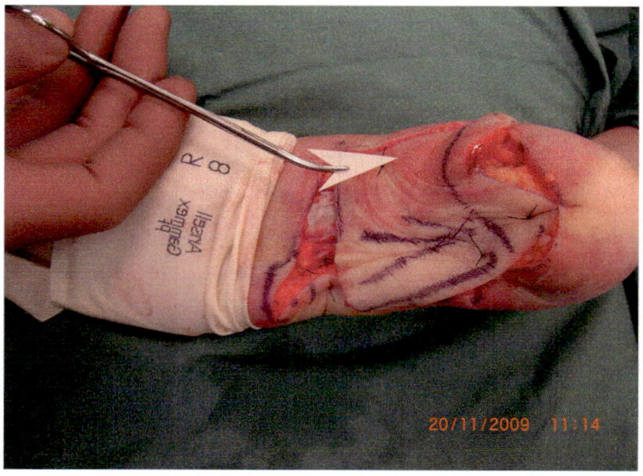

Fig. 5.115 On the release of tourniquet: note the reactive hyperaemia evident through the medial side of the Keystone indicating the medial plantar arterial supply is the predominant input and on the lateral side the lateral plantar input would have been divided to allow rotation advancement of the Keystone over the calcaneum

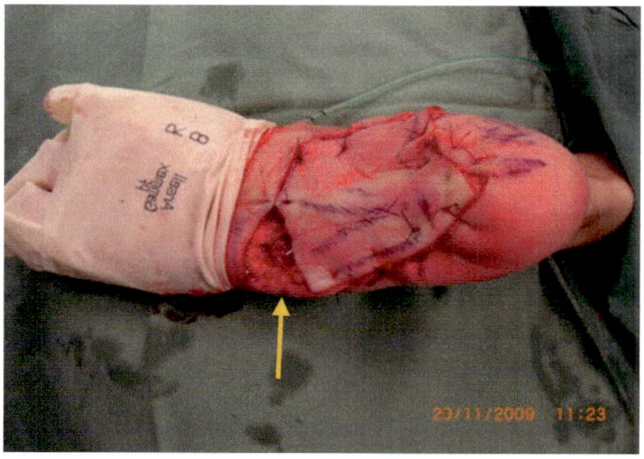

Fig. 5.116 Staged repair: the arrow indicates the site of planned skin grafting site for closure for the secondary defect. Fortunately, mobilisation of local plantar tissues eliminated the need for grafting and the wound was closed directly without any tension causing any vascular impedance. The hyperaemic appearance at 20 min (timestamp on image) is unchanged

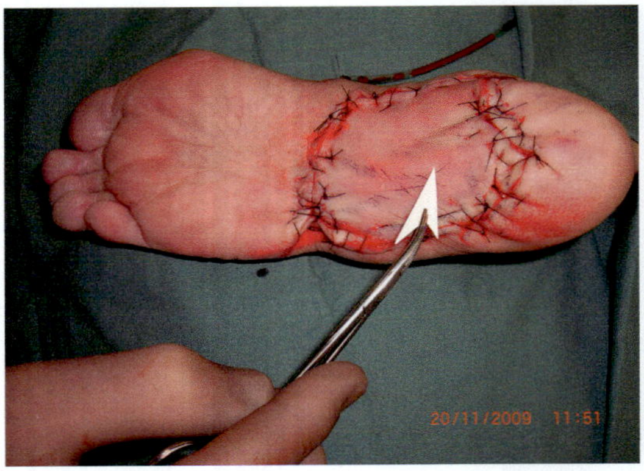

Fig. 5.117 Closure completed without grafting with Redi-vac drainage. Reactive hyperaemia (arrowed) is quite noticeable and the secondary defect at the base of the 5th metatarsal has been closed directly without any vascular embarrassment

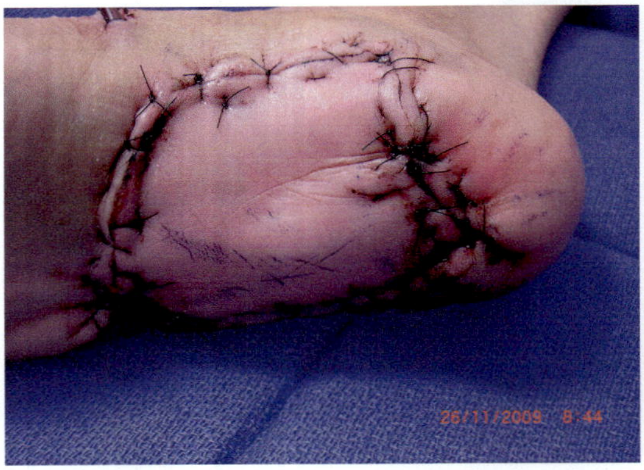

Fig. 5.118 Appearance at 5 days. The closure repeated using a 3-phase surgical technique of locking mattress sutures at the points of maximum tension and then further mattress sutures to gain wound closure and finally a continuous nylon throughout to achieve epidermal seal

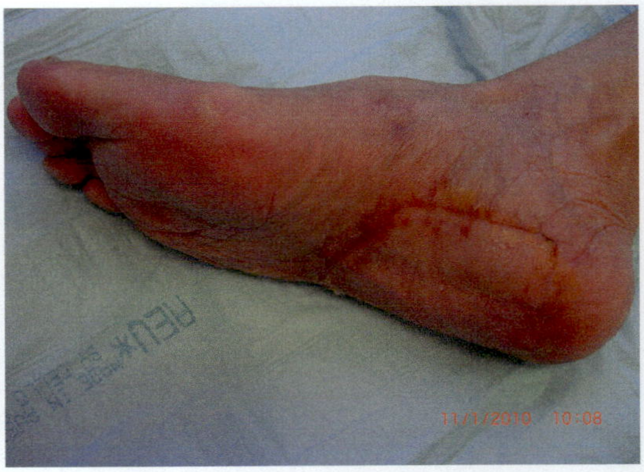

Fig. 5.119 The appearance at 1 month following staged removal of sutures with intact sensation obvious when the heel is palpated (see video)

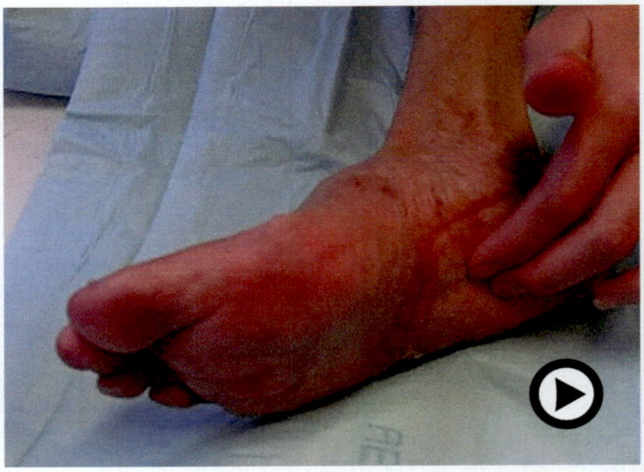

Fig. 5.120 Postoperative in hospital – patient perspective sensory recovery (▶ https://doi.org/10.1007/000-b5x)

In summary, this simple plantar Keystone supplying sensate tissue to the heel from the medial plantar Keystone is superior to any sural nerve reversal for plantar innervation and the vascular embarrassment a regular finding [4]. All the P.A.C.E.S. characteristics were again exemplified and the patient walked normally.

5.1.24 Case 69: Calf Keystone Repair – A Complicated Reconstruction Following a Transverse Biopsy Orientation and Not Longitudinally

Melanoma of calf Clark level III 1.3 mm. Re-excision with fixed pathology specimen 73 × 35 × 10 mm (see Figs. 5.121, 5.122, 5.123, 5.124, 5.125, and 5.126).

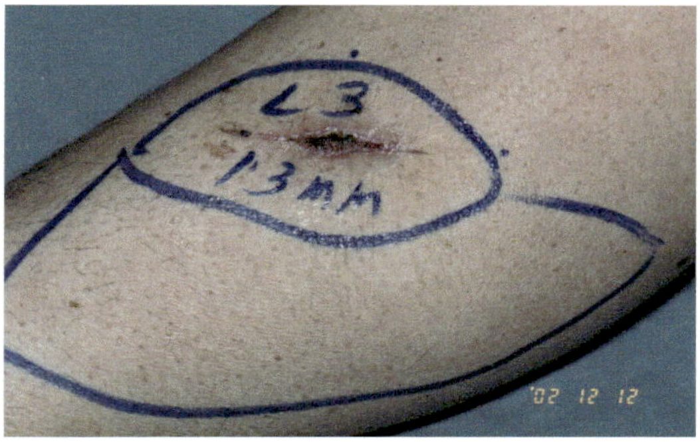

Fig. 5.121 73 × 35 × 10 mm defect including fascia of the calf muscle

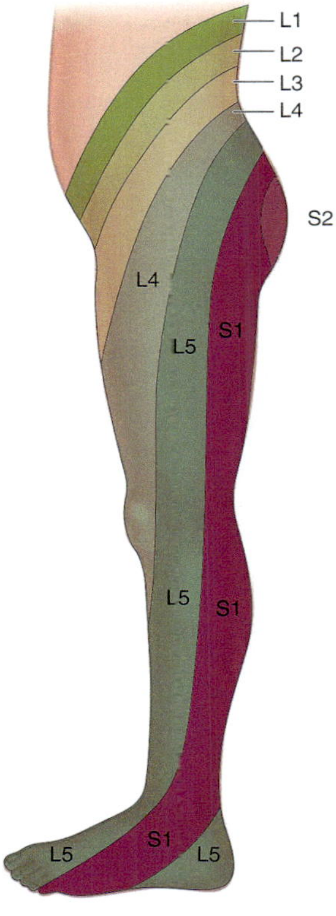

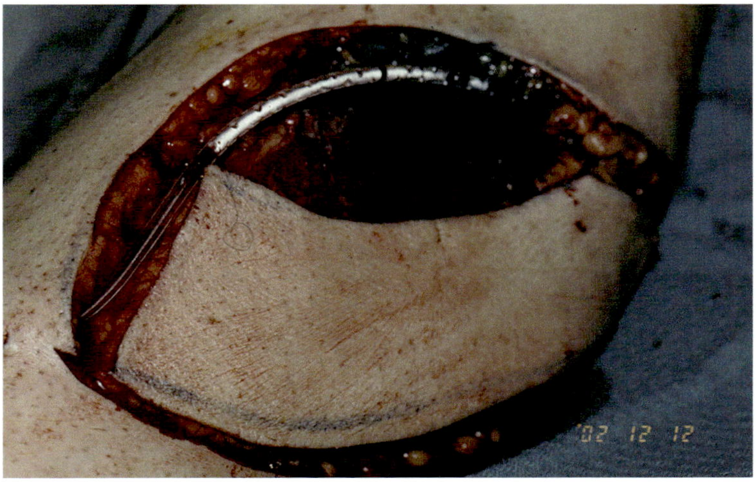

Fig. 5.122 Keystone island flap inferolateral to the melanoma defect. Planned closure over the calf muscles using the Keystone principle of direct apposition without the need for skin grafting and the muscle bulk provides a cushion of the gastrocnemious muscle allowing direct closure. A single Redi-vac tubing bent into a L-shape to drain two surgical sites. Note the reactive hyperaemia – pink – confirming the presence of random perforators

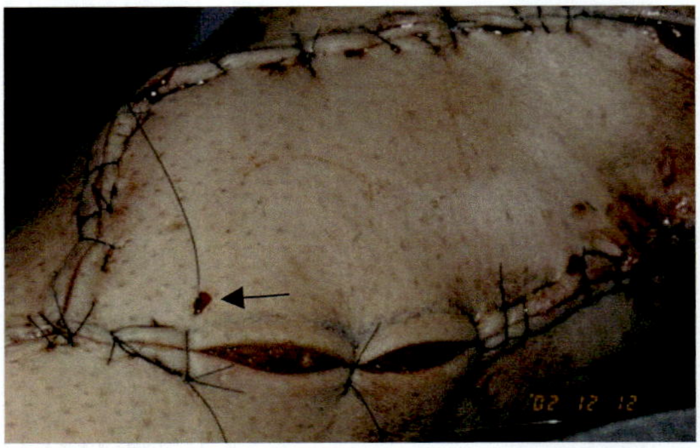

Fig. 5.123 The Red Dot Sign (arrowed) is more confirmation of reactive hyperaemia and based on random perforators. The Red Dot Sign bleeds more on the flap side rather than the inserted margin on the insertion of sutures. The 3-phase suture technique is again applied once stabilising locking mattress sutures align the tissues

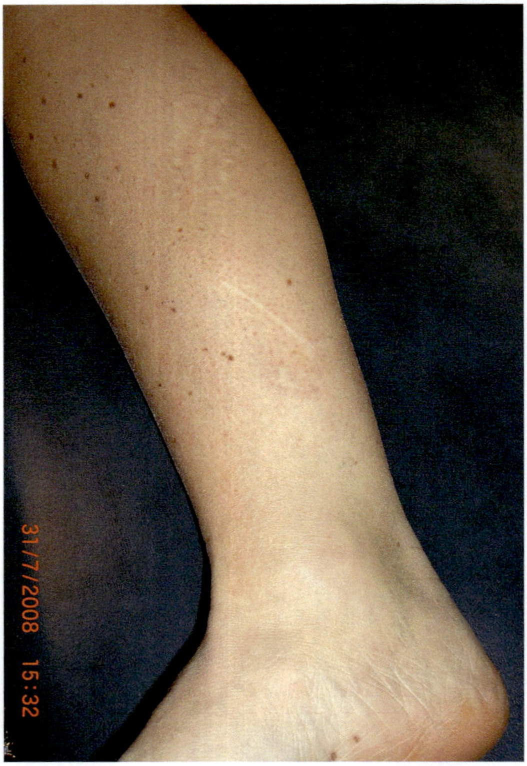

Fig. 5.124 Three years postoperative appearance with the scar barely discernible following the standard 3-phase suture technique and staged removal

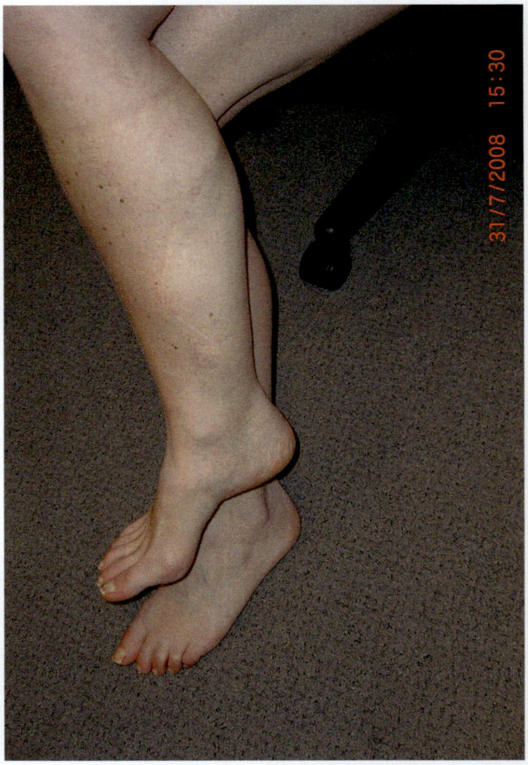

Fig. 5.125 On direct view at 3 years with the P.A.C.E.S. characteristics all evident. The patient was an athlete and enjoyed the pain-free surgical manoeuvre producing an aesthetic outcome without restraint on the type of summer clothing she chose to wear without restricting her jogging

In summary, the P.A.C.E.S. characteristics are all evident and the patient, an athlete, in full functional recovery.

5.1.25 Case 70: Another Calf Melanoma Restricted by a Poor Biopsy Orientation

Melanoma R calf Clark level IV. Tumour-free interval of 5.5 years with an acceptable aesthetic outcome (see Figs. 5.127, 5.128, and 5.129).

In summary, the P.A.C.E.S. characteristics are still evident in spite of the increased tension necessary for closure because of that biopsy orietation, not being in the dermatomal alignment.

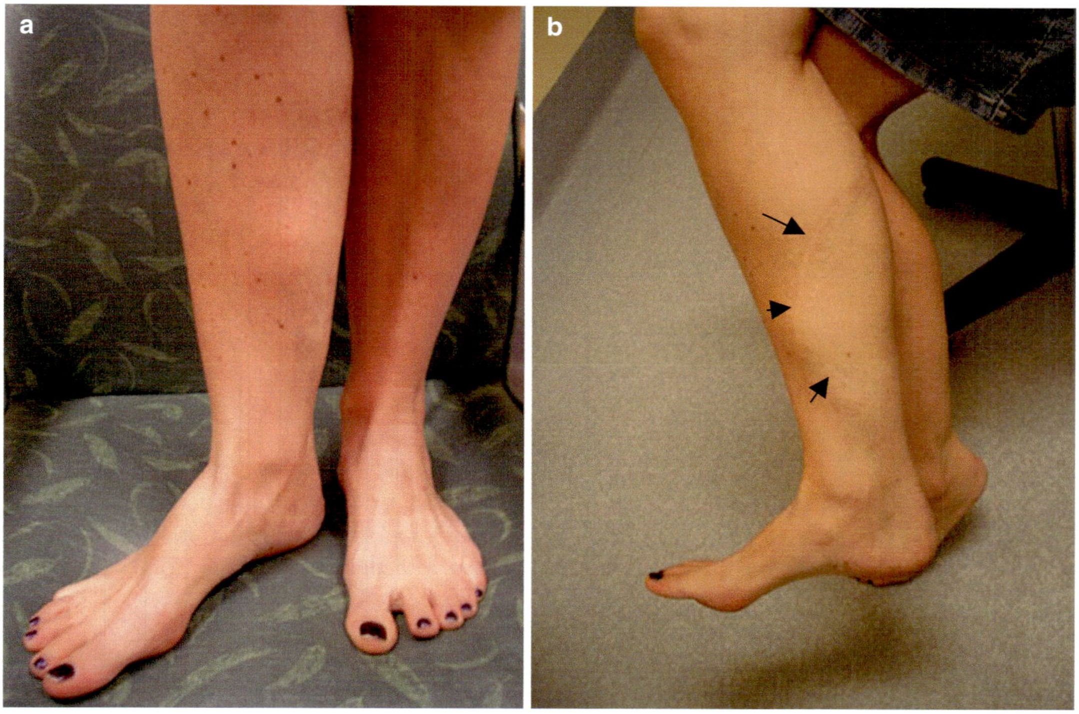

Fig. 5.126 (**a**) Aesthetic appearance. (**b**) Scar indiscernible

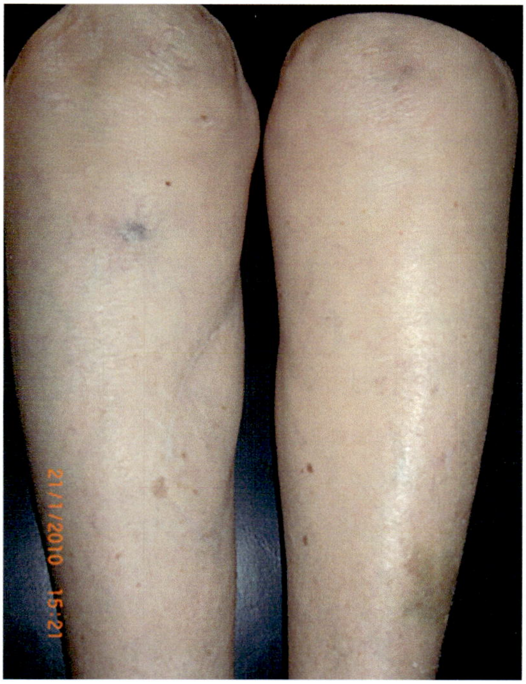

Fig. 5.127 The biopsy orientation in the oblique manner and this was the feature that necessitated an oblique Keystone, not quite aligned within the dermatomal precinct

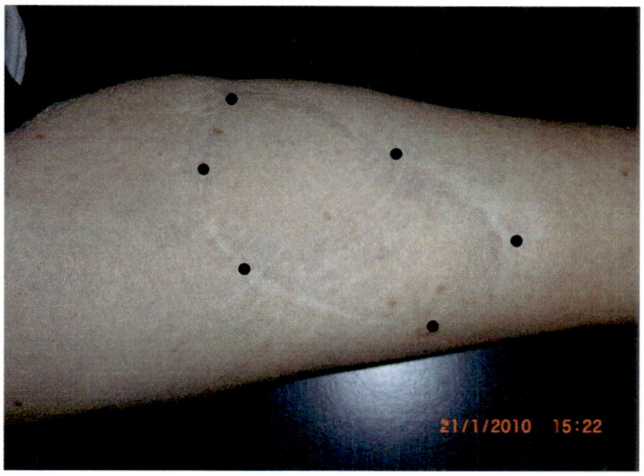

Fig. 5.128 Outline of the Keystone scar, barely discernible which allows the patient to wear summer clothing with her knees exposed. The cratiform deformity produced by skin grafting makes an obvious comparison

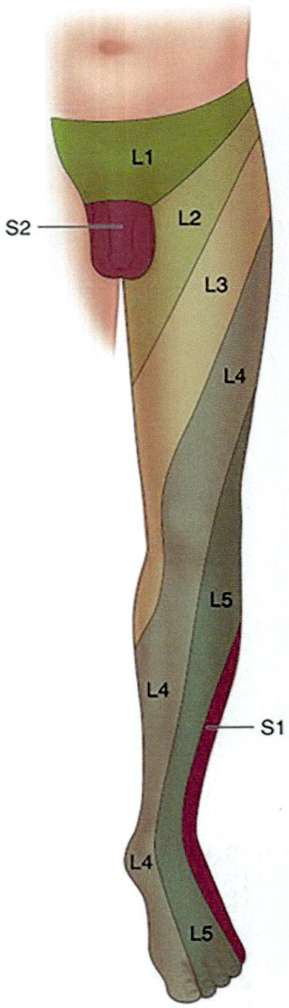

Fig. 5.129 The dermatomal mark out is the guide for the location of the random perforators coming through the fascia

5.1.26 Case 71: Recurrent Melanoma of the Calf Following Previous Excisions and Grafting Producing Chronic Lymphoedema Including a Groin Dissection

Split skin graft Clark level IV melanoma L calf then dissemintation into the groin with nodal secondaries. Lymphadectomy followed by radiation and subsequent lymphodema of the L lower limb in this 55-year-old female (see Figs. 5.130, 5.131, 5.132, 5.133, 5.134, 5.135, 5.136, 5.137, 5.138, and 5.139).

In summary, because of the delay in healing aggravated by the ongoing peripheral oedema, the design of bilateral Keystones has been dispensed with and a YIN YANG [5] design variant is now my preference.

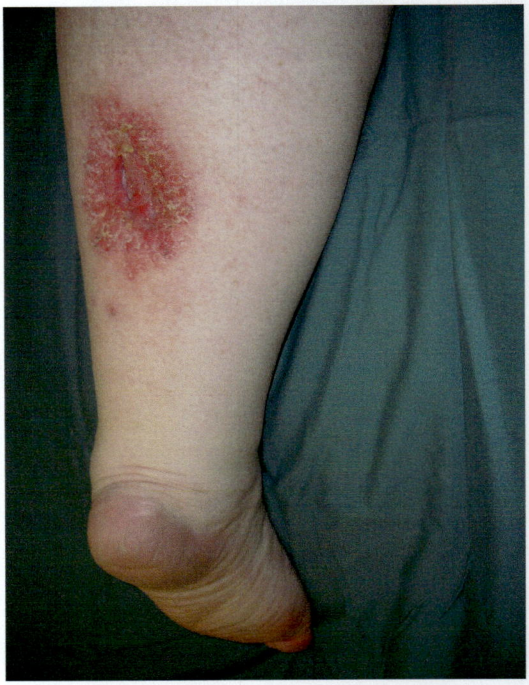

Fig. 5.130 The quality of life after 9 months having to shower in a plastic bag because of the lymphoedema leaking around the graft site

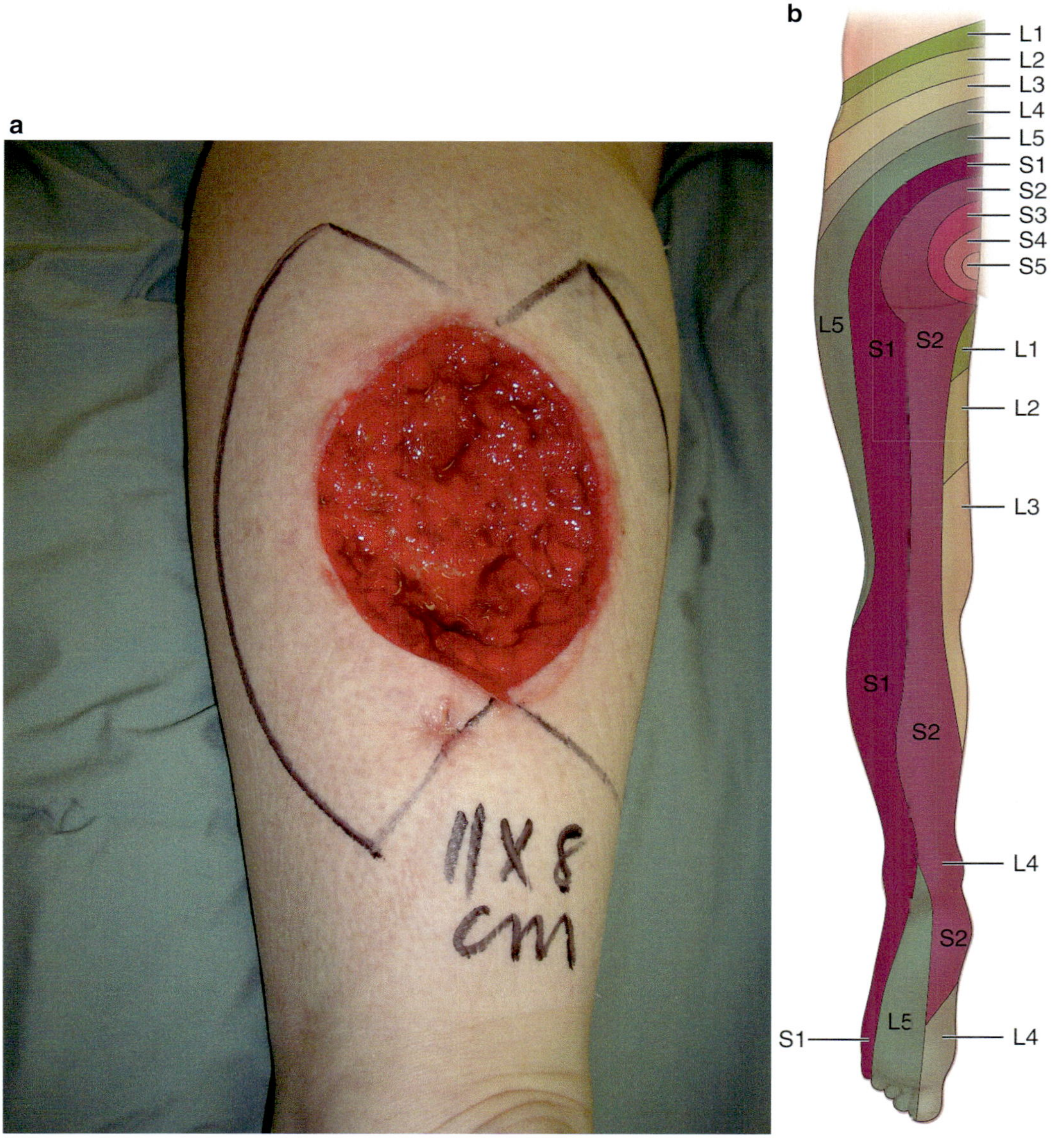

Fig. 5.131 Re-excision of the melanoma creating a surgical defect 11 × 8 cm with the mark out of a double Keystone flap reconstruction

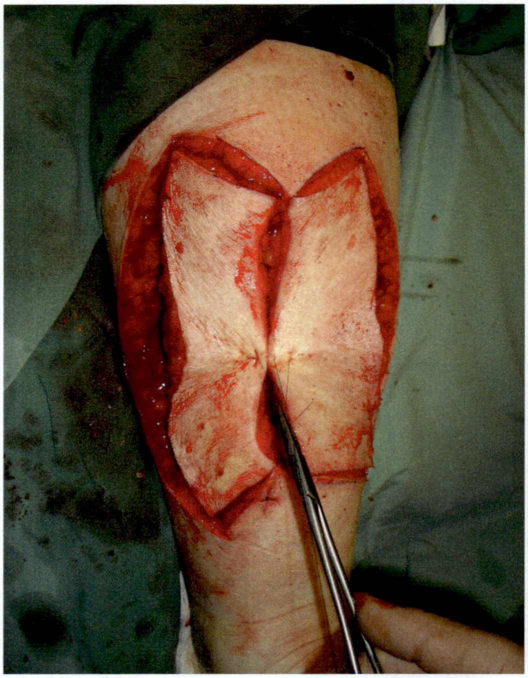

Fig. 5.132 Double Keystone flap apposition. Because of the tension evident and slow healing phase with odema, my preference now is to use a Yin Yang design with the apex of one flap crossing the calf into the inferior limit of the other

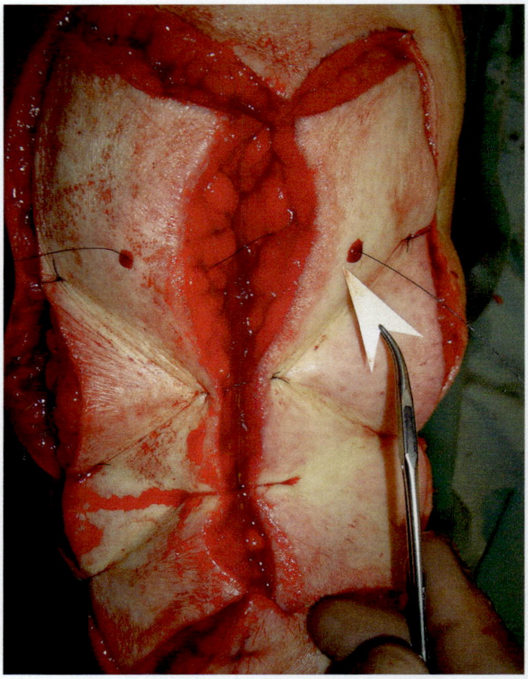

Fig. 5.133 Double Red Dot Signs (arrowed) indicating the hyperaemic vascular phase and integrity, yet tension is evident, based on supra and infrafascial random perforator circulation of the lower calf region

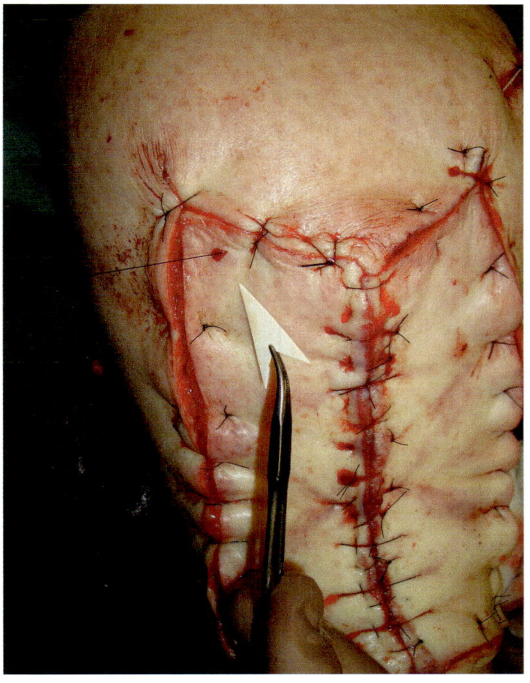

Fig. 5.134 Full closure and proximal Red Dot Sign using the staged 3-phase suture technique of locking mattress sutures at the points of maximum tension, ordinary mattress for wound apposition and a continuous nylon for epidermal seal

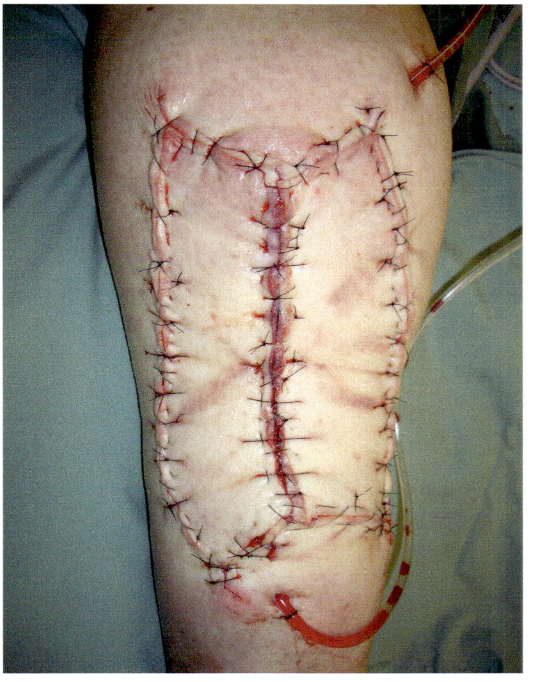

Fig. 5.135 This patient has a delayed wound management because of tension and lymphoedema present in the lower limb. Wound and tensional closure is evident in this epidermal apposition technique here. However, because of this delay in healing, up to 6 weeks, such defects in future are more easily closed using the double Keystone but with a Yin Yang design variant. However, healing was achieved eventually after some weeks with the appearance below

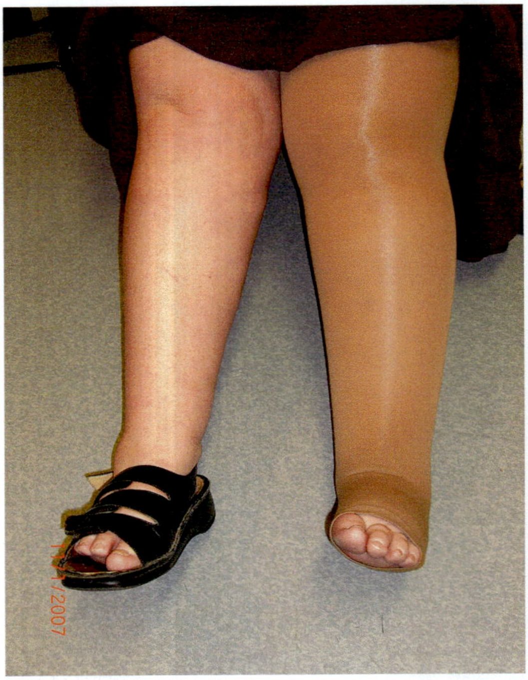

Fig. 5.136 Wearing support stockings, a consequence of the previous radiation of the groin after lymphadenectomy with a healed wound achieved. The lymphoedema continued to resolve with the help of vascular support stockings

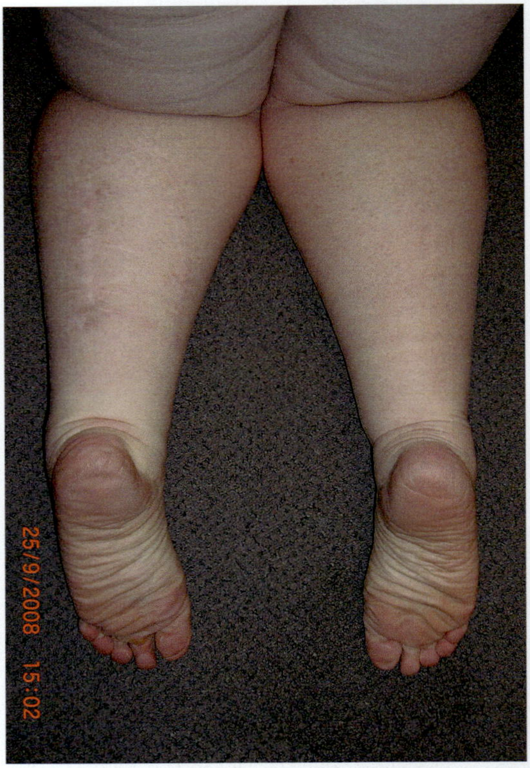

Fig. 5.137 Postoperative appearance at 12 months an aesthetic outcome for an otherwise cratiform skin grafting defect

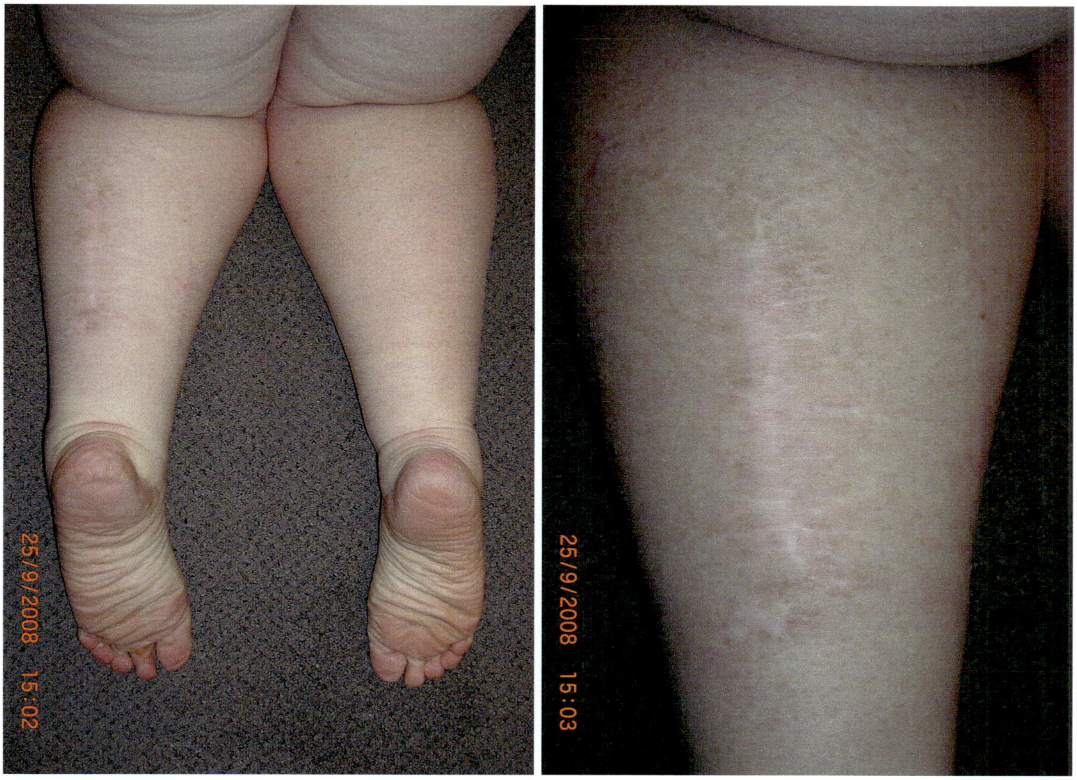

Fig. 5.138 Postoperative appearance at 12 months. The P.A.C.E.S. acronym all apply but what was particularly noteworthy was the continuing resolution of oedema, helped by wearing vascular support stockings. The observational factor is the good clinical outcome, could it be that the lymphatic channels in the Keystone allow oedema to settle by opening up, similar to the vascular hyperaemia, when one sees the Red Dot Sign in the early clinical phase

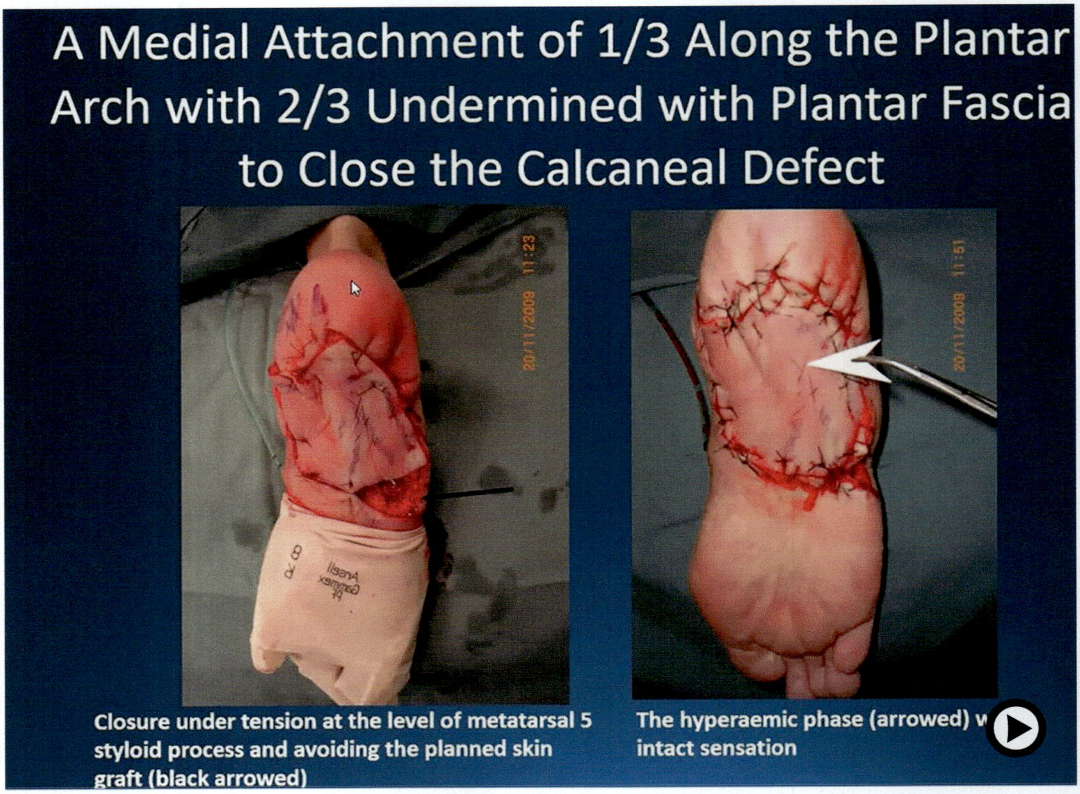

Fig. 5.139 Lower limb (▶ https://doi.org/10.1007/000-b6b)

References

1. Marenco F, et al. Cutaneous melanoma metastases arising on a split-skin graft donor site. Dermatol Surg. 2009;35(8):1282–5.
2. Behan FC, Rozen WM, Tan S. Yin-Yang flaps: the mathematics of two keystone island flaps for reconstructing increasingly large defects. ANZ J Surg. 2011;81:574–5.
3. McLean NR, Boorman JG. Secondary malignant melanoma arising in a contralateral thigh donor site. Br J Plast Surg. 1989;37(3):386–7.
4. Gill NA, Hameed A. The sural compendium: reconstruction of complex soft-tissue defects of leg and foot by utilizing the posterior calf tissue. Ann Plast Surg. 2012;69(2):203–8.
5. Behan FC. Keystone perforator island flap in lower limb reconstruction. Aust J Plast Surg. 2021;4(2):105–7. https://doi.org/10.34239/ajops.v4n2.34.1. Audio visual presentation

Conclusion/Summary

6

Contents

The Keystone concept emphasizes the role of the dermatome precincts and the intrinsic neurocutaneous vascular supply of the human skin [1–35]. These flaps are robust all over the body and vascular complications are rare. However, in diabetics type II and the immunocompromised, sometimes vascular complications occur with tight closures. The 3-phase technique of sutures simplifies closure in spite of elements of tension existing in wound apposition. Blood vessels and lymphatic vessels follow nerves, so the Keystones are based on random multiple arterial perforators, their venae comitantes and the fine vascular networks that accompany nerves, all within the dermatomal mark outs and embryological observation. It Keystone is a very straightforward flap to raise quickly, safely and will often avoid the need for more complex, time-consuming, risky and more expensive methods of repair. In this Atlas of 71 cases ranging from head to toe all feature singularly or collectively Keystone closure characteristics of P.A.C.E.S. and have achieved a sound and reliable repair are presented in.

Dr Frederick J. Menick wrote in 1998 about the interface of aesthetic and reconstructive surgery in facial reconstruction. Distant tissue does not match facial skin in colour, texture or thickness. Nor does it have facial shape. The subunit approach employing loco-regional tissue in contrast improves the aesthetic reconstructive result. Herein lies the useful option of the Keystone for facial reconstruction using loco-regional techniques for repair (Fig. 6.1).

Supplementary Information The online version contains supplementary material available at https://doi.org/10.1007/978-3-031-39868-1_6. The videos can be accessed individually by clicking the DOI link in the accompanying figure caption or by scanning this link with the SN More Media App.

F. Behan, *Atlas of Keystone Reconstructive Technique in Melanoma Management*,
https://doi.org/10.1007/978-3-031-39868-1_6

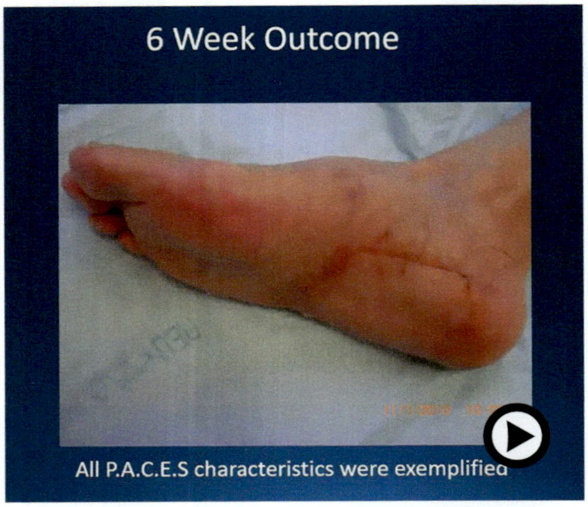

Fig. 6.1 Conclusion (▶ https://doi.org/10.1007/000-b6c)

References

1. Behan et al. Vascular basis of laterally based forehead island flaps and their clinical applications. In: Transactions of the 2nd Congress of the European Section of the International Confederation of Plastic and Reconstructive Surgery. Madrid, The Angiotome concept, 1973
2. Behan FC. Dashboard dislocations. Br J Hosp Med. 1937;1(9):363.
3. Behan FC, et al. Reconstruction of plantar pad after degloving injury of foot. Surg Gynecol Obstet. 1973;137(6):971–4.
4. Behan F, et al. Subungual malignant melanoma difficulty in diagnosis. Br Med J. 1974;1(5903):310–2.
5. Behan FC, Wilson JSP. The principle of the angiotome a system of linked axial pattern flaps. In: Transactions of the 6th International Congress on Plastic and Reconstructive Surgery, Paris, 1975
6. Behan FC. The fascio-cutaneous Island flap: an extension of the angiotome concept. Aust N Z J Surg. 1992;62:874–86.
7. Behan FC, et al. Fasciocutaneous island flaps for orthopaedic management in lower limb reconstruction using dermatomal precincts. ANZ J Surg. 1994;64(3):155–66.
8. Behan FC, et al. Island flaps, including the Bezier type in the treatment of malignant melanoma. ANZ J Surg. 1995;65(12):870–80.
9. Behan FC. The Venous Island Conduit (VIC) flap for ring avulsion injuries. J Hand Surg Br Vol. 1998;23(4):465–71.
10. Behan FC. The keystone design perforator island flap in reconstructive surgery. ANZ J Surg. 2003;73:112–20.
11. Behan F, Sizeland A, Porcedu S, Somia N, Wilson J. Keystone island flap: an alternative reconstructive option to free flaps in irradiated tissue. ANZ J Surg. 2006;76:407–13.
12. Pelissier P, Santoul M, Pinsolle V, Casoli V, Behan F. The keystone design perforator island flap: Part I. Anatomic study. J Plast Reconstr Aesthet Surg. 2007;60:883–7. Bordeaux, France
13. Behan F. Evolution of the fascio-cutaneous island flap leading to the keystone flap principle in lower limb reconstruction. ANZ J Surg. 2008;78:116–7.
14. Behan FC, Lo CH, Ramin S. Perforator territory of the keystone flap—use of the dermatomal roadmap. J Plast Reconstr Aesthet Surg. 2008; https://doi.org/10.1016/j.bjps.2008.08.078.
15. Behan FC, Lo CH, Shayan R. Perforator territory of the keystone flap: use of the dermatomal roadmap. J Plast Reconstr Aesthet Surg. 2009;62:551–3.
16. Behan F, Sizeland A, Gilmour F, Hui A, Seel M, Lo CH. Use of the keystone island flap for advanced head and neck cancer in the elderly—a principle of amelioration. J Plast Reconstr Aesthet Surg. 2010;63:739–45.
17. Behan FC, Rozen WM, Tan S. Yin-Yang flaps: the mathematics of two keystone island flaps for reconstructing increasingly large defects. ANZ J Surg. 2011;81:574–5.
18. Behan FC, Rozen WM, Lo CH, Findlay M. The Omega—Ω—variant designs (types A and B) of the keystone perforator island flap. ANZ J Surg. 2011;81:650–2.
19. Behan F, Findlay M, Lo CH. The keystone perforator island flap concept. Sydney, Australia: Elsevier Textbook Churchill Livingstone; 2012.
20. Behan FC, Rozen WM, Azer S, Gran P. Perineal keystone design perforator island flap for perineal and vulval reconstruction. ANZ J Surg. 2012;82:381–2.
21. Behan FC, Paddle A, Rozen WM, et al. Quadriceps keystone island flap for radical inguinal lymphadenectomy. ANZ J Surg. 2013;83:942–7.
22. Shayan R, Behan FC. Re: The keystone concept: time for some science. ANZ J Surg. 2013;83:499–500.
23. Behan F. Surgical tips and skills illustrating the keystone principle. Sydney, Australia: Elsevier Textbook Churchill Livingstone; 2014.
24. Klaassen MF, Brown E, Behan F. Simply local flaps. Cham: Springer; 2016. Chapter 11
25. Lo C, et al. Keystone island flap effects of islanding on vascularity plastic and reconstructive surgery. Global Open. 2016;4(2):e617. https://doi.org/10.1097/GOX.0000000000000607.
26. Behan FC. Keystone perforator island flap: a clinical summary of 28 melanoma cases. Aust J Plast Surg. 2018; https://doi.org/10.34239/ajops.v1i1.66.
27. Behan FC. A Keystone solution for major head and neck reconstructions. Aust J Plast Surg. 2019; https://doi.org/10.34239/ajops.v2n2.154.
28. Behan FC. Dupuytren's disease: modified keystone techniques to improve vascular dynamics in fasciectomy. Aust J Plast Surg. 2019; https://doi.org/10.34239/ajops.v2i1.134.

29. Rodriguez-Unda N, Abraham J, Saint-Cyr M. Keystone and perforator flaps in reconstruction. Clin Plast Surg. 2020;47(4):635–48. Elsevier
30. Potet P, De Bonnecaze G, Chabrillac E, Dupret-Bories A, Vergez S, Chaput B. Closure of radial forearm free flap donor site: a comparative study between keystone flap and skin graft. Wiley Head Neck 2020;42:217–223. Toulouse, France
31. Behan FC, Sizeland A. Keystone perforator island flaps in major head and neck surgery—the P.A.C.E. perspectives. World J Surg Surg Res. 2021;4:1293.
32. Behan FC. Keystone perforator island flap in lower limb reconstruction. Aust J Plastic Surg. 2021;4(2):105–7. https://doi.org/10.34239/ajops.v4n2.341. Audio visual presentation
33. Behan FC. A simple solution to mallet deformities—a patient's perspective. Aust J Plast Surg. 2022;
34. Behan FC, In association with Klaassen M. and Burton I. Atlas of extreme facial cancer, challenges and solutions: keystone flap concepts. Springer Nature; 2022.
35. Behan FC. Part D: The keystone perforator island flap. In: Blondeel M, Neligan H, editors. Perforator flaps: anatomy, technique, & clinical applications. 3rd ed. New York: Thieme Publishers; 2022. (in press).

Printed by Printforce, the Netherlands